Josué Sznitman

Respiratory Flows in the Pulmonary Acinus

Josué Sznitman

Respiratory Flows in the Pulmonary Acinus

A dissertation on respiratory airflows in the pulmonary acinus of the lung, inhalation aerosol transport, and the control of alveolar flows

Südwestdeutscher Verlag für Hochschulschriften

Impressum/Imprint (nur für Deutschland/ only for Germany)
Bibliografische Information der Deutschen Nationalbibliothek: Die Deutsche Nationalbibliothek verzeichnet diese Publikation in der Deutschen Nationalbibliografie; detaillierte bibliografische Daten sind im Internet über http://dnb.d-nb.de abrufbar.

Verlag: Südwestdeutscher Verlag für Hochschulschriften Aktiengesellschaft & Co. KG
Dudweiler Landstr. 99, 66123 Saarbrücken, Deutschland
Telefon +49 681 37 20 271-1, Telefax +49 681 37 20 271-0, Email: info@svh-verlag.de
Zugl.: ETH Zurich, Diss., 2008

Herstellung in Deutschland:
Schaltungsdienst Lange o.H.G., Berlin
Books on Demand GmbH, Norderstedt
Reha GmbH, Saarbrücken
Amazon Distribution GmbH, Leipzig
ISBN: 978-3-8381-0684-7

Imprint (only for USA, GB)
Bibliographic information published by the Deutsche Nationalbibliothek: The Deutsche Nationalbibliothek lists this publication in the Deutsche Nationalbibliografie; detailed bibliographic data are available in the Internet at http://dnb.d-nb.de.

Publisher:
Südwestdeutscher Verlag für Hochschulschriften Aktiengesellschaft & Co. KG
Dudweiler Landstr. 99, 66123 Saarbrücken, Germany
Phone +49 681 37 20 271-1, Fax +49 681 37 20 271-0, Email: info@svh-verlag.de

Printed in the U.S.A.
Printed in the U.K. by (see last page)
ISBN: 978-3-8381-0684-7

Abstract

Historically, the role of convective respiratory flows in the pulmonary acinar region of the lung has drawn comparably little attention with respect to problems pertinent to gas diffusion. Indeed, it was long thought that the nature of acinar convective flows was rather trivial due to the slow motion of airflow at these small scales. However, the pulmonary acinus, known as the gas exchange region of the lung encompassing the complex of millions of sub-millimeter alveoli, may represent a potential host for pulmonary complications and diseases. These health disorders may require, amongst other, the inhalation of therapeutic drugs typically administered in the form of aerosolized particles. Both a precise understanding of the mechanisms leading to particle deposition, whether aerosols may be recognized as a possible health risk or a therapeutic tool, as well as the need to target inhalation aerosols to specific pulmonary sites for treatment, remain ongoing challenges and depend directly on the fluid dynamics in the lung, and specifically on the microflows present in the acinar region. Furthermore, low or insufficient lung deposition of inhalation aerosols, in particular in young children, continues to burden the efficacy of such therapeutic procedures. These considerations have called altogether not only for a deepening of our understanding of the fluid mechanics pertinent to the acinar region of the lung, but also, for the potential development of novel strategies towards improved and enhanced particle deposition inside the lung.

The present thesis, which lies at the interface between engineering and medicine, is thus concerned with the role of convective respiratory flows in the acinar region of the lung, in conjunction with the transport and deposition of inhaled particles. Due to the complexity and limited accessibility of the pulmonary acinus, acinar flow characteristics remain typically difficult to assess. Hence, in a first step, we have developed computational fluid dynamics (CFD) models of the pulmonary acinus with various degrees of geometrical complexity, mimicking wall motion during breathing to gain detailed insight into the characteristics of convective acinar flows and their influence on the transport and deposition of inhaled non-diffusing micron-sized particles, representative of common inhalation aerosols. These computational studies have first shed light on the complex nature of alveolar flows which stand as a biological example of low-Reynolds number boundary driven cavity flows. Furthermore, our findings suggest that fine aerosol kinematics may be intricate as particles are influenced by the interplay between local convective flows and gravitational sedimentation processes leading to non-uniform deposition patterns and possibly long residence times within the airspace, depending on the orientation of gravity and particle size.

In a subsequent step, through means of modern experimental flow measurement techniques (i.e. Particle Image Velocimetry), we have investigated the implementation of non-invasive forcing mechanisms, namely (i) Marangoni-induced thermocapillary motion and (ii) acoustic streaming, to generate and control forced convective airflows within benchmark alveolar models. These experimental explorations are performed as a first milestone in view of future realizable medical applications which may potentially lead towards enhanced particle mixing and deposition in the acinar region of the lung.

Résumé

Historiquement, le rôle des écoulements respiratoires dans l'acinus des poumons a attiré peu d'attention en comparaison avec les problèmes liés à la diffusion gazeuse dans cette région des poumons. En effet, il fut longtemps songé que la nature des flux respiratoires dans l'acinus était plutôt banale dû aux écoulements lents qui résident à ces échelles. Néanmoins, l'acinus pulmonaire, reconnu comme étant la région pulmonaire responsable pour les échanges gazeux et regroupant les millions d'alvéoles, peut être potentiellement en proie à des complications et maladies respiratoires. Ces troubles de santé peuvent exiger, entre autre, l'inhalation de médicaments administrés sous forme d'aérosoles. Une compréhension détaillée des mécanismes amenant à la déposition de particules, selon que ces aérosoles soient un risque potentiel pour la santé ou plutôt un outil térapeutique, ainsi que le besoin de cibler ces particules à des sites pulmonaires spécifiques continuent tout deux de représenter un défi actuel et dépendent directement de la dynamique des fluids appliquée aux poumons et en particulier aux écoulements à échelle microscopique dans l'acinus des poumons. En outre, une déposition d'aérosoles faible voire insuffisante, en particulier chez les enfants en bas âge, continue d'être un fardeau contre l'efficacité de ces procédures térapeutiques. L'ensemble de ces considérations appellent donc à un approfondissement généralisé des connaissances de la mécanique des fluides relative à l'acinus des poumons, mais aussi au développement potentiel de nouvelles stratégies consacrées à l'amélioration et l'augmentation de la déposition d'aérosoles dans les poumons.

La thèse ici présente, qui repose à l'interface entre les sciences de l'ingénieur et la médecine, est consacrée principalement au rôle des écoulements respiratoires dans l'acinus des poumons, en relation avec le transport et la déposition de particules inhalées. Dû à la complexité de l'acinus et la difficulté d'accessibilité à cette région des poumons, les caracteristiques des ecoulements pulmonaires dans l'acinus sont typiquement difficile à évaluer. Ainsi, dans une première étape, nous avons développé des simulations numériques de la dynamique des fluides dans un nombre de modèles de l'acinus à complexité variée. Ces simulations imitent le mouvement rythmique des parois pulmonaires au cours de la respiration afin d'établir la structure et les caractéristiques propres aux écoulements convectifs dans l'acinus pulmonaire, et leur influence sur le transport et la déposition de particules non-diffusantes à l'échelle du micron, représentatives d'aérosoles térapeutiques inhalés. Les simulations présentées ont pour but d'éclaircir la nature complexe des écoulements alvéolaires, représentatifs d'un exemple biologique d'écoulements dans des cavités à bas nombre de Reynolds, entraînés par des mouvements de translation de parois. En outre, nos résultats suggèrent que la cinématique du mouvement d'aérosoles fins est délicate puisque les particules sont influencées par l'interaction entre les écoulements convectifs locaux et les processus de sédimentation dû au champs gravitationel. Ces interactions mécaniques conduisent à des champs de dépositon non uniformes ainsi que des temps de résidences potentiellement importants dans l'espace acinaire, en fonction de l'orientation du champs gravitationel et de la taille des particules.

Dans une étape suivante, à travers l'utilisation de techniques modernes expérimentelles de visualization d'écoulements (Particle Image Velocimetry), nous avons étudié l'implémentation de mécanismes de forcement non invasifs, en particulier (i) le mouvement de convection thermocapillaire de Marangoni et (ii) l'écoulement acoustique, afin de générer et contrôler des écoulements forcés dans des modèles de référence d'alvéoles pulmonaires. Ces explorations expérimentelles sont entreprises tel un premier jalon en vue d'applications médicales à venir qui pourraient potentiellement conduire vers l'augmentation du mélange et de la déposition d'aérosoles dans la région acinaire des poumons.

Acknowledgements

I am amazed to realize that four years have already passed by since I first started my PhD at the Institute of Fluid Dynamics. At the time, I was convinced that I was engaging in a new step in life, in particular in one that would bring me closer to fulfilling a kid's dream to design one day automobiles, and therefore learn on the way about aerodynamics. In a nutshell, this is perhaps the most truthful reason why I initially began looking at fluid mechanics. Four years later, the picture has slightly changed. Indeed, I have no plans on abandoning the field of fluid mechanics (yet!) and I certainly hope to contribute in some way in the years to come to the development and understanding of this fascinating field. However, my years as a PhD student have opened my eyes towards new topics, ones which have eventually convinced me that a scientific career would suit both my personality and my intellectual interests (and maybe I could be just as well content appreciating fancy cars parked on the street). So here I am, a few weeks away from defending my doctoral thesis, a PhD on the topic of respiration. I am myself still astounded.

The work I present here is a reflection of the moral, intellectual (and yes financial) support I have received over the last years from a constellation of people. I am indebted to my PhD supervisor, Prof. Thomas Rösgen, for giving me the freedom of thought to venture out, find my way, and discover my passion for fluid mechanics. I have learned much from you. I would like to thank very warmly Prof. Urs Frey (Inselspital, Universität Bern) and PD Dr. Johannes H. Wildhaber (Kantonspital Fribourg) for introducing me to the fascinating world of pulmonary medicine. This thesis is the outcome of our joint interdisciplinary effort through the support of the Swiss National Science Foundation (SNF). If I've learned with conviction one thing during this period, it is that research is a highly nonlinear field and quite unpredictable.

I would like to thank several other people for contibuting throughout the different stages of my work. I first thank Prof. Peter Niederer (Institute of Biomedical Engineering, ETH Zurich) for his support and giving me the opportunity to lecture in his Biofluidmechanics' course. This has been a particularly wonderful experience for me. I am grateful to Prof. Peter Gehr (Head of the Institute of Anatomy, Universität Bern) for our fruitful discussions and the immense support I have received throughout my research. I am thankful both to PD Dr. Johannes C. Schittny (Institute of Anatomy, Universität Bern) and Dr. Akira Tsuda (Harvard School of Public Health) for the challenging and collegial collaboration we have forged together. Finally, I would like to thank warmly the students whom I have helped supervise during my PhD. They have been the backbone for much of the success of my research. I hope I was able to teach them as much as they have brought me. Thanks to Fabian and Thomas Heimsch ("my genius twins"), Sebastian Schmuki, Retto Sutter, Simon Frey, David Altorfer, and T.-H. "John" Ho (Imperial College, London).

I would like to add some special words for my family to share my appreciation and love for them. I have been truly spoiled. Mom, although you probably don't understand most of the equations written here and we all know that any quote from Richard Feynman can put you to sleep instantly, you continue being an irreplacable moral and emotional pillar in my life. Dad, I realize how some of the work I've published should bear your name. Raphael and I stay amazed by the fact that not only do you understand what we do, but you actually help us with it. Your scientific and fatherly advice is a blessing. Raphael, needless to say how important you are to me, irrespective of geographical location or time zone. I just never imagined we'd end up speaking so much about science together. I look forward to your success. Finally, I thank my beloved one. Sharon, you are an amazing wife and friend to me. Thank you for giving me courage, ambition and believing in me. As you know, I am not a real engineer. I just like books.

I often ask myself whether I have gained after this intense and intellectually stimulating time of my life a deeper understanding of fluid mechanics. I like to hope so. However, I am much more convinced today that the more I learn, the more I realize how little I know.

Josué Sznitman
November 2007

Contents

Notation

Nomenclature

A	cross-sectional area [m^2]
Bo	Bond number
c	speed of sound [m/s]
Ca	Capillary number
C	specific volume excursion; chapter 3: concentration
C_D	drag coefficient
Co	Courant number
d,D	diameter [m]
$D_{O_2,air}$	diffusion coefficient of O_2 in air [m^2/s]
$\underline{e}$	unit vector
E	energy [J]
f	frequency [Hz]
$\underline{f}$,$\underline{F}$,	force [N]
g	gravitational acceleration [m/s^2]
h	height; sedimentation distance [m]
H	gravity number
k	Boltzmann's constant [K^{-1}s^{-2}m^{2}kg]; chapter 8: mode
l,L	length [m]
M	dimensionless frequency parameter
Ma	Mach number
m	mass [kg]
$\underline{n}$	unit normal vector
n	number of deposited particles
N	total number (particles, airways, etc.)
p	pressure [Pa]
P	acoustic power [V]
P_n^m	associated Legendre functions
Pe	Peclet number
P_d	deposition parameter
$\dot{Q}$	volume flow rate [m^3/s]
r,θ,ϕ	spherical coordinates
r,R	radius [m]
R	universal gas constant; resistance [kg/m^{4}s]
Re	Reynolds number
s	edge length [m]
S	surface area [m^2]

St	Strouhal number
Stk	Stokes number
t	time [s]
T	breathing period [s]; temperature [^{o}K]
T_s	sedimentation time [s]
$\underline{u}$	velocity field [m/s]
u, v, w	Cartesian velocity components [m/s]
U	velocity [m/s]
V	volume [m^3]; speed [m/s]
W	work [Nm]
We	Weber number
Wo	Womersley number
$\underline{x}$	Cartesian coordinates [m]
x, y, z	Cartesian coordinates [m]
X_n^m,Y_n^m,Z_n^m	surface harmonics
z	(acinar) airway generation

Greek Symbols

α	opening half angle [rad]; chapter 7: phase shift [rad]
β	length scale expansion factor
χ	solid spherical harmonic
δ	boundary layer thickness [m]
Δ	infinitesimal increment; chapter 4: root-mean-square displacement [m]
ϵ	displacelement [m]
η	total number of alveoli in subacinus
γ	adiabatic constant; appendix A: surface elasticity [N/m^3]
Γ	surfactant concentration [%]
λ	sinusoidal displacement function; chapter 10: eigenvalue
Λ	alveolar dimension [m]
μ	dynamic viscosity [kg/m · s]
ν	kinematic viscosity [m^2/s]
ω	angular frequency [rad/s]; chapters 3 and 10: vorticity [s]
$\underline{\Psi}$	stream function vector
ψ	stream function
Φ	solid spherical harmonic
ρ	density [kg/m^3]
σ	surface tension [N/m]; chapter 10: spatial eigenvector
τ	shear stress [Pa]; chapter 4: particle relaxation time [s]
θ	chapter 10: temporal eigenvector

Subscripts

0	initial ($t = 0$)
a	air

ac	acinus
alv	alveolus
ae	aerodynamic
B	buoyancy
$conv$	convective
d	duct
d, D	drag
$diff$	diffusion
e	entrance
f	film
l	liquid
m	mouth
min	minimum
max	maximum
n	new; normal
o	old
p	particle
P	Poiseuille
pl	pleural
pp	peak-to-peak
r	radial
R	real
rel	relative
s,$sett$	settling
s	surface
se	sedimentation
t	terminal; total
te	thermodynamic
tp	transpulmonary
w	wall

Abbreviations

CFD	computational fluid dynamics
HFOV	high frequency oscillatory ventilation
FFT	fast Fourier transformation
FRC	functional residual capacity
PIV	particle image velocimetry
POD	principal orthogonal decomposition
RMS	root-mean-square
TLC	total lung capacity
TV	tidal volume
XTM	X-ray tomographic microscopy

Chapter 1

Introduction: Aim of Work

The present thesis is principally concerned with the role of convective respiratory flows in the acinar region of the lung, in relation with the transport and deposition of inhaled particles. The pulmonary acinus, otherwise known as the gas exchange region of the lung, constitutes the complex of densely packed alveoli (encompassing $\geq 90\%$ of total lung volume) which guarantee oxygen and carbon-dioxide exchange with blood capillaries across the alveolar membranes. In particular, this region may represent a potential host for pulmonary complications or diseases, which may require, amongst other, the inhalation of therapeutic drugs typically administered in the form of aerosolized particles using various types of existing inhalation devices. However, both the precise understanding of the mechanisms leading to acinar particle deposition, whether aerosols may be recognized as a possible health risk (e.g. pollutants) or a therapeutic tool, as well as the need to target inhalation aerosols to specific pulmonary sites such as the acinus [9, 129], remain ongoing challenges. Moreover, for successful inhalation therapy, heterogeneous if not low or insufficient lung deposition of inhalation aerosols, in particular in infants and children [226], continues to burden the efficacy of such therapeutic procedures in the treatment of pulmonary diseases including asthma, chronic obstructive diseases, cystic fibrosis, etc. Indeed, these procedures depend directly on the fluid dynamics (i.e. respiratory airflows) present in the lung, and specifically on the microflows present in the acinar region. Hence, the general considerations mentioned above call not only for a deepening of our understanding of the fluid mechanics pertinent to the acinar region of the lung and the transport of aerosols, but also for the potential development of novel strategies towards improved and enhanced particle deposition inside the lung. This latter question may involve in the future a departure from traditional methodologies largely based on the selection of aerosol particle size coupled with the limited flow controllability through patients' breathing patterns.

The aim of the present work is, thus, twofold. Due to the complexity and limited accessibility of the pulmonary acinus, acinar flow characteristics remain typically difficult to assess directly. Hence, in a first step, we have developed computational fluid dynamics (CFD) models of the pulmonary acinus to gain detailed insight into the structure and characteristics of convective acinar flows and their influence on the transport and deposition of inhaled non-diffusing micron-sized particles, representative of common inhalation aerosols. In a subsequent step, through means of modern experimental flow visualization techniques (i.e. Particle Image Velocimetry), we have investigated the implementation of non-invasive forcing mechanisms, namely (i) thermocapillary motion and (ii) acoustic streaming, to generate and control forced convective flows within benchmark alveolar models. These experimental explorations are performed as a first milestone in view of future realizable medical applications which may potentially lead towards enhanced particle mixing and deposition in the acinar region of the lung in combination with the use of state-of-the-art inhalation devices. We outline and summarize the structure of the thesis in what follows.

1.1 Thesis Outline

The present work constitutes in principle an interdisciplinary effort between the fields of engineering and medicine, or physiology. Hence, prior knowledge of very distinct, yet somehow related topics such as lung biology and fluid mechanics is paramount for an adequate understanding of the subject. For this reason, *Part I* lays down for the reader the general frame of work, with an introduction to the basics of lung anatomy, as well as to respiratory fluid mechanics and the mechanics of inhaled particles. This first part of the thesis is intended to give both the engineer and the physiologist (or clinician) an adequate background and the mathematical tools necessary to understand the research presented here.

- *Chapter 2* introduces the reader with a general description of the structure and function of the lung, exploring for the purpose of the present thesis relevant anatomical features of the gas exchange region (i.e. the pulmonary acinus). In particular, we include within a historical context a short survey of existing alveolar models and describe subsequently the functional role for lung stability and clearance of the aqueous liquid layer lining present at the alveolar surface. Finally, a brief overview of the basic properties of the mechanics of breathing are explored using energy considerations.
- *Chapter 3* lays down the governing equations of fluid (i.e. air) motion inside the respiratory tract. In particular, characterisitc dimensionless numbers including the Reynolds (Re), Strouhal (St), and Womersley (Wo) numbers are introduced and estimated along the branching airways to assess the relative role of transient, convective and viscous terms. This analysis is followed by the evaluation of airflow resistance and pressure drop along the airway tree. Pertinent to the pulmonary acinar region of the lung, the different forms of the equations of creeping motion (i.e. where airflows are very slow) are then derived. In particular, the relative roles of convection and diffusion mechanisms for gas transport in the acinar region are considered, while the influence of the aqueous liquid layer lining on the continuous phase gas flow is derived using a simple one-dimensional steady-state model for fluid flow. Finally, an extensive review of the relevant literature pertinent to acinar fluid dynamics is surveyed.
- *Chapter 4* is intended to give the reader the basic mathematical tools needed to understand the mechanics governing the motion of inhaled particles. In particular, an overview of the principal mechanisms for aerosol transport and deposition is given. Specifically, these include (i) gravitational sedimentation, (ii) inertial impaction, and (iii) Brownian diffusion. The reader is then exposed to the existing clinical strategies employed to target deposition inside the lung. Finally, a simple analytical approach is followed to derive the approximate time scales necessary for particle deposition inside a model alveolus, depending on the transport mechanism considered.

Part II focuses on elucidating the detailed nature and role of airflows in the acinus and, in particular, within alveolar cavities. For this purpose, we implement computational fluid dynamics (CFD) simulations of respiratory flows in models of the pulmonary acinus. Specifically, three distinct models of the acinus are developed to resolve detailed transient acinar flow structures as well as to determine the transport of inhaled micron-sized particles.

- *Chapter 5* introduces the most basic, yet relevant acinar model developed: namely, a simple alveolated duct. This study both confirms previous findings [97, 270] and illustrates that under wall motion mimicking quiet breathing, alveolar flow topologies may be complex, illustrating recirculating regions, where flows are governed by the interplay between ductal shear flow occuring over the alveolar opening and radial motion induced from the basic wall motion. In particular, under self-similar breathing conditions, alveolar flow patterns may be entirely determined by the location of the alveoli along the acinar tree. In essence, alveolar flows constitute a biological example of low-Reynolds boundary driven cavity flows. The present findings are published in: J. Sznitman, F. Heimsch, T. Heimsch, D. Rusch, and T. Rösgen, "Three-dimensional convective alveolar flow induced by rhythmic breathing motion of the pulmonary acinus," *ASME J. Biomech. Eng.* 129: 658-665, 2007.
- In *chapter 6*, a novel space-filling model of the pulmonary acinar tree is developed based on the original description of lung structure by Fung [71]. Detailed particle trajectories and deposition efficiencies, as well as acinar flow structures, are investigated under different orientations of gravity. The space-filling acinar model is particularly well suited to capture the influence of bulk kinematic interaction between ductal flows and alveolar flows on aerosol transport. In particular, we find the existence of intricate trajectories of fine 1 μm aerosols spanning over the entire acinar airway network, which cannot be captured by simple alveolar models. In contrast, heavier 3 μm aerosols yield trajectories characteristic of gravitational sedimentation, similar to those observed in the simple alveolated duct. For both particle sizes, however, particle inhalation yields highly non-uniform deposition. While larger particles may deposit within a single inhalation phase, finer 1 μm particles exhibit long residence times over multiple breathing cycles. These findings are published in: J. Sznitman, S. Schmuki, R. Sutter, A. Tsuda, and T. Rösgen, "CFD investigation of respiratory flows in a space-filling pumonary acinus model, CA Brebbia ed., In: *Modelling in Medicine and Biology VII, WIT Transactions on Biomedicine and Health*, Vol. 12, pp. 147-156, 2007.
- *Chapter 7* is principally concerned with the implementation of novel, high-resolution (isotropic voxels of 1.43 μm^3) imaging techniques (i.e. synchrotron-based X-ray Tomographic Microscopy (XTM) [253]) to reconstruct, in a first step, 3D alveolar airspaces and perform, subsequently, respiratory flow simulations under moving wall boundary conditions. The resulting alveolar flow patterns in the alveolar sacs are governed by creeping radial motion and are fundamentally time-independent, confirming findings obtained using the above geometrical models. Despite limitations in the image reconstruction schemes due both to intrinsic noise and low intensity contrast in the raw data, the feasibility of the present CFD simulations using reconstructed 3D XTM geometries opens the path towards future, more realistic aerosol kinematics and deposition studies in the pulmonary acinus. The present findings were presented in: J. Sznitman, F. Heimsch, D. Altorfer, JC. Schittny, and T. Rösgen, "Alveolar flow simulations during rhythmical breathing motion in reconstructed XTM acinar airspaces," In: *Proceedings of the 5th World Congress of Biomechanics, 29 July-4 August 2006, Munich, Germany*, D. Liepsch ed., Medimond Inter. Proc., pp. 601-605, 2006.

Part III gathers results obtained from our experimental flow visualization investigations aimed at exploring the implementation of non-invasive flow forcing mechanisms in benchmark models of alveoli. The present experiments were motivated by the potential enhancement of particle mixing and deposition inside the acinar region of the lung using non-invasive convective flow forcing.

- In *chapter 8*, we look at an original family of boundary-driven cavity flows occurring at a fluid-

fluid interface, in analogy to the thin aqueous liquid layer lining at the alveolar surface. Particle Image Velocimetry (PIV) is used to study the structure of internal convective flows observed inside millimeter-sized thin liquid shells (i.e. soap bubbles). Results reveal that the shell exhibits slow motion described by local sporadic "bursts" due to surface tension gradients. The resulting internal flows exhibit similarities with classic setups of low-Reynolds number boundary-driven cavity flows at solid-fluid interfaces. Under thermal forcing, Marangoni induced flow motion in the liquid shell may yield (quasi) steady-state flow recirculation inside the soap bubble cavity. In *chapter 10*, these forced flows are captured by considering analytical solutions of the creeping motion equations in the region interior to the sphere. While it seems probably unlikely to use such techniques in a straightforward medical application for the enhancement of acinar gas flows for increased alveolar depositon, our findings may give further insight on flows induced at the interface between two fluids, where surface tension effects play an important role. These findings were presented in J. Sznitman, and T. Rösgen, "PIV investigation of internal recirculating flows in thin liquid shells," *Proceedings of the 12th International Symposium on Flow Visualization, 10-14 September 2006, Göttingen, Germany.*

- Finally, in *chapter 9*, flow visualizations are presented for acoustic streaming inside transparent hemispherical elastic cavities (~ 5 mm in diameter) oscillating in an acoustic field. Streaming flows are visualized using Particle Image Velocimetry (PIV) and diverse flow fields are encountered for a range of excitation frequencies (3–50 kHz). While the generation of such flows relies on viscous mechanisms at a solid-fluid boundary, in the bulk of the fluid, however, flow patterns are steady and inviscid. Analytically, the measured planar flows may be captured from the general solution of the creeping motion equations inside a sphere, as described in *chapter 10*. The present boundary-driven cavity flows may enhance particle fluid transport mechanisms, leading ultimately to potential fluid mixing applications and perhaps the development of medical applications used for non-invasive enhancement of aerosol lung deposition. The present findings are published in: J. Sznitman, T.H. Ho, and T. Rösgen, "PIV investigation of internal acoustic streaming inside elastic cavities". *Proceedings of the 7th International Symposium on Particle Image Velocimetry, 11-14 September 2007, Rome, Italy*; J. Sznitman, and T. Rösgen, "Acoustic streaming flows in a cavity: an illustration of small-scale inviscid flow," *Physica D*, 2008, in press; and J. Sznitman, and T. Rösgen, "Acoustic streaming visualization in elastic spherical cavities," *J. Visualization*, 2008, in press.

Part I

An Overview of Lung Anatomy and Respiratory Fluid Mechanics

Chapter 2

A Description of the Lung

To understand the fluid dynamics of respiration, and in particular respiratory flows in the smallest units of the lung (i.e. alveoli), it is essential to gain a basic understanding of the structure and function of the lung. In this introductory chapter, we first give a brief overview of the anatomy of the airway tree. For our purposes, we describe in some detail the structures of the distal regions of the lung (i.e. pulmonary acini which are composed of millions of alveoli) and introduce some of the models postulated over the course of history which describe the alveolar geometry. We elaborate on the existence of an aqueous liquid lining layer at the surface of the airways, containing amongst other pulmonary surfactant crucial for lung stability. This lining layer is essential for clearance mechanisms (e.g. clearance of deposited particles on airway walls) through the motion of beating ciliated cells on conducting airways (similar to tiny hairs), and gives rise to surface tension gradient driven motion in the acinus. Finally, an understanding of fluid mechanics in the lung requires an exposure to the essentials of respiratory mechanics. We describe, here, basic notions on the mechanics of breathing, including the importance of pressure–volume diagrams to introduce stress-strain relations for the lung and derive quantitative values for surface tension acting at the liquid/air interface.

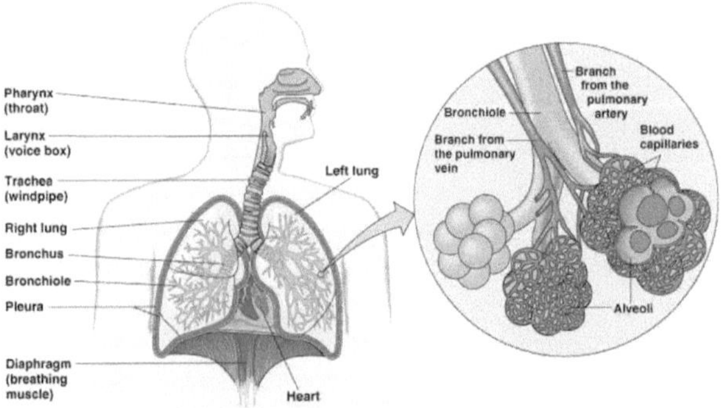

Figure 2.1: Schematic illustration of the respiratory tract. Copyright 2004 Pearson Education, Inc.

2.1 The Airway Tree

To exchange oxygen and carbon dioxide within the body, blood and air must be brought into close contact over a large surface area, nearly the size of a tennis court (approximately 130 m^2), in the human lung [282]. For this to happen in an orderly fashion, a system of branched airways that have their origin in the trachea is constructed to connect all of the ~ 300 million alveoli, which constitute the gas exchanger, to the outside air.

In the human and mammalian lung, the airways are built as dichotomous (dividing into two parts) trees (Figs. 2.1 and 2.2). In the human lung, this goes on for approximately 23 generations, and since the number of branches doubles with each generation, there will be approximately 2^{23} (or 8 million) end branches, generally called alveolar sacs. This, of course, remains an average value as the number of branching generations needed to reach the alveolar sacs is quite variable (from about 18 to 30). This variability results from the fact that the airway tree forms a space-filling tree whose endings must be homogenously distributed in space and reach into every corner and gap in the available space which is determined by the form of the chest cavity into which the lung develops. Some spaces are filled rapidly and the airways cannot continue to divide, whereas in other regions more branches are needed to fill the space.

There is, however, a marked difference in terms of the degree of irregularity in the airway branching pattern: in the human lung, the airway branching is to some extent symmetric (Fig. 2.3(a)), but in other mammalian lungs (Fig. 2.3(b)) the branching pattern is quite asymmetric. This difference has largely to do with the shape of the space that must be filled. In the human lung that space is nearly "spherical" whereas in most quadrupedal animals, the lung is longer and narrower.

Of approximately 23 generations of airways, the first 14 proximal airways are purely conducting pipes built as smooth-walled tubes to distribute convective airflow into the lung. This design ends more or less abruptly when the airways reach lung parenchyma, the complex of alveoli that are arranged as a foam-like sleeve on the surface of peripheral airways (Fig. 2.4(a)). Roughly speaking, this is the region of the airway tree where oxygen diffusion plays an important role in the supply of oxygen to the gas exchange surface (we will later look at the role of diffusion for oxygen transport more quantitatively).

The airway tree is thus divided into two major functional zones (Fig. 2.5(a)): the first (approximately)

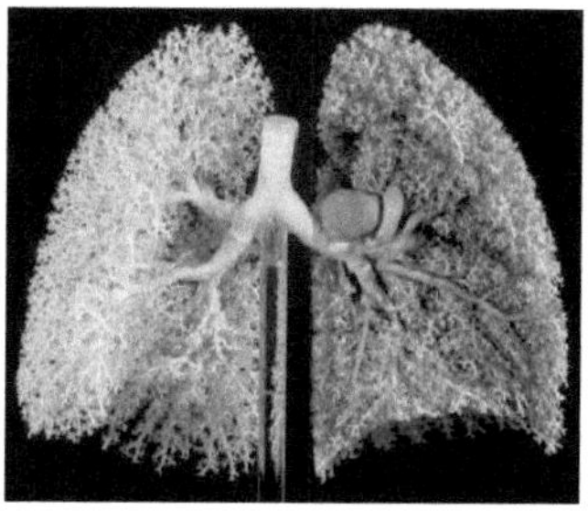

Figure 2.2: Cast of human bronchial tree. Arteries and veins are shown in red and blue [281]. With kind permission of Springer Science and Business Media.

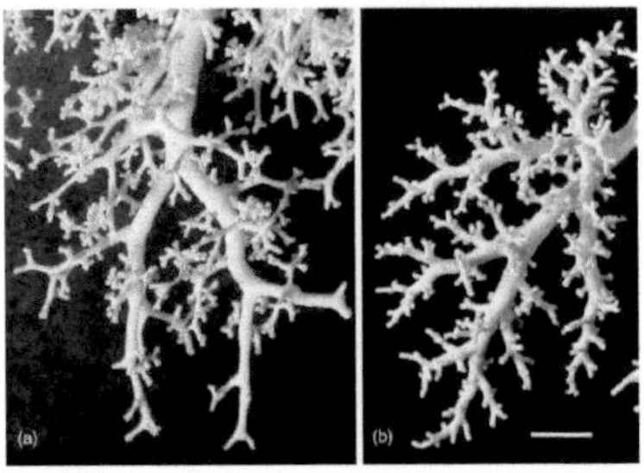

Figure 2.3: Casts of peripheral conducting airways of (a) human lung, (b) rat lung [284]. With permission from Elsevier Publisher.

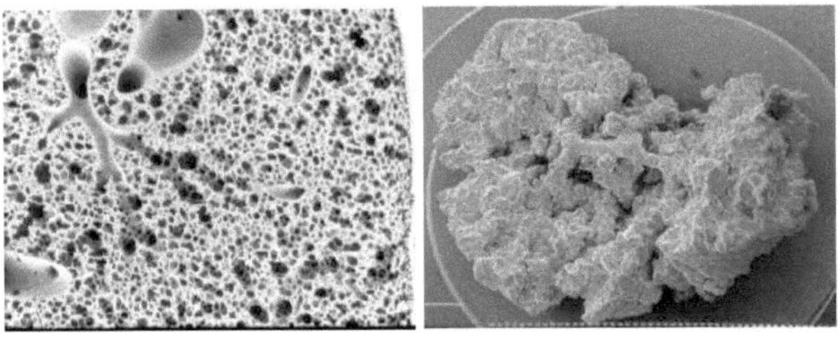

(a) (b)

Figure 2.4: (a) Transition from conducting to acinar airways in scanning electron micrograph. The sequence of branched alveolar ducts following on transitional bronchiole is seen from inside [284]. With permission from Elsevier Publisher. (b) Partly dissected acinus from human lung showing transitional and respiratory bronchioles as well as alveolar ducts and sacs [90]. With kind permission from John Wiley & Sons, Inc.

14-16 generations are designed as conducting airways where air flows by convection; this is followed by about 8 generations of acinar airways where axial channels (called "alveolar ducts") are wrapped around by a sleeve of alveoli with gas exchange tissue on their surface.

2.2 Structure of the Gas-Exchanger

The pulmonary gas exchanger forms in the walls of the alveoli that contain a dense capillary network. Here oxygen and carbon dioxide are exchanged between air and blood with great efficiency because of the intense contact between these two media over a very large surface and across a very thin barrier (approximately 3–4 μm [156]). The driving force for gas exchange is the partial pressure difference for oxygen between alveolar air and capillary blood. This can only be maintained if the capillaries are

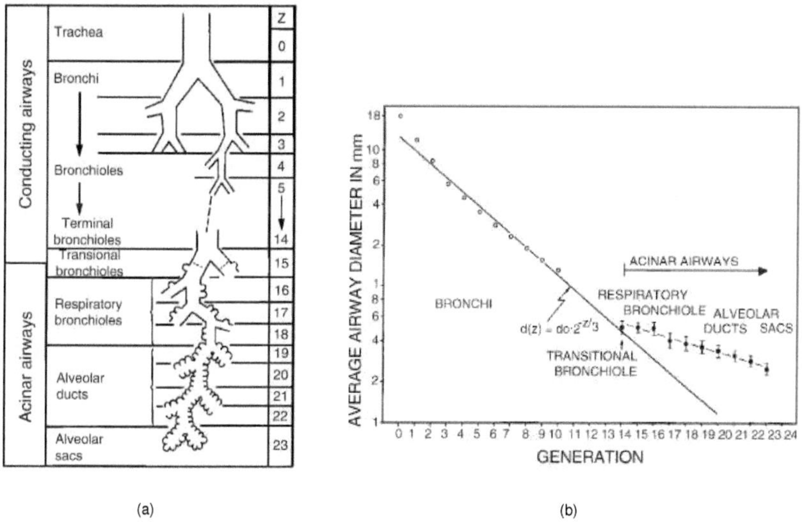

Figure 2.5: (a) Model of human airway system assigned to generations of symmetric branching from trachea (generation 0) to acinar airways (generations 15-23), ending in alveolar sacs. Modified after Weibel [281]. With kind permission of Springer Science and Business Media. (b) Average airway diameter in a symmetric model of human airways [90]. With kind permission from John Wiley & Sons, Inc.

perfused at a high rate, and the alveolar air continuously replenished with oxygen.

In order to allow efficient ventilation of the gas exchange surface, alveoli are arranged around the ducts and form a tightly packed sleeve of cup-like chambers that all open onto one duct. Adjacent alveoli are separated by septa (dividing membranes) that contain the capillary network. By this arrangement, the alveolar surface area available for gas exchange is approximately five times larger than the surface of the duct.

The capillary network is also related to the conducting blood vessels. It appears as a continuum of flat networks within the connected inter-alveolar septa, similar to a knitted "sheet", with which arterioles and venules are connected, thus allowing the perfusing blood to spread broadly over the alveolar surface [73]. Capillaries are contained within the inter-alveolar septa and exchange gases with two adjacent alveoli (Fig. 2.6). Furthermore, as alveolar septa form a three-dimensional maze after the pattern of soap bubbles [281] or honey combs [57], the capillary network follows that geometry and also forms a three-dimensional complex of inter-connected flat network units (Fig. 2.6(a)).

We open a short parenthesis to introduce a useful terminology, the "pulmonary acinus", commonly employed to describe the gas-exchange region of the lung. We will use this expression again in later topics on respiratory fluid dynamics. The pulmonary acinus is the terminal unit of the respiratory airways that are directly associated with the gas exchanging surface. The most precise definition is that the pulmonary

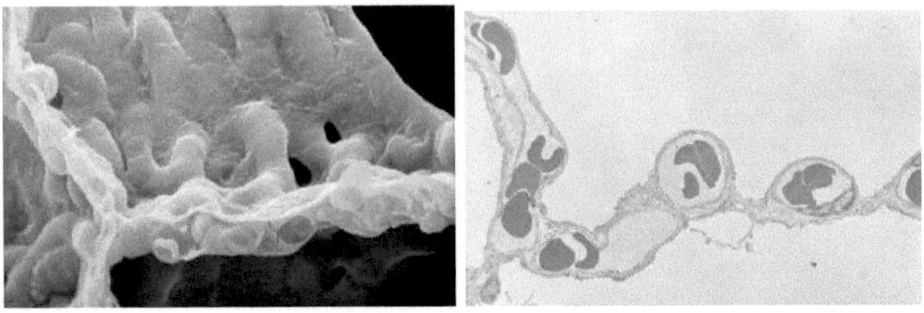

(a) (b)

Figure 2.6: Fine structure of the alveolar septum in human lungs shown in a scanning electron micrograph (a) and a thin section (b). Note the thin tissue barrier separating the blood cells from the air [284]. With permission from Elsevier Publisher.

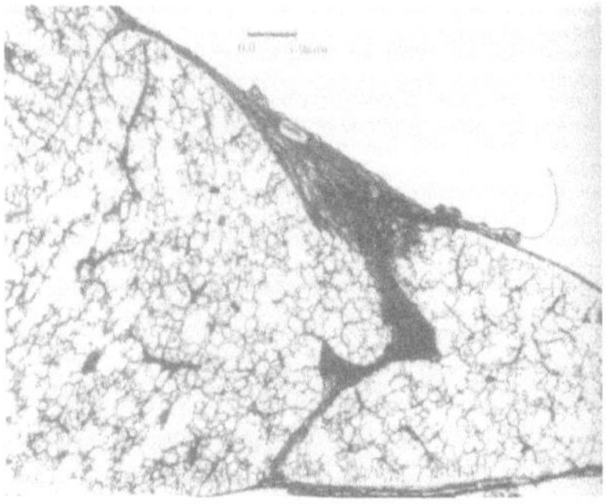

Figure 2.7: Histological photograph of alveolar ducts in a thick section (150 μm) of human lung [148]. With kind permission of Springer Science and Business Media. Curvature of alveolar mouths is evident.

acinus comprises the branched complex of alveolated airways that are connected to the same first order respiratory or transitional bronchiole (Fig. 2.5(a)). Since the acinus is a tree-like structure, this definition would identify the transitional bronchiole as the stem of the acinus [90]. An example of a complete acinus is illustrated in Fig. 2.4(b). Estimates place the total number of acini at 30'000 in an average adult human lung (total lung volume is on the order of 6 l). This space accounts for well over 90% of the total lung volume, while the conducting region of the lung (also known as the "dead space" as it does not participate in gas exchange) only holds approximately 150 ml of air.

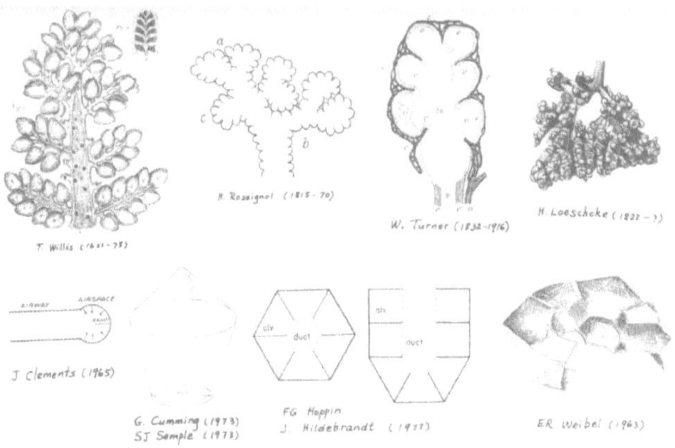

Figure 2.8: A series of well-known acinar models developed through history [72]. With kind permission of Springer Science and Business Media.

2.3 Models of Alveoli and Alveolar Ducts

From both an anatomical and fluid dynamics perspective, one must begin with a precise description of the geometric structure of the acinus. Hence it is necessary to have a mathematical model of the alveolar ducts and alveoli. Looking at histological photographs (Fig. 2.7), one gets the impression that alveolar ducts are bounded by curved edges, but it remains difficult to obtain a three-dimensional model. Hanson and Ampaya [92] reconstructed a region of postmortem human lung wall by wall, and obtained a great deal of data but nevertheless the mathematical model remains to be constructed.

Pulmonary researches have long engaged in model building. Miller [158] reviewed the history of the development of concepts of the structure of the alveoli and alveolar ducts from Malpighi (1661) [145] to Loeschke (1921) [140]. New results have been added by Orsos (1836) [170], Weibel (1963) [281] and Mercer *et al.* (1987) [155]. Some of these alveolar models are illustrated in Fig. 2.8. Those in the upper rows visualize alveoli as bunches of grapes, where each alveolar wall has an "inside" and "outside". On the inside there acts the alveolar gas pressure. On the outside, the pressure is presumably the pleural pressure (which will be described again when looking at the mechanics of breathing, section 2.5). This model culminates in that of von Neergaard (1929) [279], as shown in Fig. 2.8 from Clements [31], where the importance of surface tension on the stability of the lung was asserted. However, one difficulty the model leads to is shown in the top left corner of Fig. 2.9. If two soap bubbles were blown at the end of two tubes, where the tubes are connected and open to each other, then at equilibrium, the smaller bubble would have collapsed[1]. Similarly, if a human lung were considered as 300 millions bubbles connected in parallel to an airway, then one would conclude that at equilibrium all but one alveolus will be collapsed, unless the surface tension is zero, or the elastic force overwhelms the surface force. Obviously, the lung does not work in such fashion and the alveolus bubble model is both a misconception of anatomy and

[1] Laplace's formula, Eq. (A.13) from Appendix A, states that the pressure in the smaller bubble is higher than in the large one. Hence the gas in the smaller bubble will flow into the larger one.

misapplication of physics, as noted recently by Prange [196]. The major fault of this model is that it ignores the fact that an alveolar wall is an interalveolar septum. The inside of one alveolus is the outside of another alveolus. The pressure difference across each septum is negligibly small. A septum must be a minimal surface, one whose mean curvature is zero.

Other illustrations in Fig. 2.8 show the models of alveolar duct described by Weibel [281], Cummings & Semple [36], and Hoppin & Hilderbrandt [105], who did not describe the rules of how these units are organized into an airway tree that fills the entire space of the lung. To meet the space-filling requirement, Fung (1988) [71] proposed a model and validated it against available morphometric data. This model is based on the assumptions that all alveoli are equal and space filling before they are ventilated. Furthermore, all alveoli are ventilated to ducts as uniformly as possible, and they are reinforced at the edges of the ventilation holes (i.e. alveolar mouths) for structural integrity, and distorted by lung weight and inflation according to the theory of elasticity [71]. We will come back in more detail to the space-filling description of the acinus by Fung (1988) in section 6 to develop a computational fluid dynamics (CFD) model.

2.4 The Liquid Lining Layer

The aqueous substrate which covers the surface of the conducting airways consists of water, ions, sugars, proteins, proteoglycans, glycoproteins, and lipids [205]. It originates from the airway epithelium and

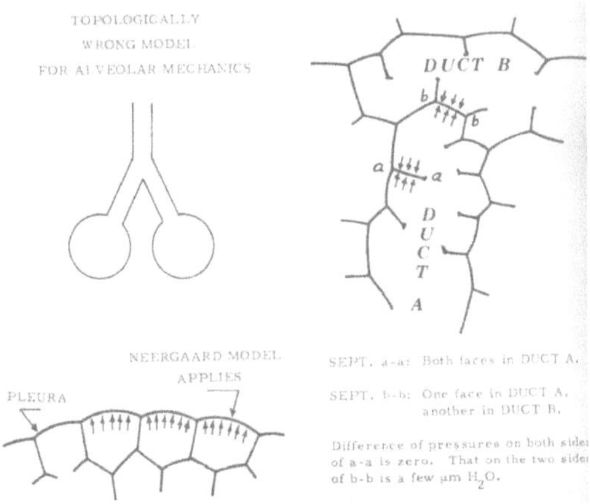

Figure 2.9: Topological structure of pulmonary alveoli. *Top left*:Topologically wrong model for alveolar mechanics. *Top right*: Schematic of the typical arrangement of interalveolar septa. Septum a-a: Both sides are in the same alveolar duct; the net pressure difference between the two sides is zero. Septum b-b: One side is in duct A, the other side in duct B; the difference in the pressures acting on the two sides is on the order of a few μm H_2O. *Bottom left*: Equilibrium of pulmonary pleura, to which von Neeergard's model applies. From Fung [70]. With kind permission of Springer Science and Business Media.

the submucosal glands [113]. Apparently, there is substantial variation in mucus thickness and the aqueous liquid layer lining is reported to vary from 10–12 μm in the trachea to 2–5 μm in the bronchi and finally 0.1 μm in the peripheral airways [75]. In particular, Bastacky *et al.* [8] claim that the liquid lining in the acinus is continuous, with a mean thickness varying from 0.14 μm over flat sections up to 0.89 μm in areas of greater concavity. Thus, it appears that the geometry of the aqueous layer is highly dynamic and that movements of liquid across the airway wall and along the airway tree are important factors in establishing the thickness of the lining layer.

The aqueous lining layer is thought to consist of two phases: a less viscous sol phase (periciliary fluid) surrounding the beating cilia and, above, a more viscous gel phase, the mucus blanket [141]. The periciliary phase is regarded as a continuous aqueous layer of relatively low viscosity, with its depth maintained at a little less than the ciliary length. This allows the ciliary tips to penetrate into the overlaying, more viscous gel phase during the propulsive (effective) strokes and claw the mucus forward to transport all sorts of particles including cells, cell debris, and dust contained in it towards the pharynx [118]. The existence, thickness and continuity of the gel phase are debated with respect to the different airway compartments and between different species [104, 296]. On the one hand, mucus has been reported to be non-continuous and to be present as streaks, flakes or plaques in large rat airways and human bronchi [275]. On the other hand, mucus has been described as a superficial continuous layer in several species [243].

Gil and Weibel [82] demonstrated for the first time the existence of an osmiophilic layer covering the bronchiolar fluid. In addition, they showed the continuity between bronchiolar and alveolar linings. More recently such a film was also demonstrated in the trachea and large airways [77, 131]. Figure 2.10 represents a transmission electron micrograph (TEM) showing an osmiophilic film at the air-liquid interface in a horse trachea. The existence of a surfactant film at the air-liquid interface in the trachea and large airways is supported by the following additional evidence. The surface tension in large accessible airways has been measured in vivo by placing oil droplets onto trachea or bronchi of anaesthetized mammals. The surface tension of $\approx$ 30 mN/m at the air-liquid interface in horses indicates the accumulation of surface

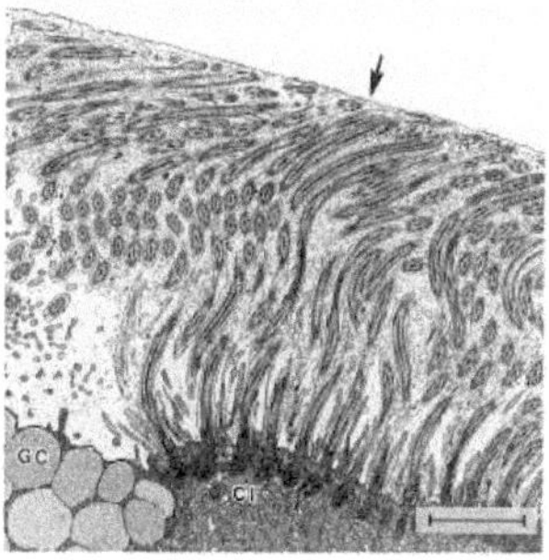

Figure 2.10: Transmission electron micrograph of normal horse trachea after fixation. The air-liquid interface is covered by an osmiophilic film (arrow). The aqueous lining layer surrounds and covers the cilia. GC, goblet cell; CI, ciliated cell. Bar = 2 μm [229]. With permission from Elsevier Publisher.

active molecules at this interface [111]. Without an accumulation of such molecules, the surface tension of the aqueous phase would be much higher, between 45 and 60 mN/m.

2.4.1 Mechanical Functions of Pulmonary Surfactant

Pulmonary surfactant stabilizes the gas exchange region of the lung by reducing the surface tension at the air-liquid interface of the pulmonary alveoli, particularly during expiration. Measurements of lung volume obtained during the controlled inflation/deflation of a normal lung show that the volumes obtained during deflation exceed those during inflation, at a given pressure. This difference in inflation and deflation volumes at a given pressure is called hysteresis and is due to the presence of surfactant (as will be discussed in greater detail in section 2.5). Surfactant decreases the surface tension part of elastic recoil as originally observed by von Neergaard [279]. If the lungs did not secrete surfactant, this surface tension would be much higher preventing the lungs from inflating normally, as is the case in premature infants suffering from infant respiratory distress syndrome (RDS). The normal surface tension for water is 70 dyn/cm (70 mN/m) and in the lungs it is $\approx$ 25 dyn/cm (25 mN/m). However, at the end of the expiration, compressed surfactant phospholipid molecules decrease the surface tension to very low, near-zero levels. Pulmonary surfactant thus greatly reduces surface tension, increasing compliance[2] and allowing the lung to inflate much more easily, thereby eliminating the work of breathing. It reduces the pressure difference needed to allow the lung to inflate. The reduction in surface tension also reduces fluid accumulation in the alveolus as the surface tension draws fluid across the alveolar wall.

As the alveoli increase in size, the surfactant becomes more spread out over the surface of the liquid. This increases surface tension effectively slowing the rate of increase of the alveoli. This also helps all alveoli in the lungs expand at the same rate, as one that increases more quickly will experience a large rise in surface tension slowing its rate of expansion. It also means the rate of shrinking is more regular as if one reduces in size more quickly the surface tension will reduce more so other alveoli can contract more easily than itself.

[2]Compliance is the volume change per unit of pressure change across the lung (see section 2.5).

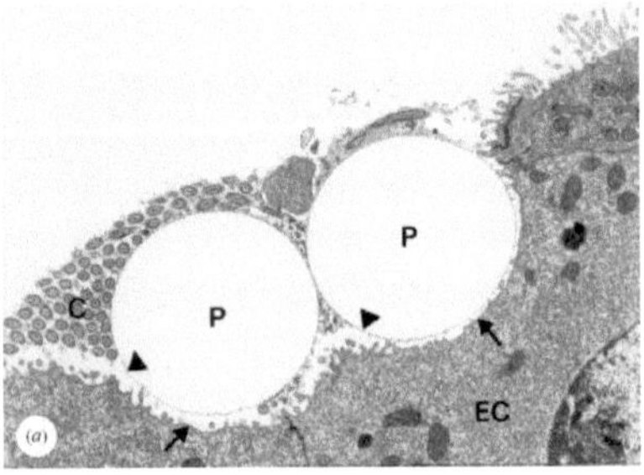

Figure 2.11: Transmission electron micrograph of the airway epithelium of a hamster. It shows two polystyrene particles (P) of a test aerosol, 6 μm in diameter, deposited on the airway wall and subsequently displaced into the aqueous liquid lining layer. Note the indentation (arrows) into the epithelial cells (EC) and the cilia (C) surrounding the particles. From Gehr *et al.* [74]. With kind permission from the Royal Society.

The entire stabilization process described above is the principal and well-known mechanical function of pulmonary surfactant. In contrast, the mechanical functions of airway surfactant are not as well established. One of the functions is particle transport from the alveoli to the ciliated airways by a surface tension gradient [193, 247]. Pulmonary surfactant is produced in the alveolar region by Type II epithelial cells. Direct measurement of surface tension in alveoli demonstrate periodic variations between 0 and 25 dyn/cm during breathing [6]. By comparison, surface tension in the trachea remains relatively constant near a value of $\approx$ 30 dyn/cm [76]. Consequently, a time-mean surface tension gradient exists with the potential to transport liquid out of the lung periphery via the airway liquid layer. Although the origin of this gradient is not fully understood, it is likely due to a variety of factors, including the localized production of surfactant in the alveolar zone, degradation, reabsorption or fouling of surfactant along the airway tree, transepithelial liquid flux, and ventilation [60].

Another important mechanical function of airway surfactant is particle translocation towards epithelium airways. After their deposition in the airspaces of the lung, particles are wetted and displaced towards the epithelium by the surfactant film during the retention process [229]. Pulmonary surfactant promotes the displacement of particles from air to the aqueous phase and the extent of particle immersion depends on the surface tension of the surface active film. The lower the surface tension the greater is the immersion of the particles into the aqueous subphase. Mathematical analysis of the forces acting on a particle deposited on an air-fluid interface shows that for small particles ($<$ 100 μm), the surface tension force is several orders of magnitude greater than forces related to gravity [228]. Thus, even at the relatively high surface tension obtained in the airways (32 $\pm$ 2 dyn/cm), particles will still be displaced into the aqueous subphase. Particles in peripheral airways and alveoli are likely below the surfactant film and submerged in the subphase. Figures 2.11 and 2.12 illustrate the complete immersion of deposited particles under the aqueous lining layer.

2.4.2 Retention and Clearance of Particles

Inhaled particles may be deposited in the conducting airways or they may enter the gas exchange region of the lungs. By definition, deposition of particles is terminated as soon as they touch the walls of the airspaces. Following deposition, retention and clearance processes begin.

Clearance of insoluble particles from the airspace surfaces in the lungs has two predominant phases.

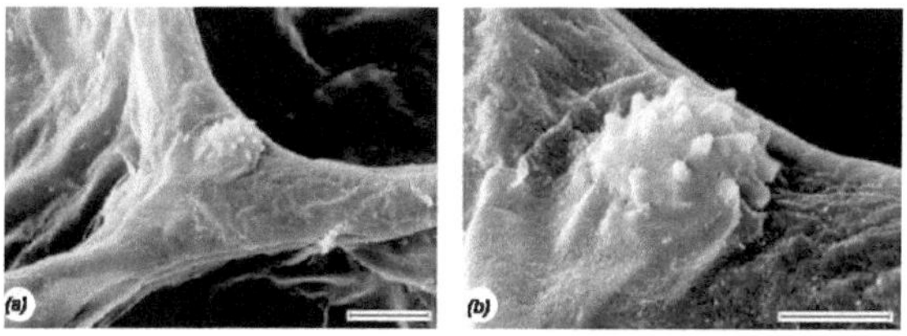

Figure 2.12: Scanning electron micrograph of puffball spores deposited on alveolar surfaces. (b) is a close-up of (a). The spore is completely covered by the surface lining layer and its topography is visible through the thin layer. Bar = $5\ \mu$m in (a) and bar = $2\ \mu$min (b). From Geiser *et al.* [78]. Used with permission from the American Physiological Society.

The first phase, which is rapid, applies to particles deposited on the surfaces of conducting airways. This phase, which is mediated by mucociliary activity (larynx, trachea, bronchi and bronchioles are covered with beating cilia and mucus that is driven toward the throat and swallowed), is usually completed in 24–36 hours but may take longer [246, 249].

In the alveolarized regions of the respiratory tract, the clearance of insoluble particles is extremely complex [124]. Alveoli are not covered with mucus and have no ciliated cells. Clearance of some particles deposited in the gas-exchange region is thus much slower in comparison and may last for months and up to years. The major clearance mechanisms are solubilization, engulfment and transport by macrophage cells [256], movement into the lymph system followed by transport to nymph nodes, and possibly movement to the mucus-coated airways were they are transported to the throat for swallowing.

If the respiratory tract is healthy, the clearance of insoluble particles will generally be multiphasic, with a faster clearance of those particles deposited on mucus-coated regions and much slower clearance for those deposited in alveoli. Figure 2.13 shows typical clearance curves for insoluble particles in normal (healthy) humans and clearance curves for several species.

2.5 Mechanics of Breathing

The lung is enveloped in a membrane–the *pulmonary* (or *visceral*) *pleura*. The internal surface of the thoracic cavity is lined with another membrane–the *parietal pleura* (Fig. 2.14). These two membranes are joined together at their edges and enclose a space known as the *pleural cavity*. Normally, the volume of the pleural cavity is small: the spacing between the pulmonary and parietal pleura is only a few μm. This space is filled with a fluid whose pressure is the *pleural pressure*, p_{PL}. The pulmonary pleura is acted on one side by p_{PL}, and on the other side by the *alveolar gas pressure*, p_{ALV}, and the stress from the lung tissue. The difference of the pressures, $p_{ALV} - p_{PL}$, is responsible for inflating the pulmonary pleura as a balloon, and is called the *transpulmonary pressure*, p_{TP}. The tendency to inflate is resisted by the stresses in *pleura* and *lung parenchyma* (lung parenchyma occupies about 90% of the total lung volume and consists of the alveoli, alveolar ducts and sacs, and capillary blood vessels, arterioles, and

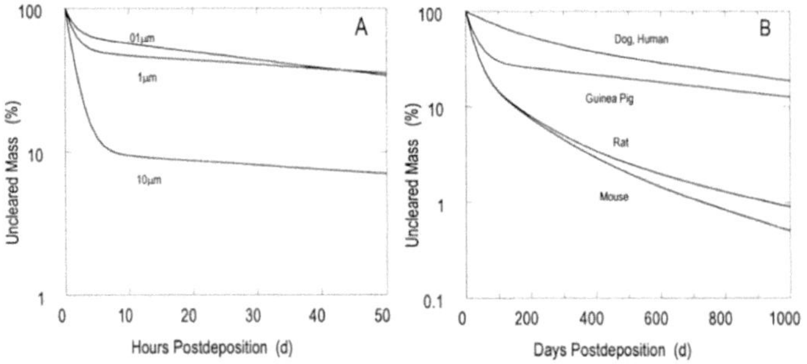

Figure 2.13: Clearance curves for (A) insoluble particles inhaled by humans [291] and (B) curves for 1 to 3 μm diameter particles for dogs, humans, guinea pigs, mice and rats [109]. With permission from Elsevier Publisher.

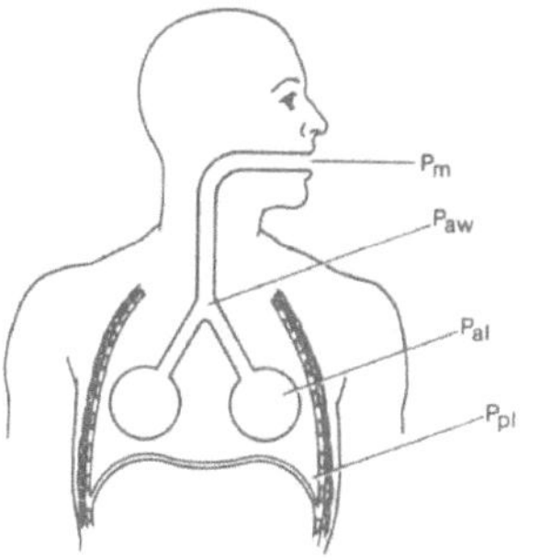

Figure 2.14: Schematic of human chest and lung. From Fung [70]. With kind permission of Springer Science and Business Media.

venules). To understand lung inflation, we will look at macroscopic pressure-volume curves of the lung. On the other hand, the movement of gas from the mouth to the alveoli and vice versa depends on the difference of the pressure at the mouth, p_M, and the pressure in the alveoli p_{ALV}. The pressure p_M is usually atmospheric. This leaves p_{PL} and p_{ALV} as the principal variables for ventilation. In normal breathing, p_{PL}, p_{ALV} and the flow vary with time.

The lung is, for most part, a passive mechanical system that functions in a continuously expanded state. When the chest wall expands, the lung expands, and when the respiratory muscles relax, the lung contracts, but transpulmonary pressure, p_{TP}, remains positive over the entire respiratory cycle. The pressure-volume behavior of the lung is its basic mechanical property, and this can be measured directly. Indeed, static mechanical properties of the lung and chest wall are conventionally expressed with pressure-volume (PV) curves, which describe the deformation (volume change, ΔV) in response to an applied force (pressure change, ΔP). The ratio $\Delta V/\Delta P$ provides an index of the relative ease with which the tissue can be deformed, and is termed *compliance*. The higher the compliance, the easier the deformation under conditions in which airflow is zero (static).

Typical PV curves of the adult lung are shown in Fig. 2.15. The saline PV curve in this figure was recorded during inflation-deflation with liquid (normal saline solution). It reflects the stress-strain characteristics of pulmonary tissue in the absence of air/liquid surface tension forces. The inflation and deflation limbs are virtually superimposed, indicating that there is little hysteresis during tissue expansion and contraction. Tissue relaxation follows the path of tissue deformation.

The extent to which air inflation and deflation curves are displaced to the right (increased pressure) of the liquid curves is traditionally accepted as the force or pressure required to overcome surface tension at the air/liquid interface [250, 251]. Whereas these differences vary among experiments and experimental technique, the curves in Fig. 2.15 are representative of experiments performed under static conditions. In this case, the deflation curve of the air PV diagram is virtually superimposable on the saline curves at volumes that exceed *functional residual capacity*[3] (FRC) and at lesser volumes to P0 (i.e. $P = 0$ in Fig. 2.15). Consequently, surface tension is predictably at or near zero, and lung recoil is essentially a function of tissue elastic recoil in these regions.

[3]The volume of gas in the lung after normal normal expiration.

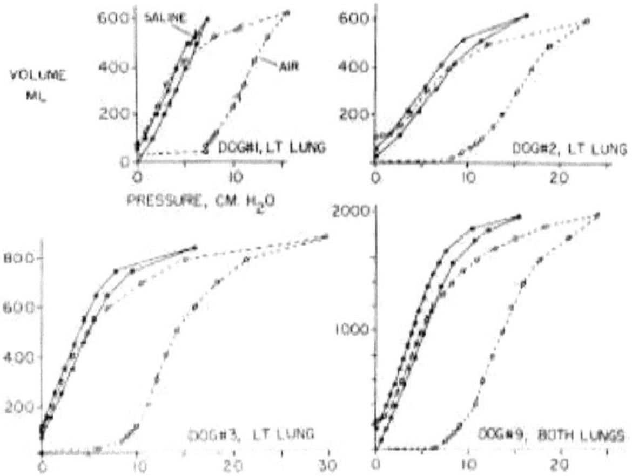

Figure 2.15: Air (dashed) and liquid (solid) PV curves of adult dog lungs inflated from the degassed state. From Mead *et* al. [153]. Used with permission from the American Physiological Society.

2.5.1 Inflation and Deflation

The initial segment of the inflation curve represents aeration of conducting airways Fig. 2.15. The onset of aeration of peripheral lung units (i.e. acinus) is marked by the bend ("knee") in the curve, followed by rapid volume gain as pressure is increased to Pmax (see Fig. 2.15). The high pressures required to aerate peripheral units (at high expanding pressures, the lung is stiffer–compliance is reduced since the slope $\Delta V/\Delta P$ decreases–) may be related to the Laplace equation (Eq. (A.14), see Appendix A).

Pressure reduction from Pmax results in progressively rapid reduction of volume in the adult lung. The deflation curve is displaced to the left of the inflation curve because the opening phenomenon is not reversed. That is, most airways and alveoli remain open at P0. Reinflation of the lung from P0 to Pmax produces an inflation curve similar to the previous deflation curve (not shown here). This suggests that once the airspaces are open, both elastic and surface forces are reversible. In fact, the extent to which the reinflation curve may be displaced to the right of the deflation curve indicates the extent to which airspaces may have closed during the preceding deflation [69].

Patency of airspaces at P0 may be explained by several mechanisms. Large airway structure is maintained by cartilage, and peripheral airways are tethered by direct fibrous continuity with the connective tissue network [217]. Connective tissue traction among peripheral units (mechanical interdependence) is given as the principal mechanism for maintaining airspace potency [152]. Whereas airways remain open at P0, they can be made to collapse at subatmospheric pressure [144]. Conversely, peripheral units do not collapse under similar conditions, the so-called intrinsic resistance of alveoli to atelectasis[4] [22].

[4]Atelectasis is the collapse of part or all of a lung. It is caused by a blockage of the air passages (bronchus or bronchioles) or by pressure on the lung.

2.5.2 Energy Analysis of the Pressure-Volume Curve

Analysis and modelling are needed to separate the contributions of surface tension and tissue forces to lung recoil and to describe how surface area of the lung changes with lung volume and surface tension. Wilson [288, 289] introduced a method to evaluate surface tension on the alveolar walls of a lung. The method is based on energy consideration.

If the differences between recoil pressure of air and saline-filled lungs is caused by surface tension, as described above, the value of surface tension in the air-filled lung might be deduced from this difference. Previous attempts to do so have relied on the assumption that the tissue component of recoil at any lung volume is equal to the recoil pressure of the saline-filled lung at that volume and that the surface area of the lung is a function of lung volume alone, independent of surface tension [7, 274]. The data show that surface area decreases with increasing surface tension at given lung volumes. This implies that surface tension causes an internal deformation, and thus the tissue component of recoil may be affected by surface tension. Instead, a method for deducing surface tension may be adopted where these assumptions are replaced by the statement that the energy of the lung is minimum at equilibrium [288].

The total energy of an air-filled lung, E, is assumed to be the sum of the elastic energy stored in the tissue and the surface energy. The tissue energy is itself composed of two parts, namely the sum of the energy of a saline-filled lung (in which the surface tension can be ignored), U_S, and the additional strain energy associated with the distortion of the alveolar wall caused by the imposition of the surface tension when the lung became air-filled, $\Delta U(V, S)$. S represents the total area of the alveolar walls and V represents the lung volume. It is assumed that U_S is a function of V alone, and ΔU is a function of two independent variables V and S. The surface energy depends on the surface tension σ and is given

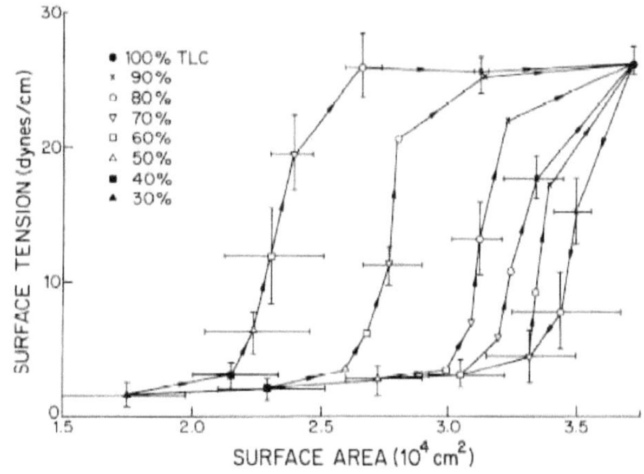

Figure 2.16: The surface area–surface tension relationship of rabbit lung as a function of lung size. TLC=total lung capacity. From Wilson (1982) [289]. Used with permission from the American Physiological Society.

by $\int \sigma dS$. Thus,

$$E = U_S(V) + \Delta U(V, S) + \int_0^S \sigma dS. \tag{2.1}$$

At a fixed lung volume, the equilibrium state of the lung structure minimizes the total energy. Hence, the partial derivative of E with respect to S must be zero at the equilibrium state:

$$\frac{\partial E}{\partial S} = \frac{\partial \Delta U}{\partial S} + \sigma = 0. \tag{2.2}$$

If the lung volume is increased by dV, the work done by the transpulmonary pressure $p_{TP} = p_A - p_{PL}$ is $(p_A - p_{PL})dV$, whereas the energy is increased by dE. These two must be equal such that:

$$p_A - p_{PL} = \frac{dE}{dV} = \frac{dU_S}{dV} + \frac{\partial \Delta U}{\partial V} + \frac{\partial \Delta U}{\partial S}\frac{dS}{dV} + \sigma \frac{dS}{dV}. \tag{2.3}$$

The sum of the last two terms vanishes on account of Eq. (2.2). The first term on the right-hand side, dU_S/dV, can be identified as the recoil pressure of the saline-filled lung p_S. Therefore, Eq. (2.3) is reduced to the following form:

$$p_A - p_{PL} - p_S = \frac{\partial \Delta U}{\partial V}. \tag{2.4}$$

Differentiating Eq. (2.2) with respect to V and Eq. (2.4) with respect to S and eliminating $\partial^2 \Delta U/\partial V \partial S$, one obtains:

$$\frac{\partial \sigma}{\partial V} = -\frac{\partial (p_A - p_{PL} - p_S)}{\partial S}. \tag{2.5}$$

Then an integration yields Wilson's equation [288]:

$$\sigma = -\int_{V_S}^{V} \frac{\partial (p_A - p_{PL} - p_S)}{\partial S} dV, \tag{2.6}$$

where V_S is the volume of the saline-filled lung at which the surface tension vanishes. The integrand in Eq. (2.6) is a function of the alveolar area A and lung volume V, and can be determined experimentally. Hence, Eq. (2.6) can be used to calculate $\sigma(V, S)$.

Bachofen *et al.* [5] and Gil *et al.* [81] fixed rabbit lungs by perfusing fixatives through pulmonary blood vessels, then prepared histological slides from which the surface area of the alveolar walls was measured by stereological methods. They obtained the surface area of alveolar walls in air-filled, saline-filled, and detergent-rinsed and then air-filled rabbit lungs inflated to various percentages of total lung capacity. From these data, Wilson & Bachofen [290] derived $p_A - p_{PL} - p_S$ and V_S as functions of V and S and calculated σ as a function of S. Their results are shown in Fig 2.16. It may be seen from the figure that the calculated values of the surface tension decrease to less than 2 dyn/cm (1 dyn/cm = 10^{-3} N/m) as surface area decreases along the deflation limb of the pressure-volume curve. Surface tension increases very steeply with surface area on the inflation limbs, reaching a limiting value just under 30 dynes/cm.

Chapter 3

Elements of Fluid Mechanics in the Respiratory Tract

To answer many questions about respiration as well the fate of inhaled aerosols in the respiratory tract, it is necessary to first understand the motion of fluid which occurs in the airway tree. In the present chapter, we make a number of informative statements about the general nature of fluid dynamics in the respiratory tract. In particular, we look at the equations governing fluid (i.e. air) motion in the pulmonary airway tree and introduce the dimensionless parameters adequate to investigate respiratory flows in the airways. We derive a simple model describing viscous resistance and pressure drop along the airway tree and discuss briefly the relative importance of each with respect to the regions of the lung (i.e. conductive and respiratory). Finally, we consider specifically gas flow in the pulmonary acinar region. We first derive the suitable equations of creeping motion and look at the roles of convection and diffusion for gas transport. A simple analytical model is then developed to evaluate the influence of the liquid layer lining on gas flow before reviewing in some detail the literature pertinent to acinar fluid mechanics.

3.1 Incompressibility

For a pure fluid (e.g. oxygen, nitrogen, etc.), the flow can normally be considered incompressible if the Mach number, defined as the ratio of the fluid speed, U, to sound speed[1], c, yields $Ma = U/c < 0.3$, and the temperature differences, ΔT, in the fluid are small relative to a reference temperature [182]. For typical inhalation conditions, this requires velocities less than approximately 100 m/s and temperature differences of less than about 30 K, both conditions normally being satisfied during breathing [66].

Because gas (i.e. air) in the lung is not a pure substance, but instead contains varying amounts of oxygen and carbon dioxide, the assumption of constant density associated with incompressibility could be violated even if Ma or ΔT are small. However, nitrogen makes up over 75% of the density of air, and is not exchanged across the lung epithelium under ambient conditions, so that variations in the content of oxygen or carbon dioxide of gases in the lung is not expected to significantly alter the density of air in the lung. Therefore, for modelling purposes, the fluid dynamics of the bulk gas motion in the lung can be reasonably approximated as an incompressible flow of air under most circumstances [47].

[1] For an ideal gas, $c = \sqrt{\gamma RT}$, where γ is the adiabatic constant, R the universal gas constant and T the gas temperature.

3.2 Dimensionless Analysis of the Equations of Fluid Motion

Assuming incompressible flow of air, consideration of Newton's second law for fluid motion (i.e. conservation of momentum) results in the Navier-Stokes equations:

$$\frac{\partial \underline{u}}{\partial t} + (\underline{u} \cdot \nabla)\underline{u} = -\frac{1}{\rho}\nabla p + \nu \nabla^2 \underline{u} + \underline{f}, \tag{3.1}$$

where $\underline{u}$ is the velocity field, t the time, ρ the density of the fluid, and $\nu = \mu/\rho$ is the kinematic viscosity of the fluid (μ is the dynamic viscosity). Here, $\underline{f}$ represents externals force acting on the fluid (e.g. gravity), whose contributions to the continuous airflow phase are assumed to be negligible in the following analysis (note that gravity will be included when considering aerosol kinematics). The incompressibility condition states that the fluid is divergence-free such that:

$$\nabla \cdot \underline{u} = 0. \tag{3.2}$$

If we non-dimensionalize the momentum equation, Eq. (3.1), using a characteristic velocity, U, length, L, and time scale T during breathing (if the flow is unsteady), such that [66]:

$$\underline{x}' = \frac{\underline{x}}{L}; \quad t' = \frac{t}{T}; \quad \underline{u}' = \frac{\underline{u}}{U}; \quad p' = \frac{p}{\rho U^2},$$

we obtain the following dimensionless momentum equation:

$$\frac{1}{St}\frac{\partial \underline{u}'}{\partial t'} + (\underline{u}' \cdot \nabla')\underline{u}' = -\nabla' p' + \frac{1}{Re}\nabla'^2 \underline{u}'. \tag{3.3}$$

Here, the Reynolds, Re, and Strouhal, St, numbers are defined, respectively, as:

$$Re = \frac{UL}{\nu}, \tag{3.4}$$

$$St = \frac{UT}{L}. \tag{3.5}$$

The dimensionless parameters above determine the importance of the unsteady term, $\left(\frac{1}{St}\frac{\partial \underline{u}'}{\partial t'}\right)$, and the viscous term, $\frac{1}{Re}\nabla'^2\underline{u}'$, relative to the nonlinear convective term, $(\underline{u}' \cdot \nabla')\underline{u}'$. In particular, Re illustrates how important the viscous term is relative to the convective term, while St relates how important the unsteady term is relative to the convective term. Hence, for very high Reynolds numbers, i.e. $Re \gg 1$, we may be able to neglect the viscous term (leading to a formulation of the inviscid Euler equations [182]), while for low Reynolds numbers, i.e. $Re \ll 1$, we may be able to neglect the convective term. Similarly, for high St numbers, we may be able to neglect the unsteady term relative to the convective term. Thus, the values of Re and St are important quantities in determining which effects need to be included if we are to model and understand the fluid dynamics in the respiratory airways.

3.2.1 A Simplified Symmetrical Lung Geometry

By considering simplified geometrical models of the respiratory tract, we can estimate Re and St in the various generations of the airway tree. One of the most well known of these lung models is the symmetric model proposed by Weibel [281], also referred to as the Weibel A model, which despite its simplifications has been used extensively in modelling airflow in the lung [32, 33, 166, 300, 301]. The Weibel A model assumes that each generation of the lung branches symmetrically into two identical daughter branches, where generations 0–16 are the tracheo-bronchial region, while generations 17–23 make up the alveolar region (see Fig. 2.5(a)). The assumption of symmetric branching simplifies the analysis dramatically, but is not entirely accurate since the diameters and lengths of daughter airways can be quite different from each other in actual human lungs (as seen in section 2.1). Several lung models do in fact include some asymmetry in the branching structure [106–108]. Note, however, that the frequency distribution of bifurcation asymmetry is a monotonic function that decays rapidly with increasing asymmetry, with symmetric bifurcations being the most common [191], such that the assumption of symmetrical branching can be quite reasonable for the present purposes.

The diameters and lengths of the alveolated airways in the alveolar region of the Weibel A model are known to be too small and also to start at too high a generation number [66]. A revised model which accounts for these facts (see Fig. 2.5(b)) is given by Haefeli-Bleuer and Weibel [90]. In addition, the original Weibel A model corresponds to a lung volume of 4.8 l, while an average adult male has a lung volume of approximately 3 l at functional residual capacity (FRC). Hence, it is usual to scale the lengths and diameters of the Weibel A model by a factor of (FRC/4.8 l)$^{1/3}$ to account for this fact. The Weibel A model is also known to underpredict the diameters of the tracheo-bronchial airways. Phillips *et al.* [192] analyze the measurements from casts taken by Raabe *et al.* [198] and suggest more realistic values for airway diameters. A symmetric lung geometry based on their airway data and the alveolar data of Haefeli-Bleuer and Weibel [90] is given by Finlay *et al.* [67] and is shown in Table 3.1. For comparison purposes, a Weibel A model scaled to an FRC of 3 l is also shown. Note that the above descriptions of lung geometry are all based on measurements made with normal lungs. Subjects with lung disease, such as asthma, cystic fibrosis, emphysema, etc., may have parts of their lung that differ substantially from the normal geometry. Such properties remain, however, beyond the scope of the present analysis.

As may be seen from Table 3.1, dimensions of the airways range over an order of magnitude $O(> 100)$, with the trachea little over 10 cm long and acinar ducts < 1 mm short. In the conducting region of the lung (Fig. 2.5(b)), the diameter $D(z)$ of airways falls gradually with each generation z of dichotomous branching according to:

$$D(z) = D(0) \cdot 2^{-z/3}, \tag{3.6}$$

where $D(0)$ is taken as the diameter of the trachea. The above relation is also known as the Hess-Murray law, first formulated by Hess for blood vessels [98] and then developed further by Murray [162]. In the respiratory region (acinus), however, the diameter of acinar airways falls less steeply than that of conducting airways and is thus larger than the prediction from the Hess-Murray law (see Fig. 2.5(b)). This property of the acinus may be explained in part by considering optimization processes in the design of the peripheral airways with respect to airflow resistance [149]. In particular, a perfectly optimal bronchial tree, as would be determined by the Hess-Murray law, is dangerously sensitive to fluctuations or physiological variability (e.g airway constrictions due to asthma, bronchitis, etc.). While the morphology of the human bronchial tree is indeed close to providing maximal efficiency in assuring air distribution with minimal viscous dissipation, real bronchi and acinar airways are a little larger than optimal (i.e. they occupy a slightly larger volume than is strictly necessary). This gives the system a safety margin with respect to resistance.

For a simplified symmetric dichotomous bifurcating tree, the number of airways at each generation z is expressed as:

$$N(z) = 2^z. \tag{3.7}$$

Table 3.1: Dimensions of the Weibel A lung geometry [281] scaled to a 3 l lung volume, compared to the symmetric lung geometry used by Finlay *et al.* [67]. Generation 0 corresponds to the trachea. The thick lines in the table indicate the border between the alveolar and tracheo-bronchial regions in the model.

Generation	Finlay *et al.* airway length (cm)	Scaled Weibel A model airway length (cm)	Finlay *et al.* airway diameter (cm)	Scaled Weibel A model airway diameter (cm)
0	12.46	10.26	1.81	1.54
1	3.61	4.07	1.41	1.04
2	2.86	1.62	1.12	0.71
3	2.28	0.65	0.86	0.48
4	1.78	1.09	0.71	0.39
5	1.13	0.92	0.57	0.30
6	0.9	0.77	0.45	0.24
7	0.83	0.65	0.36	0.20
8	0.75	0.55	0.29	0.16
9	0.65	0.46	0.22	0.13
10	0.56	0.39	0.16	0.11
11	0.45	0.33	0.12	0.093
12	0.36	0.28	0.092	0.081
13	0.28	0.23	0.073	0.07
14	0.22	0.2	0.061	0.063
15	0.13	0.17	0.049	0.056
16	0.11	0.14	0.048	0.51
17	0.091	0.12	0.039	0.046
18	0.081	0.1	0.037	0.043
19	0.068	0.085	0.035	0.04
20	0.068	0.071	0.033	0.038
21	0.068	0.06	0.03	0.037
22	0.065	0.05	0.028	0.035
23	0.073	0.043	0.024	0.035

Therefore, the total cross-sectional area, $A_t(z)$, at any generation z, then follows as:

$$A_t(z) = N(z)\pi\frac{D^2(z)}{4} = \frac{2^{z/3}\pi D^2(0)}{4}, \tag{3.8}$$

such that the total cross-sectional area of the airways increases extremely rapidly, in particular in the respiratory zone (Fig. 3.1(a)).

3.2.2 Reynolds and Strouhal Numbers in the Respiratory Tract

Intuitively, the result for $A_t(z)$ suggests that the air flow velocity, $\overline{U}$, will then rapidly fall with each deeper airway generation z. This is a direct consequence of applying at each airway generation the continuity

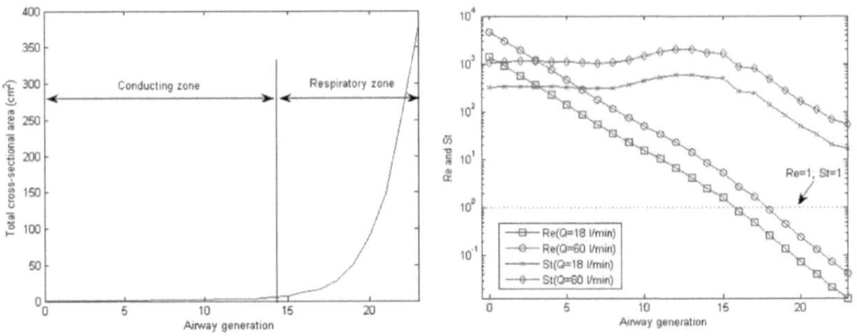

(a) (b)

Figure 3.1: (a) Total cross-sectional area of airways plotted against lung generation using a symmetric lung geometry from Finlay *et al.* [67] (Table 3.1). (b) Reynolds (Re) and Strouhal (St) number plotted against generation number for two flow rates.

equation, Eq. (3.2), such that:

$$U(z) = \frac{U(0)}{2^{Z/3}}, \tag{3.9}$$

from which Re values may be estimated, using Eq. (3.4). Figure 3.1(b) illustrates Re and St values for the idealized lung model geometry proposed by Finlay *et al.* [67] for tidal breathing (flow rate $\dot{Q}$ =18 l/min) and for a typical single breath pattern ($\dot{Q}$ =60 l/min) using an inhaler (metered-dose inhaler or dry powder inhaler). Several results follow from this data. First, it can be seen that Re values are quite high in the upper airways and conversely very low deep in the lung. Internal flows become turbulent at high Reynolds numbers (typically $Re > 2000$), and are laminar at low Reynolds numbers. In the upper and central airways there exists the possibility that turbulence may be present, while absent in the deeper regions of the lung. In fact, experimental observations do indicate the presence of turbulence in the upper airways and trachea (i.e. the laryngeal jet produces much of this turbulence), but the turbulence produced in this region decays rapidly as it is convected deeper into the lung [242, 273]. Even if turbulent production occurred distal to the larynx by shear in the boundary layers of the first few generations, such turbulence would not exist long enough to be convected significantly into daughter generations. While it is reasonable to expect that turbulence is produced in extrathoracic airways which may be convected into the first generations of the lung, it is safe to assume that flow is laminar distal to these upper regions.

In the upper regions of the lung, St is quite high and unsteadiness is thus expected to a play a large role in the fluid mechanics of respiration (Fig. 3.1(b)). In contrast, in the distal regions of the lung, $Re \ll 1$ such that the role of inertia through the convective terms is negligible. Although $St \sim O(1)$, unsteadiness is not necessarily important. Indeed, St compares the unsteady term to the convective term and if the latter one is small (i.e. $Re \ll 1$), then $St \sim O(1)$ indicates that the unsteady terms are small as well.

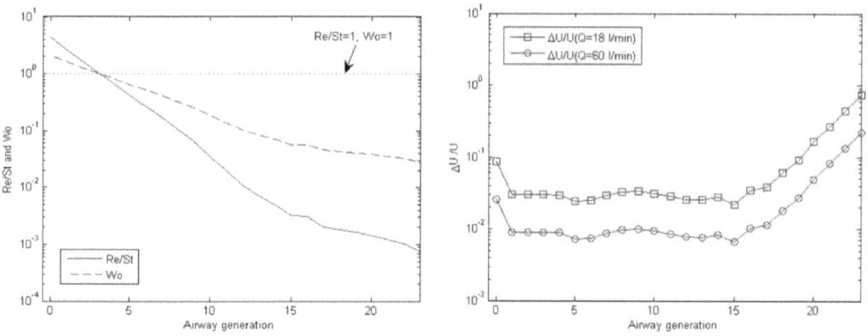

(a) (b)

Figure 3.2: (a) Ratio of Reynolds number to Strouhal number, Re/St, as well as Womersley number, Wo, plotted against lung generation using an idealized lung geometry from Finlay *et al.* [67] (Table 3.1). (b) Parameter $\Delta U/U$ indicates the importance of unsteadiness within each airway generation ($\overline{U} \approx U/(T/4)$ with $T = 5$ s).

3.2.3 Womersley Number and Unsteadiness

If the Reynolds numbers are small, one would ideally compare directly the unsteady terms with the viscous terms, since the viscous terms become dominant in the Navier-Stokes equations at low Reynolds numbers. Hence, multiplying Eq. (3.3) with Re yields:

$$\frac{Re}{St}\frac{\partial \underline{u}'}{\partial t'} + Re(\underline{u}' \cdot \nabla')\underline{u}' = -Re\nabla' p' + \nabla'^2 \underline{u}', \tag{3.10}$$

where the ratio, $Re/St = D^2/T\nu$, is illustrated in Fig. 3.2(a) and represents a measure of the importance of the unsteady term compared to the viscous term. In the acinar region as well as in distal regions of the tracheo-bronchial tree, the unsteady terms are much smaller than the viscous terms. Alternatively, the Womersley number, Wo, defined as:

$$Wo = \left(\frac{Re}{St}\right)^{1/2} = D\left(\frac{f}{\nu}\right)^{1/2}, \tag{3.11}$$

is often used to measure the importance of the unsteady term compared to the viscous term (Fig. 3.2(a)), where $f = 1/T$ is the breathing frequency (Hz). The parameter Wo appears originally in the solution for laminar sinusoidally oscillating flow in a circular pipe [292].

Combining the results seen in Figs. 3.1(b) and 3.2(a), we observe that unsteady terms are small compared to either convective terms (which are important in proximal generations of the tracheo-bronchial tree, following Re) or viscous terms (which are important in the alveolar region, again based on Re). Consequently, in the airways distal to the oropharynx where flow is inherently unsteady and turbulent, the unsteady terms in the Navier-Stokes equations can be neglected to approximate the fluid dynamics of respiration. However, the analysis above is based on using an average value of the unsteady term to estimate its magnitude. In reality, depending on the instant, t, considered during a breathing period, the unsteady term may be much larger than its average value (e.g. at flow reversal between inhalation and exhalation). Thus, when writing the dimensionless Navier-Stokes equations (Eq. (3.3)), an average value is not adequate for all times, t, during breathing. Instead, if dU/dt has a characteristic value $\overline{U}$ and we use it to non-dimensionalize the unsteady term in Eq. (3.3) at times, t, when dU/dt takes the value $\overline{U}$, we then obtain [186]:

$$\epsilon \frac{\partial \underline{u}'}{\partial t'} + (\underline{u}' \cdot \nabla')\underline{u}' = -\nabla' p' + \frac{1}{Re}\nabla'^2 \underline{u}', \tag{3.12}$$

where

$$\epsilon = \frac{D\overline{U}}{U^2}. \tag{3.13}$$

In the above equation, the value U must be used which is characteristic of the flow field at time, t, when dU/dt takes on the value $\overline{U}$. The value of the parameter ϵ gives an indication of the importance of the unsteady term relative to the convective term that can be used at different times, t, during breathing. Defined as such, the parameter ϵ is most meaningful in the extrathoracic and upper tracheo-bronchial regions since we know that the convective term is important there. In the distal airways including the acinus, the parameter ϵRe gives an indication of the importance of the unsteady terms relative to the viscous terms. Note that when calculating Re, the value of U which occurs at the same time, t, as the chosen value $\overline{U}$ should be used.

Examining the flow at a time, t, when the velocity $U = 0$, while $dU/dt = \overline{U} \neq 0$, the parameter ϵ goes to infinity (as well as ϵRe) such that the unsteady terms are very important at the time, t, considered. Therefore, at times when the velocity is small or zero, and the rate of change is conversely large, the unsteady terms in the Navier-Stokes equations cannot be neglected. This occurs at the start of a single inhalation and during flow reversal between inhalation and exhalation in tidal breathing. To accurately capture fluid dynamics at these times and in particular the kinematics and deposition of inhaled aerosols, the unsteady terms must be included (although the time over which unsteadiness is important is only a small portion of the tidal breathing cycle).

In the above analysis, we have considered only the equations of fluid motion, and have neither considered the equations of particle motion nor the boundary conditions governing the problem. If we consider the boundary conditions governing the deposition of a particle in a particular lung generation, it is easy to see that a particle carried by the fluid is only present in a given generation for an average time $\Delta t = L/U$, where L is the length of a generation and U is the average value of the fluid over the time the particle is in the generation considered. As suggested by Finlay [66], to decide whether unsteady fluid motion is important, one may ask whether the velocity of the fluid changes significantly during the time Δt. If not, the particle experiences an effectively steady velocity field and the solution of the steady problem may be used to predict particle deposition in this airway generation.

During the time Δt, the fluid may undergo a velocity change:

$$\Delta U = \overline{U}\Delta t, \tag{3.14}$$

where $\overline{U}$ is a typical value of dU/dt while the particle is in a particular generation. The residence time of the particle can be approximated as follows:

$$\Delta t = \frac{L}{U}. \tag{3.15}$$

Therefore, the parameter

$$\frac{\Delta U}{U} = \frac{\overline{U}\Delta t}{U} = \frac{L\overline{U}}{U^2} \tag{3.16}$$

may be seen to determine whether or not unsteadiness in the fluid motion is important for determining particle deposition. Values of $\Delta U/U$ are illustrated in Fig. 3.2(b) with $\overline{U} = U/(T/4)$ and T =5 s. Small values of $\Delta U/U$ indicate that a particle sees little variation in the velocity field while travelling through that generation, such that deposition in the generation considered is expected to be similar to that predicted from using a steady velocity profile equal to the value of the velocity at that time in the breathing cycle. In contrast, if $\Delta U/U$ is large, one should use an unsteady velocity to predict particle deposition. For typical tidal breathing ($\dot{Q}$ =18 l/min), unsteady effects may be of importance in the alveolar region of the lung (Fig. 3.2(b)), while for single breath pattern ($\dot{Q}$ =60 l/min), unsteadiness may only be of importance in the last generation or so. Such properties will be shown in detail when looking at aerosol kinematics in computational fluid dynamics (CFD) simulations in acinar models (see chapters 6 and 7).

3.2.4 Resistance and Pressure Drop in Branching Airways

For internal laminar flows occurring in pipes, the "entrance length", L_e, required for a flow to become fully developed with a parabolic velocity profile (i.e. Poiseuille flow) is typically given by [68]:

$$\frac{L_e}{D} \approx 0.06 Re, \tag{3.17}$$

where $Re = DU/\nu$ and U is the mean velocity. In typical bronchi, the ratio of airway lengths to diameters, L/D, is on the order of 3.5 (see Table 3.1). From the above equation, this would lead to $Re < 60$. However, this value is not found in middle and upper bronchi in average human adults, even under quiet tidal breathing conditions (see Fig. 3.1(b)). In contrast, in the human bronchi, only a short distance is available for a velocity distribution as disturbed by flow through a bifurcation to settle down again before being similarly disturbed yet once more. Hence, as shown in experiments conducted in models of human airways [188, 190], velocity profiles in a daughter branch measured at 1, 2, and 3 diameters downstream of a bifurcation (at moderate $Re = 700$) exhibit very large departures from the Poiseuille flow distribution found in the mother tube, with a strong peaking near the flow divider, that appear at once and persist for the whole length of the tube (see Fig. 1 in [188] and Figs. 4–6 in [190]). The departure from a Poiseuille distribution arises partly because on the flow divider a thin new boundary layer forms, where the velocity just outside the boundary layer is near the maximum velocity in the mother tube, and partly because secondary flows generated by curved motion of the primary flow into its new branch intensify such a peaking of the velocity on the "outside bend" of that curved motion (i.e. around the flow divider) [136]. This is schematically illustrated in Fig. 3.3 and has been reviewed in detail by Pedley [187].

If Poiseuille flow occured in all airways at all flow rates, the viscous resistance at any airway generation, z, would be given by [86]:

$$R_p(z) = \frac{1}{2^z} \frac{128\mu L(z)}{\pi D^4(z)}. \tag{3.18}$$

This may easily be derived by assuming a symmetrical dichotomous branching tree (see Eq. (3.7)) and realizing that at any generation z, the 2^z airway resistances add up in parallel (similar to a circuit). Note that $R_p(z)$ is independent of flow rate. This approximation may be valid in the smallest airways and the acinar region, where Re is small and hence L_e is very short (from Eq. (3.17)) such that a parabolic profile is valid. However, in the main and upper bronchi, it is necessary to refine Eq. (3.18) to take account of the non-parabolic velocity profile as discussed in the previous paragraph. The ratio of the real resistance

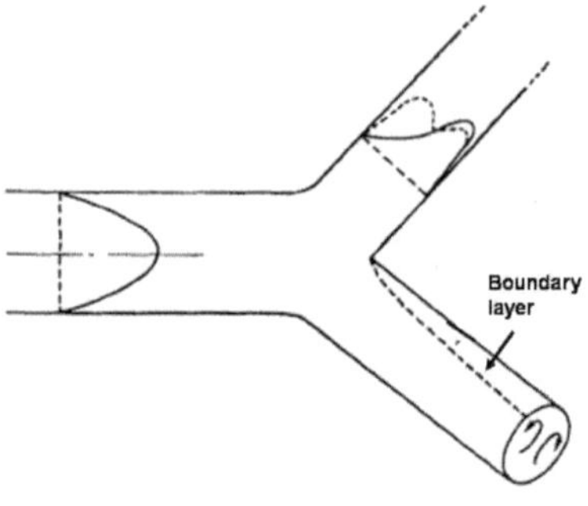

Figure 3.3: Schematic of the flow downstream of a single bifurcation with a Poiseuille velocity profile in the parent branch. Direction of secondary motions and new boundary layer indicated in lower branch. Velocity profiles in the plane of the junction (–) and in the normal plane (- -) indicated in the upper branch (adapted from [190]).

in any tube to the Poiseuille resistance in that tube is denoted by Z and formulated as [189]:

$$Z = \frac{R_R(z)}{R_p(z)} = \frac{C}{4\sqrt{2}}\left(Re\frac{D}{L}\right)^{1/2}, \tag{3.19}$$

where $C = 1.85$ is an empirical constant [188], and $R_R(z)$ is the real resistance. The dependence of $Z(z)$ on Re can be understood in terms of the idea that energy dissipation in a flow with a velocity peak very close to the wall is concentrated primarily in a boundary layer with small thickness δ, lying between the region of peak velocity and the tube wall. Velocity gradients are of the order (U/δ) leading to an energy dissipation rate of order $\mu(U/\delta)^2$ (i.e. the product of the viscosity and the square of the shear strain rate) per unit volume in a boundary layer cross-sectional area of order $D\delta$. The energy dissipation rate per unit length of tube is thus of order $\mu U^2(D/\delta)$ which itself varies as $Re^{1/2}$. If the length of the tube may be a variable multiple of D, then D/δ varies as $(ReD/L)^{1/2}$.

Thus, at generation z, the real viscous resistance depends on the flow rate and is expressed as:

$$R_R(z) = R_p(z)\frac{C}{4\sqrt{2}}\left(Re\frac{D}{L}\right)^{1/2}. \tag{3.20}$$

The expression above illustrates clearly that the real viscous resistance at any generation is no longer independent of the total flow rate[2]. The distribution of viscous resistance $R_R(z)$ is illustrated in Fig. 3.4(a) for different flow rates. At all flow rates, the resistance in the larger and middle bronchi is far greater than that predicted by Poiseuille's law. Moreover, the peak observed at the 6th generation is eliminated. As seen from the figure, the greatest resistance occurs in the first four generations, thereafter $R_R(z)$ falls steeply and the curves collapse together onto the Poiseuille resistance past approximately the 10th generation.

The viscous pressure drop, $(\Delta P)_R$, within the airways between the trachea and any generation z may be

[2]Whenever $Z(z)$ from Eq. (3.19) becomes < 1, this is unrealistic as minimum dissipation occurs in Poiseuille flow such that $Z < 1$ is unphysical. In such cases Z is replaced by 1. See discussion in [188].

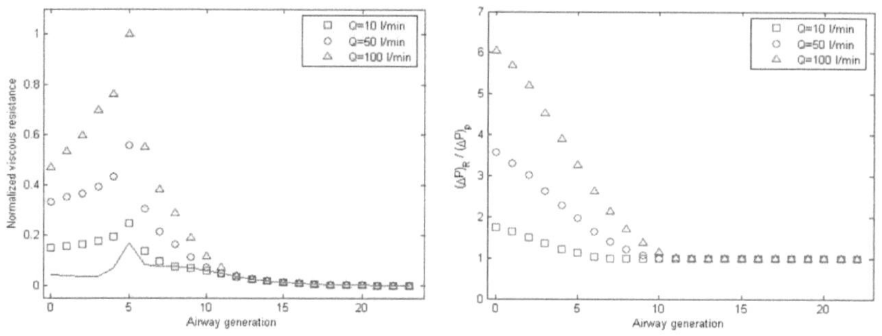

(a) (b)

Figure 3.4: (a) Variation of real viscous flow resistance (normalized with respect to the maximum peak at $\dot{Q} = 100$ l/min) along the bronchial tree at different flow rates, from Eq. (3.20). Also shown is the Poiseuille resistance from Eq. (3.18). (b) Variation of real viscous pressure from Eq. (3.21) and Poiseuille viscous pressure along the airway tree.

calculated as follows:

$$(\Delta P)_R = \dot{Q} \sum_{i=1}^{z} R_R(i), \tag{3.21}$$

where $\dot{Q}$ is the flow rate. Figure 3.4(b) illustrates the ratio, $(\Delta P)_R/(\Delta P)_p$, between real and Poiseuille pressure drops (the alveolar pressure is taken to be zero). In the larger airways, the real viscous pressure drop is much greater than that predicted by Poiseuille's law and this enhancement becomes quite intense for scenarios of heavy breathing ($\dot{Q}$ =100 l/min). Beyond the 10th airway generation, curves for the real and Poiseuille based pressure drops merge.

In summary, as the airways penetrate towards the periphery of the lung, they become more numerous but also much narrower. Intuitively, one may expect that the major part of the resistance lies in the very narrow airways since $R_p(z) \propto 1/D^4$ from Poiseuille's law (Eq. (3.18)). However, as described above, the major site of viscous resistance resides in the large bronchi, where flow patterns are in general greatly distorted, with high velocity peaks occurring in close proximity of airway walls and most of the energy dissipation occurring in the intervening high-shear boundary layers [187]. In contrast, very small bronchioles and acinar airways contribute relatively little resistance. In fact, less than 20% can be attributed to airways less than 2 mm in diameter (past approximately generation 8) [285]. This apparent paradox is reflected in the prodigious number of small airways which act in parallel rather than in series (i.e. $R_R(z) \propto 1/2^z$).

3.3 Fluid Mechanics in the Pulmonary Acinus

In this section, we introduce the equations of fluid motion suitable to describe flow phenomena in the acinar region of the lung and look at the roles of convective and diffusive mechanisms in the transport of oxygen deep in the lung. Using a simple one-dimensional steady-state model for fluid flow, we evaluate the importance of the aqueous liquid lining layer in describing airflow in the continuous gas phase. Finally, we review briefly past studies pertinent to the field of acinar fluid mechanics.

3.3.1 Equations of Creeping Motion and Stream Function

The equations of incompressible fluid motion were given in Eqs. (3.1) and (3.2). If we non-dimensionalize the variables as follows [47]:

$$\underline{x}' = \frac{\underline{x}}{D}; \quad t' = \frac{t}{T}; \quad \underline{u}' = \frac{\underline{u}}{U}; \quad (p/\rho)' = \frac{p/\rho}{\nu U/D},$$

the equations may then be written as (neglecting external forces):

$$Wo^2 \frac{\partial \underline{u}'}{\partial t'} + Re(\underline{u}' \cdot \nabla' \underline{u}') = -\nabla' \left(\frac{p}{\rho}\right)' + \nabla'^2 \underline{u}', \tag{3.22}$$

where the non-dimensionalization of the pressure, p, follows a slightly different definition as that used to obtain Eq. (3.3). From sections 3.2.2 and 3.2.3, we have seen that in the acinar region of the lung dimensionless parameters yield $Re \ll 1$ (see Fig. 3.1(b)) and $Wo \ll 1$ (see Fig. 3.2(a)), such that both the inertial and convective terms may be disregarded. Therefore, the equations of fluid motion in the acinus may be expressed as:

$$\nabla p - \mu \nabla^2 \underline{u} = 0, \tag{3.23}$$

$$\nabla \cdot \underline{u} = 0. \tag{3.24}$$

The above equations constitute the equations of fluid motion in the creeping flow regime, also referred to as Stokes flow [257]. If the divergence operator, $\nabla \cdot$, is applied to Eq. (3.23), while making use of Eq. (3.24), the momentum equation may be rewritten as:

$$\Delta p = \nabla^2 p = \frac{\partial^2 p}{\partial x^2} + \frac{\partial^2 p}{\partial y^2} + \frac{\partial^2 p}{\partial z^2} = 0, \tag{3.25}$$

which constitutes the Laplace equation for the pressure term (similar to the steady-state diffusion equation for C in Eq. (3.38)). The advantage of the above second-order differential equation stands in its unique variable p which must be solved. In Appendix B, the Laplace and creeping motion equations are solved analytically in spherical coordinates for the pressure and velocity fields around a small spherical particle (i.e. Stokes law).

Alternatively, the velocity field, $\underline{u}$, may also be expressed in terms of a scalar stream function ψ. In three-dimensional flows, the most general approach to derive the relationship between $\underline{u}$ and ψ is to consider that $\underline{u}$ is parallel or tangent to the streamline identified by the stream function ψ (thus $\nabla\psi$ is orthogonal to $\underline{u}$) and that $\underline{u}$ is equal to the curl of $\nabla\psi$ and the unit normal vector $\underline{n}$, perpendicular to the plane of $\nabla\psi$ and $\underline{u}$ (see Fig. 3.5(a)). Thus, there exists a scalar stream function, ψ, in three-dimensions such that [28]:

$$\underline{u} = \nabla\psi \times \underline{n}, \tag{3.26}$$

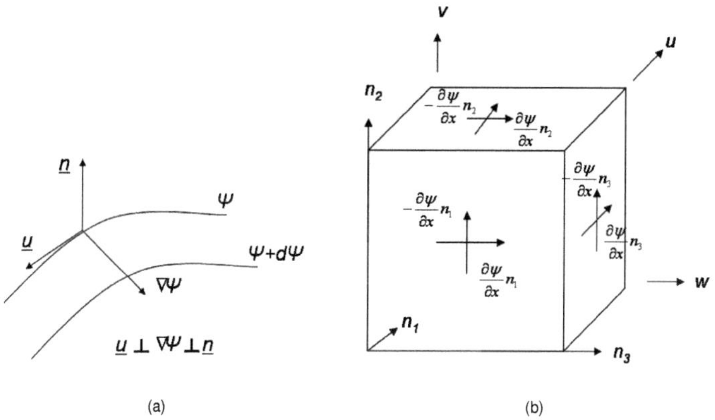

Figure 3.5: General description of the three-dimensional stream function, ψ, in cartesian coordinates.

where each velocity component, u_i $(i = 1, 2, 3)$, is given by:

$$\begin{aligned} u = u_1 &= \frac{\partial \psi}{\partial y} n_3 - \frac{\partial \psi}{\partial z} n_2, \\ v = u_2 &= \frac{\partial \psi}{\partial z} n_1 - \frac{\partial \psi}{\partial x} n_3, \\ w = u_3 &= \frac{\partial \psi}{\partial x} n_2 - \frac{\partial \psi}{\partial y} n_1. \end{aligned} \tag{3.27}$$

Consequently, we may identify the stream function vector, $\underline{\Psi}$, and its components, Ψ_i, described on each surface designated by n_i as (see Fig. 3.5(b)):

$$\underline{\Psi} = \psi_i \underline{i}_i, \quad (i = 1, 2, 3) \tag{3.28}$$

with

$$\begin{aligned} \Psi_1 &= \psi n_1, \\ \Psi_2 &= \psi n_2, \\ \Psi_3 &= \psi n_3, \end{aligned} \tag{3.29}$$

such that

$$\underline{u} = \nabla \times \underline{\Psi}. \tag{3.30}$$

Both Eqs. (3.26) and (3.30) satisfy the conservation of mass Eq. (3.24) in steady state. In two-dimensional incompressible flows, Eq. (3.27) reduces to a single stream function $\psi = \Psi_3$ and collapses to the well known form:

$$u = \frac{\partial \psi}{\partial y} n_3 = \frac{\partial \psi}{\partial y}, \tag{3.31}$$

$$v = -\frac{\partial \psi}{\partial x} n_3 = -\frac{\partial \psi}{\partial x}. \tag{3.32}$$

The deduction from Eqs. (3.26)–(3.30) has an important physical significance, in which a scalar stream function ψ is extended to the three-dimensional stream function vector $\underline{\Psi}$. As a result of the above assessments, the vorticity vector assumes the form:

$$\underline{\omega} = \nabla \times \underline{u} = \nabla \times (\nabla \times \underline{\Psi}) = \nabla(\nabla \cdot \underline{\Psi}) - \nabla^2 \underline{\Psi} = -\nabla^2 \underline{\Psi}, \tag{3.33}$$

where $(\nabla \cdot \underline{\Psi}) = 0$ arises from the geometrical property $\nabla \underline{\Psi} \cdot \underline{n} = 0$ (see Fig. 3.5(a)). Note that an irrotational ideal flow in three-dimensions can be thus described by $\nabla^2 \underline{\Psi} = 0$ in terms of the three-dimensional stream function.

Taking the curl of the momentum Eq. (3.1) and neglecting external forces, the vorticity transport equation of an incompressible fluid is given as:

$$\frac{\partial \underline{\omega}}{\partial t} - (\omega \cdot \nabla)\underline{u} + (\underline{u} \cdot \nabla)\omega = \nu \nabla^2 \omega. \tag{3.34}$$

Substituting Eqs. (3.30) and (3.33) into (3.34) leads to [56]:

$$\frac{\partial}{\partial t} \nabla^2 \underline{\Psi} - (\nabla^2 \underline{\Psi} \cdot \nabla)(\nabla \times \underline{\Psi}) + ((\nabla \times \underline{\Psi}) \cdot \nabla) \nabla^2 \underline{\Psi} = \nu \nabla^4 \underline{\Psi}. \tag{3.35}$$

The above equation constitutes a fourth-order vector partial differential equation in three unknowns Ψ_1, Ψ_2 and Ψ_3. This set of governing equations has two main advantages: the continuity equation is satisfied by $\underline{\Psi}$ independently from other variables, and the pressure, p, is eliminated. Under creeping motion, where both transient and convective terms are negligible, Eq. (3.35) may be simplified further such that $\underline{\Psi}$ satisfies the biharmonic equation:

$$\nabla^4 \underline{\Psi} = 0. \tag{3.36}$$

Neither the fourth-order differential equation above for $\underline{\Psi}$ nor its boundary conditions, which govern the spatial distribution of the stream function, contain Re such that flow patterns are independent of viscosity μ [240].

Hence, Eqs. (3.23)-(3.24) for the velocity $\underline{u}$, Eq. (3.25) for the pressure p, and Eq. (3.36) for the stream function $\underline{\Psi}$ all describe fluid motion in the creeping flow regime and govern respiratory flows in the acinar region of the lung.

3.3.2 Convection vs. Diffusion

Although the bulk of the present work is principally concerned with convective acinar flows and, in particular, their influence on the transport and deposition of inhaled aerosols, one should note, nevertheless, that convective flows in the acinus are relevant when considering the transport of oxygen. Indeed, in section 2.2 we briefly described the anatomical structure of the pulmonary acinus with respect to its principal role: to guarantee oxygen (and carbon dioxide) exchange between air and blood capillaries with great efficiency.

For gas-exchange to be efficient, an important consideration is how the blood capillary units are arranged with respect to the airways. In the mammalian lung, gas-exchange units (i.e. alveoli) are arranged as lateral chambers (Fig. 3.6(i), left). Therefore, optimized gas exchange depends crucially on ensuring adequate oxygen supply to all capillary gas-exchange units within an acinus, whether they are centrally located near the entrance or deep at the periphery of the acinus. Indeed, this condition is important because, due to dichotomous branching of the airway tree, half of the gas exchange surface of an acinus

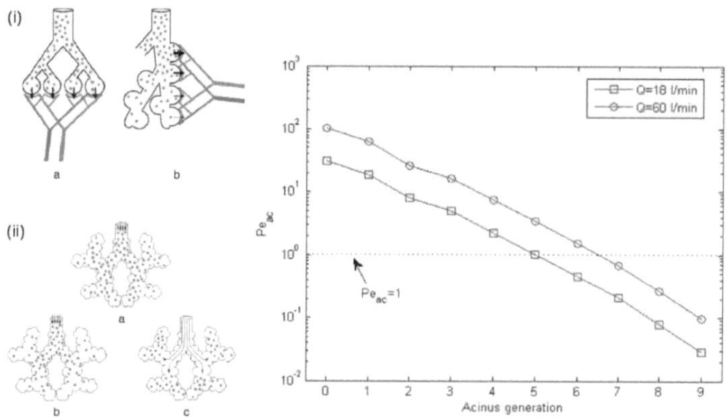

Figure 3.6: Left: (i) Models of ventilation-perfusion relationship in the pulmonary acinus (from Sapoval *et al.* [214]). Copyright (2002) National Academy of Sciences, U.S.A. (a) Parallel ventilation/parallel perfusion -which is not found in reality-. (b) A more appropriate model: serial ventilation /parallel perfusion. (ii) Possible models for the functioning of the acinus (from Sapoval *et al.* [214]). Copyright (2002) National Academy of Sciences, U.S.A. The end of the arrows schematically depicts the convection/diffusion transition. (a) For infinite diffusivity, the oxygen concentration would be uniform. (b) The real situation at rest: there is a gradient in the oxygen concentration so that the acinus works poorly. (c) During exercise: increased ventilation brings the diffusion source deeper inside the acinus; the entire acinus works with maximal efficiency. Right: Variations of the acinus Peclet number, Pe_{ac}, for an average human during tidal breathing ($\dot{Q} = 18$ l/min) and single breath pattern ($\dot{Q} = 60$ l/min) as a function of the depth in the acinar pathway (see Table 3.1).

is located in its last generation [214]. As we have seen in section 3.2.2, air flow velocity falls rapidly as air moves deeper in the airway tree (see Eq. (3.9)). This pattern continues until eventually the air flow velocity becomes smaller than the mean oxygen diffusion velocity. This transition occurs approximately at the entrance of the airways into the pulmonary acinus, as described in what follows.

In the acinar airway generations ($\sim 15 < z < 23$), oxygen will diffuse into quasi-static air ($U \approx 0$) driven by the gradient established by oxygen extraction at the alveolar surface which is transferred to the red blood cells in the capillaries. As oxygen diffuses along the acinar airways, oxygen partial pressure in air decreases. This process is important because it determines how much oxygen reaches the deepest alveoli, where the largest part of the gas-exchange surface is located. One way of illustrating the transition between convection and diffusion is through the use of a dimensionless parameter, the "acinus Peclet number", Pe_{ac} [214], which compares the mean airflow velocity, $U(z)$, at a given airway generation, z, with the mean diffusion velocity to reach deeper regions of the acinus. This dimensionless number may be expressed as:

$$Pe_{ac}(z) = \frac{U(z) \cdot \sum_{i=z}^{9} L(i)}{D_{O_2,air}}, \tag{3.37}$$

where $D_{O_2,air} \approx 0.2\text{cm}^2/\text{s}$ is the diffusivity of oxygen in air, $L(z)$ is the acinar duct length at generation

z, and there are a total of 9 acinar generations following the symmetric lung model of Finlay *et al.* [67] in Table 3.1. At any branching generation z, the distance to cross to the end of the acinus is approximated by the sum in the numerator of Eq. (3.37). One should note that the definition of the acinar Peclet number, Pe_{ac}, is slightly different from the classical Peclet number which corresponds to airflow velocity multiplied with the ratio between airway diameter and diffusion coefficient. The velocity, U, depends on the breathing regime such that for humans under exercise conditions, the air velocity may be increased by a factor of order 10 above rest along all levels of the airway tree due to the increased inhaled volume of air and the breathing frequency [282]. The resulting values for Pe_{ac} are shown on the right of Fig. 3.6 for the human lung.

One observes that the transition from convection to diffusion ($Pe_{ac} = 1$) is moved slightly deeper between tidal breathing and a single breath pattern (Fig. 3.6, right). As a result, the size of the "diffusion cell", i.e. the part of the acinus where convection can be reasonably neglected and where diffusion governs oxygen transport, will be considerably reduced under even more increased effort. This difference is schematically illustrated in Fig. 3.6(ii), (b) and (c).

Beyond the entrance of the "diffusion cell", the system will obey the stationary form of the diffusion equation (Fick's second law [65]), since convection may be neglected ($Pe_{ac} \ll 1$):

$$\nabla^2 C = \frac{\partial^2 C}{\partial x^2} + \frac{\partial^2 C}{\partial y^2} + \frac{\partial^2 C}{\partial z^2} = 0, \tag{3.38}$$

where the oxygen concentration, C, is governed by the Laplace equation . For such systems, diffusional screening is a classical phenomenon which may occur. Here, screening means that part of the oxygen that diffuses along the acinar airway is absorbed on the alveolar surfaces along the path, because a molecule starting at a diffusion source has a higher probability to hit the surface of the wall on the most accessible regions than deeper in the structure.

If oxygen diffusivity is infinite, the oxygen concentration would be uniform in the entire acinus. If alveolar membrane permeability is large, the oxygen molecules are absorbed at the very first hits and cannot reach the deeper regions. These regions would then be of no use, hence, they are *screened.* In contrast, if the membrane permeability is small, molecules will be absorbed only after many collisions with the wall. They then have a fair chance to reach the deeper regions, and the entire surface will be effective for gas exchange. These various situations are qualitatively described in Fig. 3.6(ii), (a) and (b). Two- [62] and three-dimensional models [63] solving the steady-state diffusion equation (Eq. (3.38)) have been developed to investigate the importance of diffusional screening of oxygen in the pulmonary acinus. While these remain beyond the scope of the present work, the role of convection and diffusion in the pulmonary acinus may be summarized as follows. In the acinar region, the role of convection is negligible for oxygen transport, compared to the importance of diffusion as described by Pe_{ac}. In contrast, however, convective flows may hold an essential role in the transport of non-diffusing micron-sized inhaled particles (as we will see subsequently).

3.3.3 Influence of the Liquid Lining Layer

We are interested in assessing in a simple manner the influence of the thin aqueous liquid layer lining, described earlier in section 2.4, on the continuous phase (i.e. air) flow in the acinar region of the lung. The following analysis is conducted in a simple horizontal pipe (i.e. acinar duct) of radius R, lined with a thin liquid layer of height h, with $h \ll R$ (Fig. 3.7). Neglecting the influence of gravity, the velocity profile

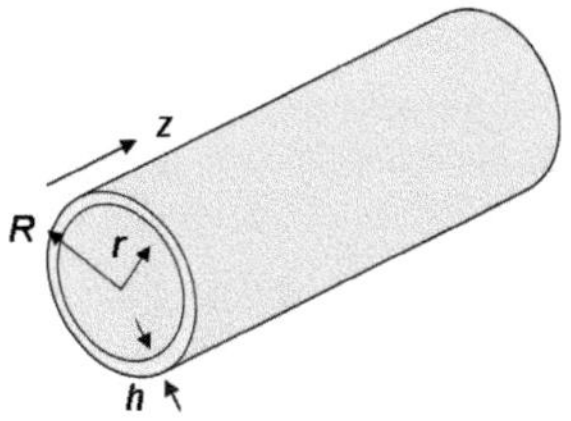

Figure 3.7: Schematic of acinar duct with thin liquid layer lining using using cylindrical coordinates (r, z).

of the gas in the acinar duct is modelled using the equations of creeping motion (i.e. 1D fully developed steady-state flow in z-direction) in cylindrical coordinates which reduce to [182]:

$$\left(\frac{\partial p}{\partial z}\right)_a = \mu_a \frac{1}{r}\frac{\partial}{\partial r}\left(\frac{\partial u_z}{\partial r}\right), \tag{3.39}$$

$$\left(\frac{\partial p}{\partial r}\right)_a = 0, \tag{3.40}$$

$$\frac{\partial u_z}{\partial r} + \frac{1}{r}\frac{\partial}{\partial r}(r u_r) = 0, \tag{3.41}$$

where the first two equations are the momentum equations in the z- and r direction, respectively, and the continuity equation is given last (the subscript a denotes air). Dropping the subscript z, and denoting the z-component of the gas (i.e. air) velocity u_a, integration of Eq. (3.39) yields:

$$u_a(r) = \frac{1}{\mu_a}\left(\frac{\partial p}{\partial z}\right)_a \left(\frac{r^2}{4} + C_1 \ln r + C_2\right), \tag{3.42}$$

where C_1 and C_2 are constants and $(\partial p/\partial z)_a$ is the pressure gradient in the axial direction. Due to axisymmetry along the z-direction, the first boundary condition is trivially given by:

$$\left.\frac{\partial u_a}{\partial r}\right|_{r=0} = 0, \tag{3.43}$$

such that

$$\frac{1}{\mu_a}\left(\frac{\partial p}{\partial z}\right)_a \left(\frac{C_1}{r}\right) = 0, \tag{3.44}$$

and therefore $C_1 = 0$. The velocity, u_a reduces to:

$$u_a(r) = \frac{1}{\mu_a}\left(\frac{\partial p}{\partial z}\right)_a \left(\frac{r^2}{4} + C_2\right), \tag{3.45}$$

where the constant C_2 must still be determined.

Similarly, flow of the liquid film in the z-direction may be described using lubrication theory for a thin film [182]:

$$\left(\frac{\partial p}{\partial z}\right)_l = \mu_l \left(\frac{1}{r}\frac{\partial}{\partial r}\left(\frac{\partial u_l}{\partial r}\right) + \frac{\partial^2 u_l}{\partial z^2}\right), \tag{3.46}$$

where the subscript l denotes the liquid film and u_l is the film velocity in the z direction. Note that in the equation above, we assume that the thin aqueous liquid layer behaves like a Newtonian fluid (e.g. water) such that its dynamic viscosity, μ_l, is constant. In reality, this liquid layer behaves as a mucus where viscosity is dependent on the applied strain rate.

Assuming no pressure gradient in the z-direction (motion may only be induced due to shear stress from the continuous gas phase flow and from surface tension gradients $\nabla\sigma$, where σ is the surface tension), $(\partial p/\partial z)_l = 0$. Furthermore, for a thin film $\partial u_l/\partial z \ll \partial u_l/\partial r$ such that the term $\partial^2 u_l/\partial z^2$ may be neglected. Therefore, Eq. (3.46) reduces to:

$$u_l(r) = C_3 \ln r + C_4. \tag{3.47}$$

The no-slip boundary condition at $r = R$ requires $u_l|_{r=R} = 0$ leading to $C_4 = -C_3 \ln R$ such that:

$$u_l(r) = C_3 \ln\left(\frac{r}{R}\right), \tag{3.48}$$

where C_3 is yet to be determined.

At the liquid-gas interface ($r = R - h$), two kinematic conditions arise:

$$u_a(r = R-h) = u_l(r = R-h), \tag{3.49}$$

$$\mu_a \left.\frac{\partial u_a}{\partial r}\right|_{r=(R-h)} + \nabla\sigma = \mu_l \left.\frac{\partial u_l}{\partial r}\right|_{r=(R-h)}. \tag{3.50}$$

The first equation represents the no-slip boundary condition at the interface. The second equation relates to the viscous shear stress at the interface. Using Eqs. (3.45) and (3.48), the no-slip condition leads to:

$$\frac{1}{\mu_a}\left(\frac{\partial p}{\partial z}\right)_a \left(\frac{(R-h)^2}{4} + C_2\right) = C_3 \ln\left(\frac{R-h}{R}\right), \tag{3.51}$$

such that

$$C_2 = \frac{\mu_a C_3}{\left(\frac{\partial p}{\partial z}\right)_a} \ln\left(1 - \frac{h}{R}\right) - \frac{(R-h)^2}{4}. \tag{3.52}$$

The boundary condition in Eq. (3.50) leads to

$$C_3 = \frac{(R-h)}{\mu_l}\left(\left(\frac{\partial p}{\partial z}\right)_a \frac{(R-h)}{2} + \nabla\sigma\right). \tag{3.53}$$

Inserting the above into Eq. (3.52), the constant C_2 yields:

$$C_2 = (R-h)\left[\frac{\mu_a}{\mu_l}\left(\frac{(R-h)}{2} + \frac{\nabla\sigma}{\left(\frac{\partial p}{\partial z}\right)_a}\right)\ln\left(1 - \frac{h}{R}\right) - \frac{(R-h)}{4}\right]. \tag{3.54}$$

The velocity of the gas, u_a, is found by inserting Eq. (3.54) for C_2 into Eq. (3.45) such that:

$$u_a(r) = \frac{1}{\mu_a}\left(\frac{\partial p}{\partial z}\right)_a \left[\frac{r^2}{4} + (R-h)\left(\frac{\mu_a}{\mu_l}\left(\frac{(R-h)}{2} + \frac{\nabla\sigma}{\left(\frac{\partial p}{\partial z}\right)_a}\right)\ln\left(1 - \frac{h}{R}\right) - \frac{(R-h)}{4}\right)\right]. \tag{3.55}$$

The above equation may be simplified by considering that $h/R \sim O(10^{-3})$, since the thickness of the liquid lining layer in the acinus is typically < 1 μm [8,75] and the radius of acinar ducts is on the order of $R \sim 100$ μm [90,281]. Furthermore, properties of the air and the aqueous lining layer yield $\mu_a/\mu_l \sim O(10^{-3})$. The above equation reduces effectively to:

$$u_a(r) = \frac{1}{4\mu_a}\left(\frac{\partial p}{\partial z}\right)_a \left(r^2 - R^2\right), \tag{3.56}$$

which is an exact formulation of the equation for Poiseuille flow in cylindrical coordinates [182]. Hence, in the acinar region, the continuous gas phase may be described to a reasonable extent using a Poiseuille formulation. Moreover, as seen above, the gas flow does not "feel" the liquid lining layer. Therefore, it is reasonable to model acinar airflows altogether by neglecting the influence of the aqueous liquid lining layer. Note that this assertion is only valid when the lining layer is very thin ($h/R \ll 1$), such as in healthy subjects.

In contrast, in subjects with respiratory diseases such as Acute Respiratory Distress Syndrome (ARDS) which may involve surfactant replacement therapy (liquid is either instilled into the airways in the form of boluses to deliver macromolecules or clinical agents into the lung) or partial liquid ventilation (a liquid with high gas solubility is used for expanding those shrunken alveoli in order to improve compliance and gas exchange), liquid may partially fill alveoli when it reaches the acinar region [280]. Furthermore, the mucous layer can become much thicker in diseases with excess secretion or reduced clearance rates of airway surface fluid. In such scenarios, the mucous layer may significantly affect the airway fluid dynamics in the conduction region (i.e. main and upper bronchi, etc.) of the lung [30,119,120]. However, such considerations lie beyond the scope of the present study.

Turning our attention to the flow in the thin liquid film, the velocity, u_l, is found by inserting Eq. (3.53) for C_3 into Eq. (3.48) such that:

$$u_l(r,z) = \frac{(R-h)}{\mu_l}\left(\left(\frac{\partial p}{\partial z}\right)_a \frac{(R-h)}{2} + \nabla\sigma\right)\ln\left(\frac{r}{R}\right). \tag{3.57}$$

Hence, flow in the thin film results from the superposition of shear stresses at the interface due to the axial pressure gradient, $(\partial p/\partial z)_a$, from the airflow and the surface tension gradients, $\nabla\sigma$, if such arise. Gradients in surface tension may be rewritten using the chain rule of differentiation [134]:

$$\nabla\sigma = \left(\frac{\partial\sigma}{\partial T}\right)\nabla T + \left(\frac{\partial\sigma}{\partial\Gamma}\right)\nabla\Gamma + ..., \tag{3.58}$$

where T is the temperature and Γ the surfactant concentration. Commonly liquids will maintain a constant value for $(\partial\sigma/\partial T)$ and $(\partial\sigma/\partial\Gamma)$. Over the range $R-h<r<R$, the function, $\ln(r/R)$, in Eq. (3.57) is nearly linear, while both the temperature and the surfactant concentration may generally be spatially dependent functions (i.e. $T(z)$ and $\Gamma(z)$). For the time being we will restrict ourselves to the results obtained for the velocity field, u_a, in the continuous gas phase (Eqs. (3.55) and (3.56)). We will revisit our analysis on the forced motion of a thin liquid film when considering experimentally induced recirculating flows in a thin liquid shell (see chapter 8).

3.3.4 Past Studies on Acinar Flows

From an engineering and fluid mechanics point of view, the acinar region of the lung has drawn considerable attention over the past half-century or so. We can loosely define two broad areas of research which have attracted scientists, whether from an engineering or a more medical/physiological background. The first area has been mostly concerned with problems relating to gas (i.e. oxygen) transport and mixing in the respiratory region of the lung (i.e. acinus). Much of the early work [25,175–177,298] has been constructed around lumped (pseudo) one-dimensional models of the lung (see "trumpet models" in Fig. 3.8, left), where the gas concentration, C, is governed by the convective-diffusive equation:

$$\frac{\partial C}{\partial t} + (U\cdot\nabla)C = D\nabla^2 C, \tag{3.59}$$

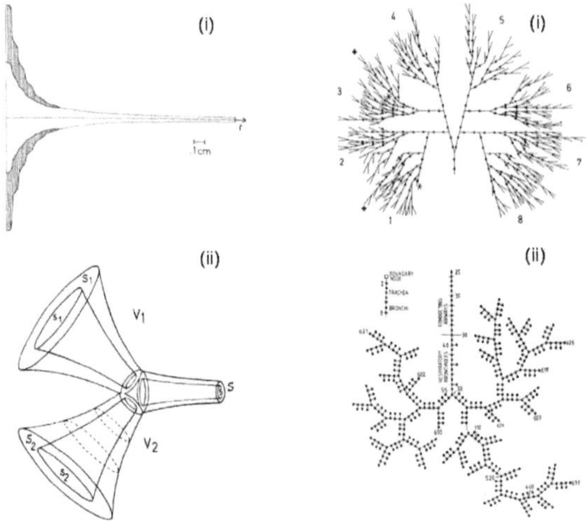

Figure 3.8: Left: (i) Trumpet model of the last pulmonary generations corresponding to the summed cross-sectional area at each airway generation, built from anatomical data of Weibel [281]. Shaded part corresponds to the volume occupied by alveoli (from Paiva [176], used with permission from the American Physiological Society). (ii) Two-trumpet model representing asymmetry where each branch (V_1 and V_2) is represented by a symmetrical trumpet, with a common stem joining at the branch. s, s_1, and s_2 refer to cross-section of conducting portions only. S, S_1, and S_2 represent total cross-sectional area including alveoli. Trumpet with shorter pathway extends from branch point to *dashed line* (from Paiva & Engel [178], with permission from Elsevier Publisher). Right: (i) Diagrammetric representation of multi-branch-point asymmetrical acinar branching model (from Paiva & Engel [179], Used with permission from the American Physiological Society). (ii) Asymmetrical model of lung represented by nodes (from Bowes *et al.* [14]), used with permission from the American Physiological Society.

where D is the diffusion coefficient. Such investigations have been reviewed in detail by Engel [58] and Paiva & Engel [180], and have been later extended to slightly more realistic models (see Fig. 3.8, right) based on asymmetric branching airways in the acinus [14, 42, 179, 277]. Later, investigations of gas transport have been complemented in geometrical models (see Fig. 3.9) depicting acinar ducts or alveolar sacs with individual alveoli [25, 46, 48, 61, 268, 269]. More recently, the existence of "diffusional screening" in the acinus due to its specific structure has been investigated in two- and three-dimensional models [62, 63], as noted earlier in section 3.3.2. Here, we only briefly mention some of the work relevant for gas transport in the acinus.

The second broad area of engineering research related to the acinar region of the lung has been aimed at understanding the nature of small-scale flows in the pulmonary acinus (often termed "acinar flows" or "alveolar flows") and their influence on the fate of inhaled particles. In the present work, we are principally concerned with this latter topic and review in more detail past investigations on the subject. Quantitatively speaking, up until recently, research concerned with gas diffusion and mixing as well as ventilation distribution in the lung has possibly been a more rewarding field, as reflected perhaps in the larger amount of publications available on the subject, compared with research aimed at understanding convective flows in the acinar region. This may also in part be due to the fact that the principle role of the pulmonary acinus is to guarantee oxygen transport into the blood stream across the alveoli, and furthermore, the role of convective flows in the acinus is indeed negligible when considering gas transport, as seen in section 3.3.2 (i.e. acinar Peclet number $Pe_{ac} \ll 1$). In contrast, however, this observation may only reflect the fact that we have discovered and begun to understand only much more recently both the complexity of convective acinar flows and their determining role in the transport and deposition of inhaled particles.

Due to the sub-millimeter dimensions (see Table 3.1), accessibility and complexity of the pulmonary acinus, detailed acinar flow characteristics have been usually difficult to assess directly. Hence, there exist only a limited number of experimental studies which have been published to date. Historically, the first attempts to study (both experimentally and numerically) such small-scale flows were initiated in the early 1970s, in models of individual alveoli mimicking terminal alveolar units (i.e alveolar sacs). The first analytical investigation to our knowledge solved the biharmonic Eq. (3.36) in cylindrical coordinates (r, θ) for quasi-steady creeping motion in simple axisymmetric models of individual alveoli (i.e. in a sphere, ellipsoid, and cylinder, similar to Fig. 3.9(a)), under the influence of wall motion simulating breathing [47]. Resulting alveolar streamlines in these terminal units exhibited simple radial-like profiles, and the authors concluded that even in the final generations of the lung, convective flows may be significant for gas transport. Similarly, a simple alveolar geometry was used soon after to model the local alveolar deposition of diffusing particles by solving numerically the convective-diffusive Eq. (3.59) using a finite-difference approach [299]. In parallel, the first experimental flow visualization study was conducted by Cinkotai [29] in a scaled-up model of an alveolus using a simple latex sac and silicone dye, by matching physiological values of $Re \sim O(10^{-4} - 10^{-3})$ in human alveoli. Here, the author observed that dyed layers injected into the model were found to be preserved over cycles during homogeneous expansion and contraction motion, suggesting that tidal and residential (i.e. FRC) fluid will mix mechanically unless the conditions of reversibility are met.

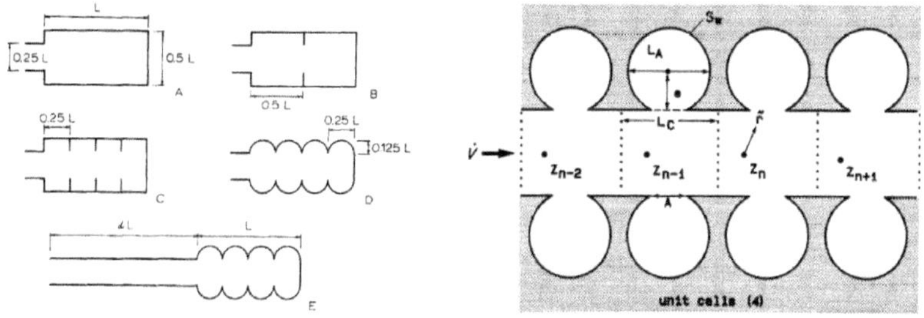

(a) (b)

Figure 3.9: Geometric models of alveolar structures employed in gas transport studies. (a) Cross sections of models of alveolar sacs (from Chang *et al.* [24], with permission from Elsevier Publisher). (b) Geometric model of alveolar duct composed of an axisymmetric central duct region and surrounding alveoli, shown in longitudinal cross section (from Federspiel *et al.* [61]). Used with permission from the American Physiological Society.

Until the pioneering work of Heyder *et al.* [99], the classical theories on acinar flows argued that the low Reynolds number airflow deep in the lung is mainly governed by acinar wall motion [187] and the principal mode of lung expansion approximately satisfies geometric similarity [3,81,83,157]. These conditions led to the conclusion that acinar flow is kinematically reversible [29,47]. This view of acinar fluid mechanics has been extended to the study of aerosol transport in the acinus, in which it has long been thought that there is little flow-induced mixing in the acinus. Consequently, for fine ($0.1-10$ μm) inhaled particles which are thought to follow the gas flow [39,267,268], most will be exhaled without being mixed with residual gas and will show negligible deposition within small airways or the acinar region [49,273]. However, Heyder *et al.* [99] were the first to demonstrate experimentally in healthy subjects that nondiffusing fine (1 μm) inhaled particles do in fact mix substantially with residual alveolar gas and deposit deep in the lung despite their low diffusivity and sedimentation rate. These observations have strongly suggested that flow-induced mixing does in fact occur in the acinar region through kinematic irreversibility.

Much of the work, both experimental and numerical, following the revealing bolus studies [44,208,227] initiated by Heyder *et al.* [99] has concentrated on elucidating the detailed nature of acinar flows and their role on the fate of inhaled particles. Among the few existing flow-visualization studies, a number of them have investigated alveolar velocity fields in scaled-up models of alveolated ducts using particle image velocimetry [116,262,265]. Without wall expansion, the flow fields are characterized by a large recirculation region within the alveolar cavity and a separation streamline separating this region from

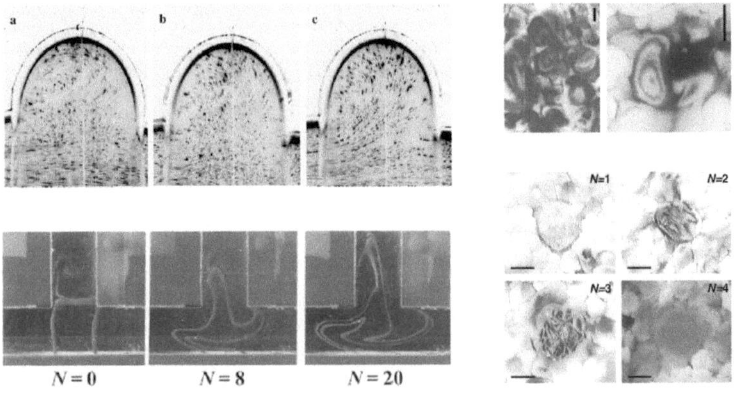

(a) (b)

Figure 3.10: (a) Top: Visualized flow fields in an expanding alveolar duct model at different values of the alveolar to ductal flow ratio (from Tippe & Tsuda [265], with permission from Elsevier Publisher). Bottom: Tracer patterns in the T-shaped junction alveolar model after N cycles (from Tsuda *et al.* [271], used with permission from the American Physiological Society). (b) Top: Alveolar recirculation pattern in rat alveolus with enlarged view (right) at $N = 1/2$ cycle (Bar $= 100$ μm). Bottom: Typical mixing pattern of two colors observed in approximately 200 μm acinar airways of adult rats after ventilatory cycles of $N = 1, 2, 3,$ and 4 (from Tsuda *et al.* [272]). Copyright (2002) National Academy of Sciences, U.S.A.

the duct flow [116, 262]. With wall expansion, the topology of the flow changes entirely. The separation streamline at the alveolar opening disappears and convective flow exchange between duct and alveolus is initiated [265]. Large recirculation flows observed in the expanding alveolus indicate the occurrence of a stagnation saddle point in the alveolar flow field (see Fig. 3.10(a), top). Such singularity point is characteristic for the occurrence of chaotic flow mixing, which in turn leads to significant increase in deposition of fine aerosols in the pulmonary acinus [265].

The remaining experimental studies have concentrated on revealing the existence of "stretch-and-fold" convective flow patterns in the acinus, which differ qualitatively from laminar flow in tubes and form part of the basis of the study of chaotic mixing [173]. Namely, over a number of breathing cycles, there is an increasingly detailed fine structure in the flow patterns, which is followed by a threshold number of cycles where the mixing characteristics qualitatively change from one with a fine but well-defined structure to one which is, in effect, completely mixed. This phenomenon is characteristic of the stretch and fold convective kinematics, during which two important characteristics emerge. First, the area over which diffusion can take place grows exponentially over cycle number, and second, the lateral or transverse distance scales from one fold to its neighbor decrease exponentially in time [19]. These properties were first shown in a large-scale acinar model consisting of a T-shaped junction of three short, straight, square ducts (see Fig. 3.10(a), bottom), where the motion of tracer dye was monitored [172, 271]. Results showed indeed that even a slight asynchrony in cyclic boundary motion of the model adjusted to match the small but finite geometric hysteresis observed in rabbit lungs [157] led to flow irreversibility with complicated swirling tracer patterns (i.e stretching of the tracer with narrowing of the separation between adjacent

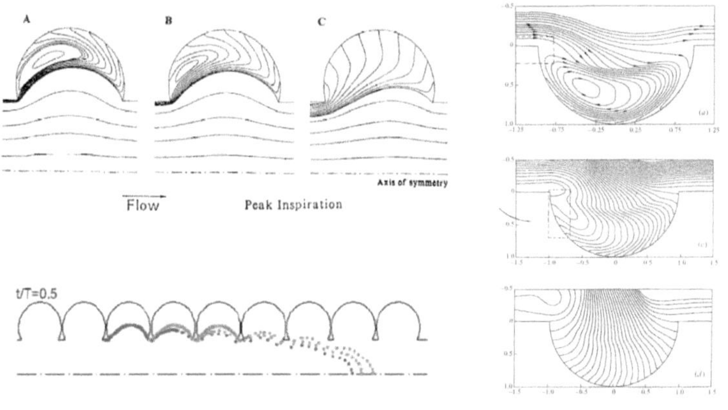

(a) (b)

Figure 3.11: (a) Top: Instantaneous flow patterns at peak inspiration in expanding alveolated duct at different values of the alveolar to ductal flow ratio (from Tsuda *et al.* [270], used with permission from the American Physiological Society). Bottom: "Massless" fluid particle tracks at different initial axial locations at the end of inspiration (from Henry *et al.* [97], used with permission from the American Physiological Society). (b) Streamline maps under different alveolar flow conditions (from Haber *et al.* [87]).

tracer lines).

Only recently, the existence of both recirculating alveolar flows and "stretch-and-fold" patterns was demonstrated in real lungs through flow visualization studies in rhythmically ventilated rat lungs [272]. Hitherto, the pioneering work of Tsuda *et al.* [272] remains to our knowledge the only attempt to reveal acinar flow characteristics in real lungs (see Fig. 3.10(b)). These important experimental visualizations have supported findings from concomitant numerical simulations [87, 270] performed to quantify the influence of structural characteristics of the acinar airways and the effects of cyclic expansion of the alveolated duct during normal breathing. Namely, these latter computational studies have showed in two- and three-dimensional models of simple alveolated ducts the existence of complex acinar flow patterns, illustrating stagnation saddle points near the alveolar openings associated with slow alveolar recirculation. Furthermore, Lagrangian tracking of "massless" fluid particles have indicated that the fluid motion may exhibit unpredictable and irreversibly stretched and folded patterns. Hence, experimental and numerical investigations performed in the last 20 years or so have both pointed towards the existence of chaotic acinar flows due to the peculiar geometry of the alveolated duct and its time-dependent motion associated with tidal breathing.

Following the findings pertinent to the complexity of acinar flows described above, acinar flow simulations have been complemented with deposition studies of micron-sized particles ($\leq 5\ \mu$m) under the influence of gravity in alveolated duct structures. A number of two- [39,40] and three-dimensional [43,95] simulations have emphasized on the importance of the geometry orientation with respect to gravity in determining deposition sites. Furthermore, deposition patterns were found to be heterogeneous, with non-uniformities in deposition between generations, between ducts of a given generation and within each alveolated duct [39]. However, these models failed to include the intrinsic boundary motion induced during rhythmic breathing. Indeed, not only does the geometrical structure of the alveolar duct itself have an important role for gravitational sedimentation [268], but also alveolar wall motion is both crucial in determining the enhancement of aerosol deposition inside the alveoli [89] and has a pronounced effect on particle residence time inside the alveolus [88]. In addition, fine (i.e. 1 μm-diameter) particles are sensitive to the detailed alveolar flow structure (i.e. recirculating flow), as they undergo gravity-induced convective mixing and deposition, as shown by Haber *et al.* [89] in a hemispherical alveolus with its opening plane located normal to the gravity field

In summary, these last 20 years have not only witnessed a major change in our understanding of acinar flow theories but also stimulated exciting new research relevant to respiratory fluid mechanics. As described above, experimental and numerical findings have contradicted the hypothesis of simple and reversible kinematics in the acinus, and have strongly suggested that kinematic irreversibility in small airways and the acinar region of the lung is a key factor in the transport and deposition of fine particles deep in the lung.

Chapter 4

Basic Aspects of Inhaled Aerosol Mechanics

Deposition is the process that causes inspired particles to be caught in the respiratory tract and thus fail to exit with expired air. Most particles that are inhaled and deposited in the lungs are typically smaller than 10 μm in diameter. Distinct physical mechanisms operate on such inspired particles to move them across streamlines of air and towards the surface of the respiratory tract. The mechanisms that contribute to the deposition of a specific particle depend significantly on the geometry of the respiratory tract and the subject's breathing pattern as well as on the particle's aerodynamic characteristics. In particular, particles may often be characterized by their aerodynamic equivalent diameter, $d_{ae} = d_p \rho_p^{1/2}$ where d_p is the particle geometric diameter. The aerodynamic diameter is the diameter of the unit density (1 kg/m^3) sphere that has the same gravitational settling velocity in air as the particle in question. The aerodynamic diameter, d_{ae}, is especially useful because it can be used to compare particles of unknown density or shape [16]. In the following sections, we will briefly introduce the three main mechanisms for particle deposition in the lung: (i) gravitational sedimentation, (ii) inertial impaction, and (iii) diffusion. A more complete description of particle deposition mechanisms is given for example by Finlay [66] and Brain & Blanchard [16].

4.1 Motion of a Single Aerosol Particle

Much of aerosol mechanics can be understood by studying the motion of a single particle in a fluid. For this reason, it is useful to look at forces and equations that govern the motion of a single, isolated, particle moving through a fluid. For our purposes, we can examine a simplified version of the trajectory of a particle in a fluid flow using two important simplifying assumptions [66]:

- the particle is assumed to be spherical;
- the particle density is assumed to be much larger than the surrounding fluid: the densities of pharmaceutical compounds are typically near that of water (i.e. $\rho_p \gg \rho_f$, where the subscripts p and f refer to the particle and the fluid, respectively).

By invoking the first assumption, we can make use of the vast body of work that has been done on the motion of spheres in fluids. One may think that this would make the problem easy to solve, but in fact it wasn't until 1983 that a relatively complete development of the equation governing the motion of a spherical particle in a flow field was made [150]. The second assumption simplifies the analysis because it results in the drag force on the particle being much larger than all the other fluid forces acting on the particle (buoyancy force, Magnus force, etc.).

4.1.1 Drag Force

Assuming that the drag force, $\underline{F}_d$, is the only non-negligible fluid force on a particle and that the only body force is gravity, the equation of motion governing the trajectory of a particle is then (Newton's second law):

$$m\frac{d\underline{u}_p}{dt} = m\underline{g} + \underline{F}_d, \tag{4.1}$$

where $\underline{u}_p$ is the particle velocity, $|\underline{g}|$ =9.81 m/s^2 is the gravitational acceleration and $m = \pi\rho_p d_p^3/6$ is the mass of a spherical particle. For a perfect sphere, the definition of the drag coefficient is given by:

$$C_d = \frac{|\underline{F}_d|}{\frac{1}{2}\rho_f u_{rel}^2 A}, \tag{4.2}$$

where $A = \pi d_p^2/4$ is the cross-sectional area of the sphere, and the relative velocity of the particle is $u_{rel} = |\underline{u}_p - \underline{u}_f|$. The drag coefficient depends on $Re = u_{rel}d_p/\nu$. Most inhaled pharmaceutical aerosol particles have a very small $d_p \sim O(10^{-7} - 10^{-5})$ and relatively low velocities u_{rel} such that $Re_p = u_{rel}d_p/\nu \ll 1$. For such cases, the drag coefficient is given by (see Appendix B):

$$C_d = \frac{24}{Re_p}, \tag{4.3}$$

which for $Re_p < 0.1$, gives a value of C_d that is accurate to within 1%. Combining the above equations for $Re_p \ll 1$, we can write:

$$\underline{F}_d = -3\pi d_p\mu(\underline{u}_p - \underline{u}_f), \tag{4.4}$$

where the negative sign arises from the fact that the drag force acts in the same direction as the velocity of the particle relative to the fluid.

Equation (4.4) is often referred to as Stokes law[1] (see Appendix B). It is derived from the Navier-Stokes Eq. (3.1) and is only valid for particle diameters that are much greater than the mean free molecular path (which in air at typical inhalation conditions is near 0.07 μm).

4.2 Settling Velocity and Sedimentation

A particle in stationary air will settle under the action of gravity and reach a terminal velocity corresponding to the (terminal) settling velocity u_t. Because the particle's velocity does not change once it reaches its settling velocity, u_t, the acceleration on the particle is zero (and therefore the net force is

[1] It is named after G. Stokes (1851) who first determined the flow field due to a rigid sphere in translational motion through a fluid for very low Re_p [257].

zero). Assuming the only forces acting on the solid, non-rotating, spherical particle are drag and gravity, the equilibrium condition yields $mg = F_d$ from Eq. (4.1).

If one assumes furthermore $Re_p \ll 1$ so that Eq. (4.4) is valid, $u_f = 0$ and $mg = \rho_p g \pi d_p^3/6$. Thus, the equilibrium condition yields:

$$u_t = \frac{\rho_p g d_p^2}{18\mu}. \tag{4.5}$$

For example, a particle of 1 μm falling through air at atmospheric pressure and body temperature has a terminal velocity of approximately 34 μm/s. In particular, particles less than 10 μm reach their terminal sedimentation velocity instantaneously (~ 1 ms).

Particles are removed from the inhaled air when their settling causes them to strike airway walls or acinar surfaces (see section 2.4.2). In the lungs, we may define a sedimentation parameter as $u_t t/L$, where L is some characteristic distance (e.g. airway diameter) and t the residence time in the respiratory tract. Intuitively, breath holding will enhance deposition by sedimentation. Sedimentation is important for particles typically larger than 0.1 μm within the peripheral airways and acini where airflow rates are slow and residence times are long [16].

4.3 Inertial Impaction

If a particle moving at velocity $|\underline{u}_p|$ is suddenly placed into still air in the absence of any external forces, its momentum carries it forward a certain distance until the resistive drag forces of the surrounding air bring it to a stop. This is analogous to what occurs when an air stream carrying a particle at velocity $|\underline{u}_p|$ makes a sudden change in direction by an angle θ as it occurs at airway bifurcations. The particle suddenly obtains a velocity of magnitude $|\underline{u}_p| \sin\theta$ at right angles to its original velocity. Hence, the particle will move across the deflecting air streamlines before it loses its original momentum and again passively follows the air streamlines in the new direction. If travelling this distance brings it into contact with a wall, the particle is assumed to deposit. For example, if a particle with $d_p = 1$ μm travels in an air stream moving at 0.2 m/s (typical of the air velocity in a bronchus), then a 30° change in the direction of flow moves the particle 0.3 μm away from its previous streamline.

Conceptually then, a particle may be carried forward by its momentum. In particular, if the fluid travels around a bend, a particle that is massive enough may not be able to execute the bend and will deposit on the wall, as illustrated in Fig. 4.1. In order to determine whether a particle will deposit by impaction, its trajectory needs to be determined, which requires solving Eq. (4.1) and integrating $d\underline{x}_p/dt = \underline{u}_p$, where $\underline{x}_p$ is a particle's position.

It is possible, however, to estimate whether inertial impaction is likely to occur without solving per se Eq. (4.1). Let us substitute Stokes law (see Eq. (4.1)) for the drag force of the fluid on the particle, and rearrange Eq. (4.1) such that:

$$\frac{d\underline{u}_p}{dt} = \underline{g} - \frac{1}{\tau}(\underline{u}_p - \underline{u}_f). \tag{4.6}$$

where $\tau = \rho_p d_p^2/18\mu$. This parameter is called the particle relaxation time and is important, as we will see shortly. Introducing dimensionless parameters, Eq. (4.1) may be expressed in non-dimensional form as:

$$Stk\frac{d\underline{u}'_p}{dt'} = \frac{u_t}{U_0}\underline{g}' - \underline{u}'_{rel}, \tag{4.7}$$

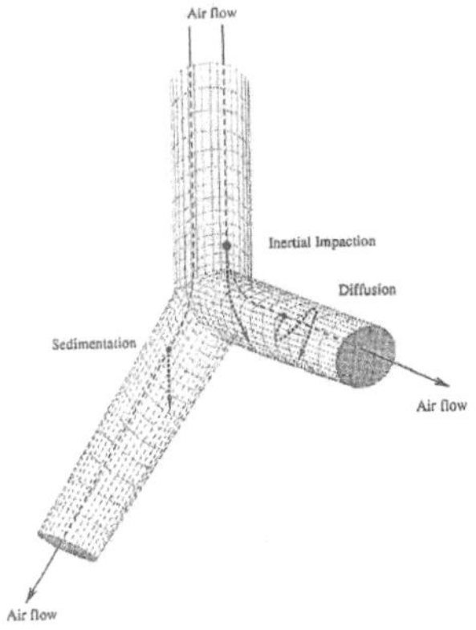

Figure 4.1: Conceptual illustration of the three main particle deposition mechanisms in the lung (from Martonen & Yang [147]).

where the variables are non-dimensionalized as follows:

$$\underline{u}'_p = \frac{\underline{u}_p}{U_0}; \quad \underline{u}'_f = \frac{\underline{u}_f}{U_0}; \quad t' = \frac{t}{D/U_0}; \quad \underline{g}' = \frac{\underline{g}}{|g|}, \tag{4.8}$$

and $\underline{u}'_{rel} = (\underline{u}'_p - \underline{u}'_f)$. We have introduced U_0 as a typical velocity of the fluid flow (e.g. mean velocity of the fluid in the lung airway where the particle is located) and D as a typical dimension of the geometry containing the fluid flow (e.g. the diameter of the lung airway). The Stokes number, Stk, is given by:

$$Stk = \frac{\tau U_0}{D} = \frac{U_0 \rho_p d_p^2}{18 \mu D}. \tag{4.9}$$

Note that Stk is analogous to the definition of the Strouhal number, St, from Eq. (3.5). Because we have non-dimensionalized Eq. (4.1), all the terms $d\underline{u}'_p/dt'$, $\underline{g}'$, and $\underline{u}'_{rel}$ are expected to be at most of order $O(1)$. The left-hand side of Eq. (4.8) will be zero if $Stk \to 0$. In the absence of gravity, however, both terms other than $\underline{u}'_{rel}$ will be zero if $Stk \to 0$. The only way for Eq. (4.8) to be satisfied in this case is if $\underline{u}'_{rel} = 0$, which implies that $\underline{u}_p = \underline{u}_f$ and therefore particle trajectories are fluid streamlines. In summary:

- for $Stk \ll 1$, particles will follow streamlines (neglecting gravitational settling);
- if $Stk \approx 1$ or larger, a particle that encounters a rapid change in direction of flow, will move relative to the fluid. In other words, particles with $Stk > 1$ will not follow rapid changes in fluid streamlines.

For *in vivo* deposition measurements, the probability of impaction is proportional to $d_{ae}^2 \dot{Q}$ where $\dot{Q}$ is the flow rate [16]. Inertial impaction is typically an important deposition mechanisms for particles with $d_{ae} > 2$ μm and may occur both during inspiration and during expiration in the extra-thoracic airways and central airway bifurcations.

4.3.1 Particle Relaxation Time and Stopping Distance

We briefly introduced above the particle relaxation time τ (see Eq. (4.9)). To understand its meaning, let us consider a particle that is placed initially with zero velocity into a fluid having a constant velocity U_0. Because of the drag on the particle, it will start moving, and will be accelerated so that after some time, t, the particle's velocity will be the same as the fluid velocity, namely $\underline{u}_p = \underline{u}_f$. Neglecting gravity, we can solve the differential Eq. (4.7) such that upon integration:

$$|\underline{u}'_{rel}| = e^{-\frac{t'}{Stk}}. \tag{4.10}$$

We see that a particle moving in a uniform flow and initially having a velocity different from the fluid surrounding it will have its velocity decay exponentially with time until it is eventually moving at the same speed as the fluid surrounding it.

The particle's velocity relative to the fluid will reach a value of $e^{-1} = 37\%$ of its initial velocity when $t' = Stk$. Thus, Stk can be interpreted as the non-dimensional time required for the particle's velocity relative to the fluid to drop to 37% of its initial value when injected into the fluid.

Conversely, the Stokes number can be interpreted as a dimensionless version of a distance termed the "stopping distance." This comes from first realizing that $\underline{u}'_{rel} = d\underline{x}'_{rel}/dt'$ and integrating Eq. (4.10) such that:

$$\underline{x}'_{rel} = Stk\left(1 - e^{-\frac{t'}{Stk}}\right), \tag{4.11}$$

where $\underline{x}'_{rel} = 0$ at $t = 0$. The "stopping distance," x_{stop}, may be defined as the separation that will occur at $t = \infty$ between a particle considered and an element of fluid that the particle started out with at time $t = 0$. This result leads to $|\underline{x}'_{rel}(t = \infty)| = Stk$. Since $x'_{rel} = x_{rel}/D$, it follows that:

$$x_{stop} = StkD. \tag{4.12}$$

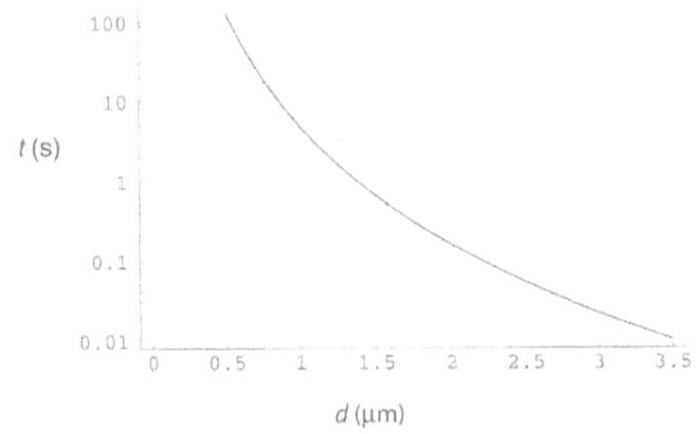

Figure 4.2: The time t above which $\Delta < 0.1x_s$, so that particle motion due to Brownian diffusion is estimated to be negligible compared to particle motion due to sedimentation (from Finlay [66]).

4.4 Diffusion

The constant random collisions of gas molecules with small aerosol particles pushes the particles in an irregular fashion called *Brownian movement.* Consider for example the motion of a particle settling in an airway under the action of gravity, shown in Fig. 4.1. Even in the absence of gravity, a particle in still air moves about in a "random walk". This is a stochastic process that allows motion in three-dimensions so that the motion of a given particle may not be actually predicted.

However, if we examine the particle motion only over times, t, that are much longer than the time between collisions with molecules, we can use a result developed by Einstein (1905) to express the root-mean-square displacement Δ of a particle [55]:

$$\Delta = \sqrt{2Dt}, \tag{4.13}$$

where the particle diffusion coefficient, D (not to be confused with the diameter D) is given by:

$$D = \frac{kT}{3\pi\mu d_p}. \tag{4.14}$$

Here k=1.38 $\times$ 10^{-23} J K^{-1} is the Boltzmann constant and T is the temperature in Kelvin. Because the diffusion coefficient, D, increases with decreasing particle size, diffusion becomes important for small particles (in contrast to gravitational settling or inertial impaction). To decide at what particle size, d_p, diffusion starts to become important, we can compare the distance, $x_s = u_t t$, a particle will settle in time t to the distance Δ that the particle will diffuse in the same time, which simplifies to:

$$\frac{\Delta}{x_s} = \frac{1}{\rho_p}\sqrt{\frac{216\mu kT}{\pi t d_p^5}}. \tag{4.15}$$

We can consider diffusion to be negligible if $\Delta/x_s < 0.1$ or so. Substituting $\Delta/x_s = 0.1$ into Eq. (4.15) allows us to solve for the time t above which diffusion will be negligible for a given particle diameter d_p. The result is shown in Fig. 4.2.

Thus, in deciding whether diffusion is an important mechanism of deposition for inhaled pharmaceutical aerosols, we must decide over what time interval we expect deposition to occur. If deposition occurs mainly during sedimentation with a breath hold, then diffusion is probably negligible for most inhaled aerosols. However, if deposition occurs mainly during inhalation while the particle is in transit through the lung, then diffusion may need to be included for particles below a few microns in diameter. For larger particles, diffusion remains unimportant.

Diffusion is certainly important for particles with diameters typically less than 1 μm. For diffusing particles that are 0.4 μm or smaller, particle size can be expressed in terms of the thermodynamic equivalent diameter d_{te}: the diameter of a sphere that has the same average diffusional velocity in air as the actual particle. The probability that a particle is deposited by diffusion is proportional to $(t/d_{te})^{1/2}$ [16]. Thus, decreasing particle size or increasing residence time in the lungs increases the chance of diffusional losses. Diffusion, like sedimentation, is most important in the peripheral airways and acini.

As particle size decreases, inertia and sedimentation become less important, but diffusion increases. A comparison of settling and diffusional displacements for a range of particle sizes is given in Table 4.1. Generally, gravity and inertia dominate transport and deposition of particles larger than 1 μm, and diffusion dominates the transport and deposition of particles smaller than 0.1 μm. Fine particles between 0.1 and 1 μm, are thought to follow gas flow while both sedimentation and diffusion are important [267, 268].

Additional mechanisms may affect particle aerodynamics and deposition. We briefly mention some of these possible mechanisms. Electric forces may cause charged particles to deposit in the respiratory tract. The surfaces of the respiratory tract are uncharged but are electrically conducting. When an electrically charged particle approaches the lung surface, the particle induces an image charge of opposite polarity on the lung surface which attracts the particle. This attraction may cause the particle to deposit. Electrostatic attraction may be an important deposition mechanism in the lung periphery for particles (especially fibers) that are charged above a certain threshold and have a diameter of $0.1 - 1$ μm [278].

In many situations, particles may experience dynamic changes in size while moving through the delivery system and the respiratory tract. Volatile droplets composed of water or Freon propellant shrink through evaporation while hygroscopic droplets, such as NaCl particles, may grow dramatically, especially as the relative humidity nears 100%. Since the relative humidity in the lungs is 99.5% beyond the upper airways, hygroscopicity has an important effect on particle size and deposition fraction. With increasing particle hygroscopicity and relative humidity, the deposition fraction minimum is shifted to smaller particle sizes [103, 161]. However, these mechanisms lie beyond the scope of the present work.

4.5 Targeting Deposition

Targeting of the respiratory tract can be of importance with therapeutic agents where efficacy is thought to depend in part on where the drug deposits in the lung. It should be noted though that such targeting will be fairly broad, for a number of reasons. First, it is not possible to adequately control the regions to which air carries aerosol in the lung. For example, one cannot target only the tracheo-bronchial region, since the pathways to some terminal bronchioles are much shorter than others and will start to fill alveolar regions before the air has even reached the terminal bronchioles in other airways. It is also impossible to have air reach only the alveolar region, since it must first travel through the extrathoracic and tracheo-bronchial regions. Second, the factors that affect deposition change gradually from region to region in the lung. For example, if particles are chosen to deposit mainly by sedimentation, such particles will deposit mainly in the alveolar regions. However, sedimentation is also operational in the small bronchioles, so that we cannot entirely avoid deposition in the tracheo-bronchial region in this manner. Finally, variations

Table 4.1: Root mean square Brownian displacement in 1 s compared to distance fallen in air ($37°$C and 100% relative humidity) in 1 s for unit density particles of different diameters. ([a]Diameter of a typical air molecule.)

	d_p (μm)	Diffusion distance in 1 s (μm)	Settling distance in 1 s (μm)
Settling greater	50	0.978	71'700
	10	2.20	2'910
	5	3.14	740
	1	7.50	33.7
Diffusion greater	0.5	11.4	9.71
	0.1	38.1	0.871
	0.05	71.4	0.382
	0.01	339	0.0689
	0.00037[a]	9'060	0.00249

between subjects in the parameters that control deposition will also broaden the regions actually reached by attempts at targeting specific lung regions.

Despite these difficulties, broad targeting is possible. In particular, if inhalation flow-rate is increased, extrathoracic deposition will increase, while total dose to the lung will decrease. Conversely, reducing inhalation flow rate will shift deposition away from the mouth-throat deeper into the lung. If inhalation flow rate is very low, impaction in the larger airways can be avoided, resulting in small airway and/or alveolar deposition, depending on particle size [20]. One should realize that it is probably unrealistic to expect patients to consistently control inhalation flow rate precisely, so that the use of specific inhalation flow rates for targeting is probably best achieved for example with a delivery device that delivers aerosols when the patient supplies a certain flow rate range [230].

Probably the most commonly used approach to targeting aerosol deposition is through particle size (combined with inhalation flow rate), with larger particles impacting and sedimenting more readily than smaller ones, while smaller ones deposit more readily by diffusion. However, inhalation volume can affect deposition, since for smaller volumes the conducting airways occupy more of the inhaled volume, resulting in a relative shift toward more tracheo-bronchial than alveolar deposition at low inhalation volumes. Finally, particle density affects deposition since impaction and sedimentation are affected by the particle's aerodynamic diameter d_{ae}.

4.6 Time Scales of Deposition Mechanisms

We are interested in formulating and estimating the principal time scales relevant for particle transport and deposition inside a pulmonary alveolus. We assume here that particles have reached the entrance ring of an alveolus. The alveolus is modelled for simplicity as a sphere of diameter $D_a \sim O(200\ \mu\text{m})$. For this problem, the following time scales may be identified:

- breathing time scale;
- convective time scale
- settling time scale;
- diffusion time scale.

During quiet tidal volume (TV) breathing, an inspiration/expiration period is on the order of $T_{tv} \approx 3-5$ s, as noted earlier in section 3.2.2. The shortest possible breathing period is perhaps reached under high-frequency oscillatory ventilation (HFOV) [245], which is an invasive mechanical ventilation technique, and can be as low as $T_{HFOV} \approx 0.033$ s.

Convective flows are generated within alveoli principally due to volume expansion/contraction during inhalation/exhalation, as we will see in detail later in our computational fluid dynamics simulations. To approximate the relevant convective time scale, we may estimate a mean velocity induced during alveolar wall expansion. An appropriate velocity scale may be given for example by the change in alveolar radius over time $r_a(t) = D_a(t)/2$. During breathing motion, we assume for simplicity that the alveolar geometry remains self-similar throughout a breathing period T. As briefly noted in section 3.3.4, this is essentially true. The alveolar radius, $r_a(t)$, may then be described by a time-dependent displacement

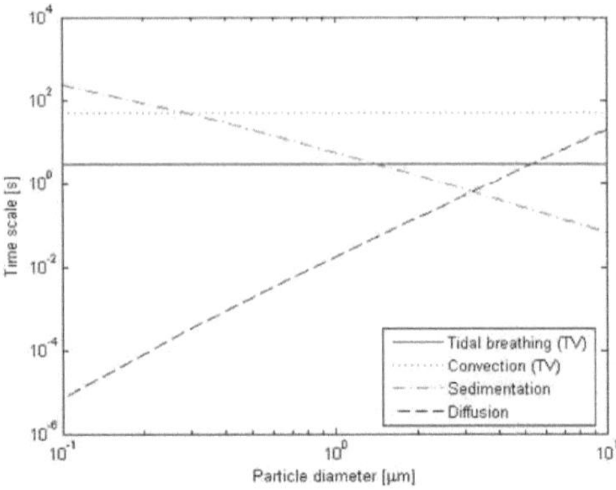

Figure 4.3: Times scales for particle deposition in an alveolus.

function:

$$r_a(t) = r_{a,0}\left[1 + \frac{\beta}{2} + \frac{\beta}{2}\sin\left(2\pi f t - \frac{\pi}{2}\right)\right], \tag{4.16}$$

where $r_{a,0} = D_a/2$ is the radius at $t = 0$, and $f = 1/T$ is the breathing frequency. For geometrically self-similar motion under quiet breathing, lung volumes change by approximately $15 - 20\%$, such that the length scale expansion factor, β, is on the order of $\sim 5\%$ (this quantity will be derived in detail in section 5.2). For oscillatory flow, the root mean square (RMS) velocity scale gives a representative estimate over the breathing cycle such that:

$$u_r|_{RMS} = \left.\frac{dr_a(t)}{dt}\right|_{max} \cdot \frac{\sqrt{2}}{2} = \frac{d_a \beta \pi \sqrt{2}}{4T}. \tag{4.17}$$

The convective time scale, t_{conv}, may then be estimated by the time needed to reach the alveolar wall by means of convective transport:

$$t_{conv} = \frac{d_a}{u_r|_{RMS}} = \frac{4T}{\beta\pi\sqrt{2}}. \tag{4.18}$$

For small particles settling to the alveolar wall, assuming $Re_p << 1$, the settling velocity, u_t, was derived in Eq. (4.5). An appropriate settling time scale is then given by:

$$t_{sett} = \frac{d_a}{u_t} = \frac{18 d_a \mu}{C_c \rho_p g d_p^2}, \tag{4.19}$$

where we've added the Cunningham correction factor for small particles, given as $C_c = 1 + 2.52\lambda/d_p$ where $\lambda \approx 0.072 \times 10^{-6}$ is the mean free path for air at $37°$C.

The Brownian diffusion time scale is found by solving Eq. (4.13) for t and substituting Eq. (4.14) and $\Delta = D_a$ such that:

$$t_{diff} = \frac{D_a^2}{2D} = \frac{3\pi D_a^2 \mu d_p}{2kT}. \tag{4.20}$$

Results for the different time scales identified are illustrated in Fig. 4.3 for particles in the range of 0.1-10 μm, which represent a wide range of inhalation aerosols characteristic sizes. As seen from the figure, for sub-micron aerosols, diffusion will dominate the deposition process within the alveolus by several orders of magnitude. For particles greater than approximately 3 μm, sedimentation will govern deposition. In the range nearby 2 μm, however, diffusion and sedimentation processes exhibit similar time scales. Note that over the entire range of particle diameters, the convective time scale, t_{conv}, is always larger than either diffusion or sedimentation. Hence, this simple analysis suggests that convection under quiet breathing may never be the leading deposition mechanism as it is always overtaken by either diffusion (for small particles) or gravitational settling (for larger particles). Furthermore, Fig. 4.3 seems to suggest that particles which have reached the alveolus entrance will deposit within one breathing period. Note that the simple analysis for time scales of alveolar deposition is by no means quantitatively precise. Rather, it serves as an initial guideline in understanding the relative importance of the different deposition mechanisms. Indeed, we will see for example in chapter 6 using computational fluid dynamics (CFD) models that, in fact, fine non-diffusing micron-sized particles may need much larger time scales spanning over multiple breathing cycles for deposition to finalize. As we will later see, such findings result from the complex interactions which may exist between sedimentation and convective mechanisms influencing aerosol transport.

The combination of the results from our simple analysis above, implying that convection time scales are always larger than diffusion or sedimentation time scales, in conjunction with findings from chapter 6, where fine particles exhibit long residence times in the bulk of the acinar airspace due to the influence of the local flow structure, suggest altogether that one possible strategy towards enhanced and increased alveolar particle deposition lies in augmenting or controlling the role of acinar convective flows, since diffusion and sedimentation processes are fixed. These considerations have stimulated our interest to investigate, in chapters 8 and 9, potential non-invasive mechanisms which can lead to forced convective flows inside benchmark models of alveoli.

Part II

Respiratory Flow Simulations in the Pulmonary Acinus

Chapter 5

Convective Acinar Flows in a Simple Aveolated Duct

Low Reynolds number flows ($Re < 1$) in the human pulmonary acinus are often difficult to assess due to the sub-millimeter dimensions and accessibility of the region. In the present computational study, we simulated three-dimensional alveolar flows in an alveolated duct at each generation of the pulmonary acinar tree using recent morphometric data. Rhythmic lung expansion and contraction motion was modelled using moving wall boundary conditions to simulate realistic sedentary tidal breathing. The resulting alveolar flow patterns are largely time-independent and governed by the ratio of the alveolar to ductal flow rates, $\dot{Q}_a/\dot{Q}_T$. This ratio depends uniquely on geometric configuration such that alveolar flow patterns may be entirely determined by the location of the alveoli along the acinar tree. Although flows within alveoli travel very slowly relative to those in acinar ducts, $0.021\% \leq \overline{U}_a/\overline{U} \leq 9.1\%$, they may exhibit complex patterns linked to the three-dimensional nature of the flow and confirm findings from earlier 3D simulations. Such patterns are largely determined by the interplay between recirculation in the cavity induced by ductal shear flow over the alveolar opening and radial flows induced by wall displacement. Furthermore, alveolar flow patterns under rhythmic wall motion contrast sharply with results obtained in a rigid alveolus, further confirming the importance of including inherent wall motion to understand realistic acinar flow phenomena. The present findings may give further insight into the role of convective alveolar flows in determining aerosol kinematics and deposition in the pulmonary acinus.

5.1 Introduction

Respiratory airflows in the human pulmonary acinus, which comprises the vast majority of the lung volume (see section 2.2), are characterized by low Reynolds numbers (typically $Re < 1$, see section 3.2.2) in sub-millimeter airways marked by the presence of alveoli [29,61,116]. Alveoli constitute the gas exchange units necessary for oxygen (and carbon-dioxide) exchange with capillary blood vessels (see section 2.2), which are embedded within the alveolar membranes. The presence of alveoli is first encountered past the terminal bronchioles distal to the trachea and located approximately at the 15th generation of the bifurcating airway tree [90,92,281]. Along the subsequent airway generations (respiratory bronchioles, alveolar ducts and sacs) which progressively decrease in dimensions while alveolar dimensions increase [90,91], clusters of alveoli become more numerous and gradually cover the acinar airways entirely. Due to the sub-millimeter dimensions and accessibility of the pulmonary acinus, acinar flow characteristics remain usually difficult to assess. Therefore, the measurement and simulation of flow phenomena in such region continue to present challenging problems. Hence, we are interested in gaining further insight into more detailed three-dimensional characteristics of convective alveolar flow patterns.

On a macroscopic level, airflow into and out of the lung is driven by pressure differences between the alveoli and the outside environment. These pressure gradients are induced by the geometrically self-similar lung expansion and contraction motion during breathing [3, 80, 83], controlled by the activity of the diaphragm muscle [167,217]. On the smaller scales, alveolar flows are governed by pressure and viscous forces, and are largely influenced by wall boundary conditions. Previous computational simulations of two-dimensional acinar flows [97, 270] have shown that low Reynolds number flows in alveoli may be kinematically irreversible due to the substantial influence of the alveolated wall structure and its rhythmical motion during respiration (see section 3.3.4). These findings have come in sharp contrast with classical theories which have commonly depicted alveolar flows as simple and reversible [29, 47]. While the role of convective acinar flow patterns may be disregarded for oxygen transport in the distal regions of the pulmonary acinus [214, 284], as described by low values of the Peclet number relating convective to diffusive lengths (see section 3.3.2), particles in the range of 0.1–10 μm, however, are generally thought to follow convective gas flow [39, 267, 268]. For these particles, characteristics of convective flow patterns in the pulmonary acinus are therefore critical in understanding and determining their motion. In particular, convective three-dimensional acinar flows can exhibit complex recirculating flow structures leading to chaotic aerosol mixing patterns. This has been shown for example in early three-dimensional alveolar flow simulations, where alveoli were modeled with a spherical cap attached at the rim to a circular opening in an infinite plane [87].

In the present study, we have carried out detailed computational fluid dynamics (CFD) simulations of flow patterns and velocity fields exhibited by the rhythmic motion of three-dimensional alveoli and airways at each generation of the pulmonary acinar tree. Based on an accurate morphometric description of the human pulmonary acinus [90, 284], under realistic breathing conditions, we employed a commercial finite volume code (CFX 5.7-1, ANSYS, INC. Canonsburg, PA, USA) to simulate three-dimensional alveolar flows in both rigid- and moving-wall alveoli. This work stands as a confirmation of and an extension to earlier results obtained for two-dimensional alveolar streamline patterns [47, 97, 270]. In addition, our results confirm the earlier findings of Haber *et al.* [87], which suggest that complex alveolar flow patterns linked to the three-dimensional nature of the flow may exist and cannot be captured by two-dimensional simulations. It is intended that this work will further contribute to the initial steps in the development toward an accurate description of convective respiratory airflow in a complete and realistic three-dimensional geometry of the pulmonary acinus.

5.2 Breathing Kinematics

The principle mode of lung expansion and contraction motion approximately satisfies geometric self-similarity (as describe above). Therefore, any length, L, in the geometry scales with the $1/3$ power of the lung volume ($L \propto V^{1/3}$), and geometric reversibility is satisfied such that any point on the wall will retrace, during expiration, the same path traveled during inspiration. We define the breathing period, T, as the time needed for a complete breathing cycle. Note that in our modeling simplification, inhalation and exhalation phases are assumed to last equally long, i.e. $T/2$. The breathing period, T, will depend on the breathing scenario considered, e.g. sedentary tidal breathing, inspiratory capacity breathing, high frequency oscillation, etc. Assuming a minimum volume, V_{min}, at the beginning of the inhalation phase ($t = 0$), which corresponds to a lung volume at functional residual capacity (FRC), and a maximum volume, V_{max}, at the end of the inhalation phase ($t = T/2$), the specific volume excursion may then be defined as:

$$C = \frac{V_{max} - V_{min}}{V_{min}} = \frac{V_{max}}{V_{min}} - 1. \tag{5.1}$$

Similarly, the specific length scale excursion (expansion) factor is defined as:

$$\beta = \frac{L_{max} - L_{min}}{L_{min}} = \frac{L_{max}}{L_{min}} - 1. \tag{5.2}$$

Following the aforementioned principle of geometric self-similarity, the following result holds true:

$$\frac{L_{max}}{L_{min}} = \left(\frac{V_{max}}{V_{min}}\right)^{1/3} = (C+1)^{1/3}. \tag{5.3}$$

Therefore, combining Eqs. (5.2) and (5.3), the length scale excursion factor reduces to:

$$\beta = (C+1)^{1/3} - 1. \tag{5.4}$$

To account for self-similar lung motion, any length scale, $L(t)$, in an acinar (or lung) geometric model is designed to expand and contract in a simple sinusoidal manner, described by a sinusoidal kinematic displacement function [97, 270]:

$$L(t) = L_0 \left[1 + \frac{\beta}{2} + \frac{\beta}{2}\sin\left(2\pi f t - \frac{\pi}{2}\right)\right] = L_0 \cdot \lambda(t), \tag{5.5}$$

where L_0 is the length scale at $t = 0$, and $f = 1/T$ is the breathing frequency. $\lambda(t)$ is the sinusoidal function defined in the brackets of Eq. (5.5) such that the length scale reaches a maximum displacement of $L_{max} = L_0(1+\beta)$ at the end of the inhalation phase ($t = T/2$). Alternatively, Eq. (5.5) may be rewritten as $L(t) = L_0[1+\beta(1-\cos 2\pi f t)/2]$. One should note, however, that in nature real tidal breathing does not exhibit a perfectly sinusoidal change of volume with time, but rather the lung illustrates a small but significant geometric hysteresis [157], as noted earlier in sections 2.4.1 and 3.3.4. Nevertheless, to the extent with which acinar flows are quasi-steady (see section 3.2.3, where $Wo < 1$), the sinusoidal breathing approximation may be adopted [47, 97, 267, 268]. The present work follows closely past studies on acinar flows [47, 87, 97, 267, 268], where airflows are generated as a result of kinematic wall displacements, rather than actual breathing mechanics simulating transmural pressure gradients. Until present, the only acinar computational fluid dynamics study to our knowledge involving direct fluid-structure interactions was recently published by Dailey & Ghadiali [37], where oscillating pressure loads (rather than oscillating wall displacements) modelling tissue motion are prescribed. However simulations were performed hitherto for a two-dimensional acinar geometry.

Table 5.1 and Fig. 5.1 illustrate the corresponding breathing parameters obtained from Eqs. (5.1) and (5.4) in an average human adult, with a total lung capacity (TLC) of approximately 6000 ml and a functional residual capacity (FRC) of 3000 ml, for different breathing scenarios.

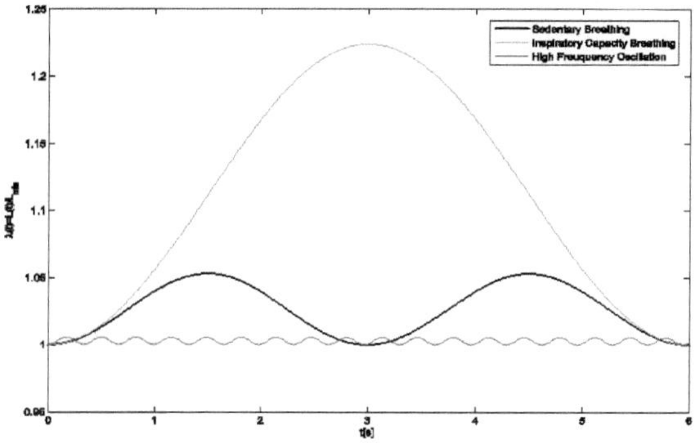

Figure 5.1: Illustration of normalized wall displacement function for different breathing scenarios.

Table 5.1: Breathing parameters in an average human adult for different breathing scenarios: sedentary tidal volume (TV) breathing, inspiratory capacity (IC) breathing, and high frequency oscillation (HFO) breathing.

Breathing scenario	T [s]	V_{min} [l]	V_{max} [l]	C	β
TV	3	3	3.5	0.167	0.053
IC	6	3	5.5	0.833	0.224
HFO	0.33	3	3.5	0.167	0.053

5.3 Alveolated Duct Geometry

In this section, we introduce the first acinar geometry investigated computationally: a single spherical alveolus placed on a cylindrical duct. The choice for this simple yet insightful model is consistent with previous alveolar flow simulations, where as mentioned earlier in section 3.3.4, alveolar geometries have been modelled as: (i) semi-circular alveolar tori on a cylindrical duct [97, 270] or alternatively as (ii) a hemispherical alveolus on a horizontal plane [87, 89]. In particular, previous results have shown that a two-dimensional geometry with spatially periodic multiple alveoli yields analogous flow patterns to those obtained for a single alveolus [267]. For such reason, we limit in the present time our three-dimensional analysis to an acinar duct with a single alveolus. The duct is modelled as a cylindrical shell with open ends, defined by a length, $l_d(t)$, and a diameter, $D_d(t)$. The alveolus is modelled by a spherical cap connected to the duct, placed arbitrarily at the center of the duct. The spherical cap is described by a radius, $r_a(t)$. Note the use of the time variable, t, for all time-dependent geometrical length scales. The opening half angle, α, defines the arc of the alveolus opening and is assumed to be constant at all acinar generations, z', and time-independent for a self-similar geometry. Clearly, modelling alveoli as spherical cavities rather than a set of open saccule, resembling a honeycomb or foam structure (see description of section 2.1), remains a simplification. Nevertheless, as we will see from the subsequent results, this simple geometry captures realistic characteristics of alveolar flows. A typical geometry of the alveolated duct is depicted in Fig. 5.2.

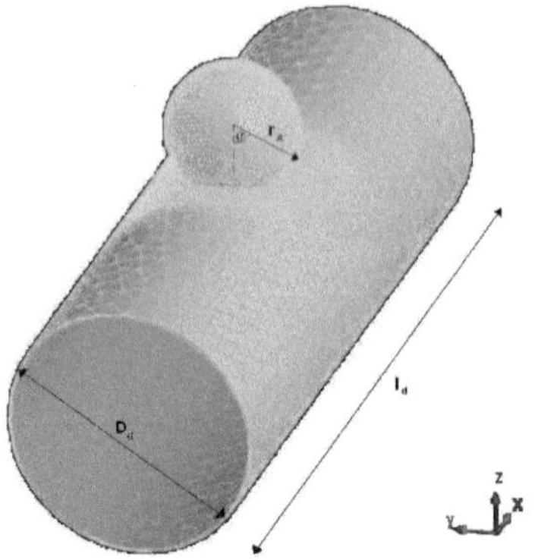

Figure 5.2: Computational mesh of alveolated duct (shown here at generation $z' = 1$). The alveolus radius is given by r_a, the airway duct diameter and length are respectively D_d and l_d. The alveolus half opening angle is denoted by α. Fine meshing is obtained within the alveolus and its near surrounding to solve accurately for the alveolar flow.

First, we must determine the opening half angle, α, for a sphere segment with radius r_a. Our approach is based on minimizing the ratio of the surface to volume of the alveolus cavity, following arguments discussed on minimizing the total energy of the lung (see section 2.5.2). Indeed, to support this idea from a mechanical point of view, one may argue, according to recent theories which assume that the strain energy resides in the alveolar walls [71], that the expansion of the lungs during inspiration is resisted by the tension across the alveolar wall membrane as well as by the surface tension induced from the thin aqueous liquid layer lining containing surfactant (i.e. a mixture of phospholipids and proteins), which covers the alveolar surface. Taking up a minimal surface for a given volume minimizes the surface tension and therefore the work needed to inflate the alveolus [90]. The volume, V_a, of the alveolar cavity (i.e. spherical cap) is given in spherical coordinates by:

$$V_a = \int_{-r_a}^{r_a \cos\alpha} dz \int_{-\sqrt{{r_a}^2 - z^2}}^{\sqrt{{r_a}^2 - z^2}} dy \int_{-\sqrt{{r_a}^2 - x^2 - y^2}}^{\sqrt{{r_a}^2 - x^2 - y^2}} dx = \frac{\pi}{3} {r_a}^3 \left((\sin^2\alpha + 2)\cos\alpha + 2 \right). \tag{5.6}$$

The surface area, S_a, of the alveolar cavity is given by:

$$S_a = \int_0^{2\pi} d\phi \int_0^{\pi - \alpha} {r_a}^2 \sin\theta d\theta = 2\pi {r_a}^2 (\cos\alpha + 1). \tag{5.7}$$

The surface to volume ratio is then given by:

$$\frac{S_a}{V_a} = \frac{6(\cos\alpha + 1)}{r_a \left((\sin^2\alpha + 2)\cos\alpha + 2 \right)}. \tag{5.8}$$

Substituting $X = \cos\alpha$ in the above yields:

$$\frac{S_a}{V_a} = \frac{6(2X-1)}{r_a\,(X^2-2X-2)^2}. \tag{5.9}$$

To minimize the ratio S_a/V_a, we solve $d/dX(S_a/V_a) = 0$ for X. This yields $X = 1/2$, such that $\alpha = \pi/3 = 60^o$. To check that $\alpha = \pi/3$ is a minimum (rather than a maximum), we substitute $\alpha = \pi/3$ into $d^2/X^2(S_a/V_a)$, which is indeed greater than zero. Therefore, $\alpha = \pi/3$ is the smallest possible value for the surface to volume ratio for a spherical cap. According to these calculations, the following results are valid:

$$\alpha = \frac{\pi}{3}, \tag{5.10}$$

$$V_a = \frac{9}{8}\pi {r_a}^3, \tag{5.11}$$

$$S_a = 3\pi {r_a}^2, \tag{5.12}$$

$$\frac{S_a}{V_a} = \frac{8}{3r_a}. \tag{5.13}$$

Note that $\alpha = \pi/3$ is consistent with values of half-opening angles investigated in previous acinar flow studies [97, 270]. Also, the alveolar volume, V_a, and surface area, S_a, have been calculated assuming that the alveolus is placed on a plane rather than on a duct such that a small region of the alveolar volume and surface is neglected. We will summarize shortly an estimation of the error induced from this difference (see also Appendix C).

Table 5.2 gives an overview of the dimensions of the alveolated duct model in dependence of the acinar generation z', following the original morphometric measurements of Haefeli-Bleuer & Weibel [90], later revisited by Weibel *et al.* [284]. In particular, the alveolar radius, r_a, has been determined based on the observation that the diameter D of a fictitious cylindrical duct laid around the alveolated duct keeps a

Table 5.2: Geometrical parameters for the duct and alveolus model at each acinar generation, z', between transitional bronchiole ($z' = 0$) and terminal alveolar sacs ($z' = 8$). Values are modified from Weibel *et al.* [284] to obtain dimensions corresponding to a lung volume at functional residual capacity (FRC) when $t = 0$. $\alpha = 60^o$ for all acinar generations.

Generation z'	Length l_d [mm]	Diameter D_d [mm]	Radius r_a [mm]
0	1.111	0.397	0.106
1	1.056	0.397	0.106
2	0.889	0.389	0.111
3	0.738	0.317	0.159
4	0.659	0.302	0.169
5	0.556	0.286	0.180
6	0.556	0.270	0.190
7	0.556	0.246	0.206
8	0.556	0.230	0.217

constant value of D =700 μm at all acinar generations. Considering Fig. 5.2, this leads to:

$$r_a(z') = \frac{D - D_d(z')}{1 + \cos\alpha}. \tag{5.14}$$

According to Eq. (5.14), Table 5.2 illustrates increasing alveolar size with acinar generation depth. This observation follows morphometical measurements of the pulmonary acinus [90, 284]. Table 5.3 summarizes the error difference between the volume, V_{alv}, of a "real" alveolus (i.e. spherical cap on a duct, see Figs. 5.2 and C.1) and the estimated alveolus volume, V_a, of a cap on a plane (see Eq. (5.11)), as discussed in Appendix C (and correspondingly the error difference between the surface area, S_{alv}, of a "real" alveolus and the estimated alveolus surface area S_a from (Eq. (5.12)). The respective errors are defined as follows:

$$E_V = \frac{V_{alv} - V_a}{V_{alv}}, \tag{5.15}$$

$$E_S = \frac{S_{alv} - S_a}{S_{alv}}. \tag{5.16}$$

As seen from Table 5.2, $E_V \leq 5\%$ and $E_S \leq 10\%$ in the first 6 or so generations of the pulmonary acinus. In the most distal acinar generations, the errors are slightly greater but remain on the order of 10%.

5.4 Human Acinar Dimensional Model

As will be seen in the subsequent sections, a dimensional model of the human pulmonary acinus is needed to determine the volume flow rates (and corresponding velocities) imposed at the entrance of individual alveolated ducts to replicate physiological breathing conditions. Table 5.4 illustrates the morphometrical model developed by Haefeli-Bleuer & Weibel [90] defining dimensional features of the acinar ducts at each acinar generation z', including total ductal volume, $S_d(z')$, volume, $V_d(z')$, and cross-sectional area $A_d(z')$. Furthermore, the acinar surface, which describes the surface area of alveoli at each generation z', is given by $S_{ac}(z')$. Note that the model assumes dichotomous symmetrical branching, as described in section 3.2.1.

Table 5.3: Numerical evaluation of alveolar volume and surface error from Eq. (5.15), following derivation in Appendix C.

Generation z'	E_V [%]	E_S [%]
0	2.22	5.31
1	2.22	5.31
2	2.39	5.60
3	4.11	8.54
4	4.51	9.21
5	4.95	9.97
6	5.38	10.73
7	6.10	11.97
8	6.62	12.87

Table 5.4: Dimensional model of acinar airways of an average human adult at functional residual capacity (FRC), adapted from Haefeli-Bleuer & Weibel [90]. Corresponding lengths and diameters of airways are given in Table 5.2.

Anatomical description	Lung generation z	Acinar generation z'	Number $N(z')$	Cross-sectional area $A_d(z')$ [mm^2]	Airway volume $V_d(z')$ [mm^3]	Acinar surface $S_{ac}(z')$ [mm^2]
Terminal bronchioles	15	0	1	0.124	0.137	4.410
	16	1	2	0.247	0.261	14.49
Respiratory bronchioles	17	2	4	0.475	0.422	42.21
	18	3	8	0.633	0.467	81.27
	19	4	16	1.143	0.753	137.96
Alveolar ducts	20	5	32	2.052	1.140	219.86
	21	6	64	3.661	2.034	416.40
Alveolar sacs	22	7	128	6.086	3.381	758.47
	23	8	256	10.652	5.918	1713.49

First, we will attempt to estimate the number of alveoli, n_a^{gen}, per acinar generation z'. As we have seen in section 2.1, the principal function of the acinus is to guarantee oxygen and carbon-dioxide exchange across the alveolar surface. Hence, since this surface area (≈ 130 m^2) is paramount for lung function, our approach to estimate n_a^{gen} is based on $S_{ac}(z')$. Using Eq. (5.12) for S_a, the number of alveoli per acinar generation z' is given by:

$$n_a^{gen}(z') = \frac{S_{ac}(z')}{S_a(z')} = \frac{S_{ac}(z')}{3\pi {r_a}^2(z')}. \tag{5.17}$$

Using the above, the number of alveoli per acinar duct follows as:

$$n_a^{duct}(z') = \frac{n_a^{gen}(z')}{N(z')} = \frac{S_{ac}(z')}{3\pi {r_a}^2(z')2^{z'}}, \tag{5.18}$$

such that the alveolar volume per generation z' is given as:

$$V_a^{gen}(z') = V_a(z')n_a^{gen}(z') = \frac{3}{8}r_a(z')S_{ac}(z'). \tag{5.19}$$

Values for $n_a^{gen}(z')$, $n_a^{duct}(z')$ and $V_a^{gen}(z')$ are given in Table 5.5 at each acinar generation z'. According to Horsfield & Cumming [106], the number of alveoli per duct should be in the range of $\sim$ 7–25, with an average of approximately 16. Comparing with values obtained for $n_a^{gen}(z')$, our model has slightly too many alveoli per duct and furthermore, $n_a^{gen}(z')$ decreases rather than increases with acinar generation. On the other hand, the average number of alveoli per duct in Horsfield & Cumming's model is in good agreement with the value obtained here, $\sum_{z'} n_a^{gen}(z')/\sum_{z'} 2^{z'} \approx 16$. Furthermore, the total number of alveoli per acinus is in good agreement with Weibel's estimated 10'000 alveoli [281], as we obtain $n = \sum_{z'} n_a^{gen}(z') = 9'086$ alveoli per acinus.

In contrast, however, the total acinar volume obtained here differs strongly with Weibel's measurement

Table 5.5: Estimated values for the number of alveoli per acinar generation, $n_a^{gen}(z')$, the number of alveli per duct, $n_a^{duct}(z')$, and the total alveolar volume per generation, $V_a^{gen}(z')$.

z'	0	1	2	3	4	5	6	7	8
$n_a^{gen}(z')$	42	137	363	432	511	721	1218	1890	3863
$n_a^{duct}(z')$	42	69	91	43	32	23	19	15	15
$V_a^{gen}(z')$ [mm³]	0.175	0.575	1.759	4.838	8.760	14.833	29.745	58.695	139.400

of ~ 93.5 mm^3 [281]. In particular, the total acinar volume, V_{acinus}, is calculated as follows:

$$V_{acinus} = V_{ducts}^{total} + V_{alveoli}^{total} = \sum_{z'} (A_d(z')l_d(z')) + \sum_{z'} (n_a^{gen}(z')V_a(z')), \tag{5.20}$$

which yields 273.294 mm^3. This difference in the total acinar volume is perhaps the biggest discrepancy our approach presents, while the total surface area of our model corresponds, in contrast, to the given total surface area by Weibel, following our original assumption. In particular, Weibel [281] measured the alveolar surface, $S_{alv}(z')$, per acinar generation z' directly from stereological methods taking the complexity of the alveolar surface into account. Consequently, our model does not provide the genuine lung or acinus volume for a given surface, because we model the alveoli as truncated spheres, which are not space filling geometries, and because the real lung surface does not consist of the straightforward sum of surfaces obtained from alveolar sphere segments. Since we rely on $S_{alv}(z')$ to calculate the number of alveoli, $n_a^{gen}(z')$, per acinar generation z', this consequently influences the total acinar volume calculated which is hence too large. In contrast to a real lung, we are dealing in our model with smooth surfaces. In particular, each alveolus has a defined radius, $r_a(z')$, and a corresponding volume, $V_a(z')$, and surface $S_a(z')$. In reality, the real surface area allocated to a single alveolus is perhaps much larger due to space-filling properties, and the fact that alveoli exhibit inter-alveolar septum, as described earlier in section 2.2. The difference between space-filling alveoli and our spherical alveoli can be pointed out by defining a factor κ which describes the ratio of acinar volume to surface, reduced to one alveolus. Therefore, taking n as the total number of alveoli in the acinus:

$$\left(\frac{V_{alveoli}^{total}}{n}\right)^{1/3} = \kappa \left(\frac{S_{alveoli}^{total}}{n}\right)^{1/2} \Longleftrightarrow \kappa = \frac{\left(V_{alveoli}^{total}\right)^{1/3}}{\left(S_{alveoli}^{total}\right)^{1/2}} n^{1/6}. \tag{5.21}$$

According to Table 5.4, $V_{alveoli}^{total}$ is given by:

$$V_{alveoli}^{total} = V_{acinus} - V_{duct}^{total} = V_{acinus} - \sum_{z'} (A_d(z')l_d(z')), \tag{5.22}$$

which yields $V_{alveoli}^{total} = 78.985$ mm^3 for Weibel's model. From Eq. (5.21), $\kappa_{Weibel} = 0.342$. In the present model, $V_{alveoli}^{total}$ is obtained as follows:

$$V_{alveoli}^{total} = \sum_{z'} (n_a^{gen}(z')V_a(z')), \tag{5.23}$$

which yields $V_{alveoli}^{total} = 258.78$ mm^3, such that $\kappa_{model} = 0.5$. The incompatibility between the values obtained for κ_{Weibel} and κ_{model} is illustrated by calculating the corresponding half-opening angle, α, needed such that $\kappa_{model} = \kappa_{Weibel} = 0.342$:

$$\kappa_{model} = \frac{{V_a}^{1/3}}{{S_a}^{1/3}} = 0.342 \Longleftrightarrow \alpha \approx 163.47^o. \tag{5.24}$$

It is easy to realize that a half-opening angle of approximately 160° does not make any physical sense. This strongly suggests that our simple alveolated duct model (e.g. Fig 5.2) is fundamentally wrong from a "macroscopic" point of view (i.e. looking at the entire acinus). In particular, it seems in principle unfeasible to fit both simultaneously the acinar volume, V_{acinus}, and the acinar surface, S_{acinus}, to the chosen alveolated duct geometry. However, we are specifically interested in investigating flow phenomena inside alveolar cavities, and alveolar radii used in our models have similar dimensions (see Table 5.2) to those measured in morphometrical studies [90, 281].

5.5 Acinar Volume Flow Rates

Due to the expansion and contraction of the entire pulmonary acinus (i.e. alveoli and ducts), a volume flow rate of air is sucked into and back out of the lungs. In our computational model of a simple alveolated duct, we must derive an expression for the volume flow rate that is sucked into an alveolus and into a duct.

The volume of an alveolus at any acinar generation z' is given in Eq. (5.11). Therefore, the alveolar volume flow rate, $\dot{Q}_a$, may be obtained as follows:

$$\begin{aligned} \dot{Q}_a &= \frac{dV_a}{dt} = \frac{d}{dt}\left(\frac{\pi}{3}{r_a}^3(t)\right) \\ \dot{Q}_a &= \frac{9\pi^2}{4}\frac{\beta}{2}f{r_a}^3\left(1+\frac{\beta}{2}+\frac{\beta}{2}\sin\left(2\pi ft-\frac{\pi}{2}\right)\right)^2\cos\left(2\pi ft-\frac{\pi}{2}\right), \end{aligned} \tag{5.25}$$

where r_a corresponds specifically to the alveolus radius at functional residual cavity (FRC). We can also calculate the volume of air, Q_a, sucked into the alveolus during an inhalation phase, from $t=0$ to $t=T/2$:

$$Q_a = \int_0^{T/2}\dot{Q}_a(t)dt = \frac{9\pi^2}{4}{r_a}^3\beta(\beta^2+3\beta+3) = V_aC, \tag{5.26}$$

where C was defined earlier as the specific volume excursion in Eq. (5.1) and V_a is given in Eq. (5.11). This result is not surprising since V_a is the minimal value for the alveolar volume and the above equation states that the inhaled volume inside an alveolus over a complete inhalation phase is simply the difference between V_{max} and V_{min}, with $V_a = V_{min}$.

Similarly, we compute the volume flow rate, $\dot{Q}_d$, produced by the volume change generated during breathing motion of a single duct. The volume of any duct is simply given by that of a cylinder, namely $V_d = \pi l_d(t){D_d}^2(t)/4$, such that:

$$\begin{aligned} \dot{Q}_d &= \frac{dV_d}{dt} = \frac{\pi}{4}{D_d}^2(t)\frac{dl(t)}{dt} + \frac{\pi}{2}D_d(t)\frac{dD_d(t)}{dt}l(t) \\ \dot{Q}_d &= \frac{3\pi^2}{4}\beta fl{D_d}^2\left(1+\frac{\beta}{2}+\frac{\beta}{2}\sin\left(2\pi ft-\frac{\pi}{2}\right)\right)^2\cos\left(2\pi ft-\frac{\pi}{2}\right). \end{aligned} \tag{5.27}$$

The volume, Q_d, sucked into the duct due to its expansion during an inhalation phase is given by:

$$Q_d = \int_0^{T/2}\dot{Q}_d(t)dt = \frac{\pi}{4}l{D_d}^2\beta(\beta^2+3\beta+3) = V_dC, \tag{5.28}$$

which is similar to the result obtained earlier in Eq. (5.26). Note that here the length l corresponds to the length of a single, isolated, acinar duct given at generation z'. We will now extend our analysis to consider the "real" volume flow rates which may exist in an acinar duct at any given generation z'. Indeed, at any generation z', a duct must supply all the distal daughter branches including their alveoli. This is schematically illustrated in Fig. 5.3 and termed "subacinus", which includes the entire sub-acinar volume (made up of airway ducts and alveoli) distal to an acinar duct considered at generation z'.

We define $\dot{Q}_T$ as the total volume flow rate at generation z'. This is formally written as:

$$\dot{Q}_T = \dot{Q}_{d,eq} + \eta \dot{Q}_A, \tag{5.29}$$

where $\dot{Q}_{d,eq}$ is given by Eq. (5.27) by replacing the single duct length l by l_{eq}. The length, l_{eq}, corresponds to the length of an equivalent duct of diameter $D_d(z')$ which has the same volume as the sub-acinar volume distal to a duct at generation z', without accounting for the alveolar volume. Namely, the equivalent duct of volume $V_{d,eq} = D_d l_{eq}$ distal to generation z' includes solely contributions from ductal airways distal to the generation considered (see schematic in Fig. 5.3). Hence, $\dot{Q}_{d,eq} = dV_{d,eq}/dt$ expresses the volume flow rate through a duct at generation, z', feeding the corresponding subacinus, considering only ductal volume contributions. Here $\dot{Q}_A$ defines the alveolar flow rate derived using an alveolar radius $r_A(z')$, such that the correct total acinar volume (93.5 mm^3 [90]) is matched. This differs slightly from $\dot{Q}_a$ (and correspondingly r_a) which is based on matching the correct alveolar surface S_{ac} given in Table 5.4. Indeed, in the present model, the derivation of ductal volume flow rates is based on matching the correct acinar volumes to replicate macroscopic phenomena, while the individual alveolar geometries follow from matching the correct alveolar surface areas. Note however that $r_a(z')$ and $r_A(z')$ have, nevertheless, similar values (compare Tables 5.2 and 5.6).

The expression $\eta(z')$ in Eq. (5.29) corresponds to the number of alveoli in the subacinus distal to generation z' and is derived from the total number of alveoli per generation, $n_a^{gen}(z')$, in Eq. (5.17). Looking at

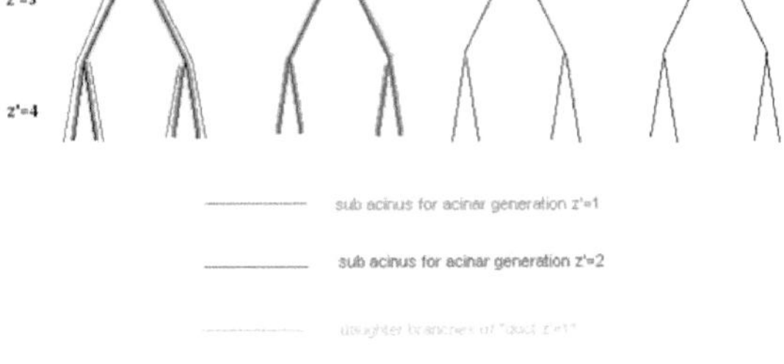

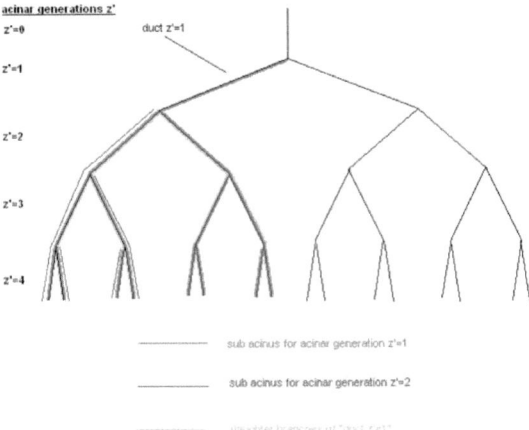

Figure 5.3: Illustration of the subacinus for different acinar generations considered.

Fig. 5.3, this expression yields:

$$\eta(z') = \frac{1}{2^{z'}} \sum_{i=z'}^{8} n_a^{gen}(i). \tag{5.30}$$

Values for $\eta(z')$ are illustrated in Table 5.6. In particular at $z' = 0$, η has to be equal to the total number of alveoli in the acinus (i.e. 9'086) since the subacinus at generation $z' = 0$ is the acinus itself. We may derive from Eq. (5.29) expressions for $\dot{Q}_d, eq$ and $\dot{Q}_A$, such that:

$$\dot{Q}_d, eq = \frac{3\pi^2}{4} \beta f l_{eq} {D_d}^2 \left(1 + \frac{\beta}{2} + \frac{\beta}{2} \sin\left(2\pi f t - \frac{\pi}{2}\right)\right)^2 \cos\left(2\pi f t - \frac{\pi}{2}\right), \tag{5.31}$$

$$\dot{Q}_A = \frac{9\pi^2}{4} \frac{\beta}{2} f {r_A}^3 \left(1 + \frac{\beta}{2} + \frac{\beta}{2} \sin\left(2\pi f t - \frac{\pi}{2}\right)\right)^2 \cos\left(2\pi f t - \frac{\pi}{2}\right), \tag{5.32}$$

which are similar to expressions obtained in Eqs. (5.27) and (5.25), respectively. Following Eqs. (5.26) and (5.28), we may define the subacinar volume, $V_{subacinus}(z')$, at any generation z', such that $Q_T(z') = V_{subacinus}(z')C$, where $Q_T(z')$ is the subacinar volume inhaled over an inhalation phase. Using results from Eqs. (5.29)–(5.32), the subacinar volume is analytically given as:

$$V_{subacinus}(z') = \frac{\pi}{4} l_{eq}(z') {D_d}^2(z') + \frac{9\pi}{8} \sum_{i=z'}^{8} \left(2^{i-z'} n_a^{gen}(i) {r_A}^3(i)\right), \tag{5.33}$$

where $l_{eq}(z')$ and $R_A(z')$ will be determined shortly.

We first derive an analytical expression from $\dot{Q}_T$ for the airflow velocity, $U(z', t)$, across a duct. Here, the velocity, $U(z', t)$, is assumed to have a bulk flow like profile such that:

$$U(z', t) = \frac{\dot{Q}_T}{\frac{\pi}{4} {D_d}^2} = U_{max}(z') \sin(2\pi f t), \tag{5.34}$$

$$U_{max}(z') = \frac{V_{subacinus}(z')}{{D_d}^2/4} \beta f. \tag{5.35}$$

For a sinusoidal wave form velocity, the root-mean square (RMS) velocity may be more appropriate, where $U_{rms}(z') = \sqrt{2}/2 U_{max}(z')$. In particular, $U(z', t) = U_{rms}(z')$ at time $t = T/8$. Hence, we define an RMS Reynolds number:

$$Re_{rms} = \frac{U_{rms} D_{d,rms}}{\nu_{air}}, \tag{5.36}$$

where ν_{air} is the kinematic viscosity of air and $D_{d,rms} = D_d(z', t = T/8) = D_d \left(1 + \frac{2-\sqrt{2}}{4}\beta\right)$.

Table 5.6: Derived values for the subacinar model. See text for details (section 5.6).

z'	0	1	2	3	4	5	6	7	8
$\eta(z')$	90862	4522	2227	1068	513	240	109	45	15
$l_{eq}(z')$ [mm]	117.35	58.12	29.71	21.62	11.57	6.08	3.10	1.53	0.56
$r_A(z')$ [mm]	0.172	0.143	0.122	0.128	0.132	0.135	0.137	0.140	0.133
$V_{subacinus}(z')$ [mm^3]	93.50	46.32	22.74	11.09	5.33	2.51	1.14	0.47	0.15

5.6 Subacinar Volume

To quantify $\dot{Q}_T$ and $U(z',t)$, the subacinar volume, $V_{subacinus}$, as well as $l_{eq}(z')$ and $r_A(z')$ must be determined. The subacinar volume is composed of the ductal volume of the subacinus considered and the volume of the alveoli located along the ducts. For modelling purposes, we construct an equivalent duct of diameter $D_d(z')$ and length $l_{eq}(z')$ which has the same volume as the subacinus considered at generation z'. Looking again at Fig. 5.3, one may derive an expression for $l_eq(z')$, such that:

$$\frac{\pi}{4}D_d(z')l_{eq}(z') = \sum_{i=z'}^{8}\left(2^{i-z'}\frac{\pi}{4}D_d(i)l(i)\right) \Longleftrightarrow l_{eq}(z') = \frac{1}{D_d(z')}\sum_{i=z'}^{8}\left(2^{i-z'}D_d(i)l(i)\right). \tag{5.37}$$

Values for $l_eq(z')$ are given in Table 5.6. To calculate now the alveolar radius $r_A(z')$, based on the total acinar volume (see section 5.5), we impose that the total acinar volume be $V_{acinus} = 93.5$ mm^3, following Haefeli-Bleuer & Weibel [90]. The total ductal volume is $V_{d,acinus} = 14.515$ mm^3 (from summing $V_d(z')$ in Table 5.4) and the ratio of alveolar volume to ductal volume is defined as:

$$\epsilon_{ac} = \frac{V_{acinus}}{V_{d,acinus}} \approx 5.44. \tag{5.38}$$

We make the assumption that the ratio ϵ_{ac} applies not only over the entire acinus but applies also at each generation z'. Clearly, this assumption is somewhat daring because it is unlikely that the ratio of alveolar volume to ductal volume in the acinus remains constant at all acinar generations z'. Nevertheless, this approach will guarantee that the entire acinar volume $V_{acinus} = 93.5$ mm^3 is maintained and a straightforward relationship may be obtained for $r_A(z')$. The number of alveoli per duct is given by $n_a^{duct}(z') = 2^{-z'}n_a^{gen}(z')$ (see Table 5.4). Therefore we may determine $r_A(z')$ by solving the following equation:

$$2^{-z'}n_a^{gen}(z')\frac{9\pi}{8}r_A(z') = \epsilon_{ac}\frac{\pi}{4}{D_d}^2(z')l(z'), \tag{5.39}$$

such that:

$$r_A(z') = \left(\frac{2^{z'+1}\epsilon_{ac}{D_d}^2(z')l(z')}{9n_a^{gen}(z')}\right)^{1/3}. \tag{5.40}$$

Values for $r_A(z')$ are given in Table 5.6 and the subacinar volume, $V_{subacinus}(z')$, is determined from Eq. (5.33) in combination with values obtained from $l_{eq}(z')$ (Table 5.6). Figure 5.4(a) illustrates a plot of the resulting subacinar volume, $V_{subacinus}(z')$, as a function of acinar generation z'.

5.7 Numerical Methods

Assuming laminar, incompressible airflow in the acinar airways [47], the governing equations are the incompressible, unsteady Navier-Stokes equations expressed as (see section 3.2 and Eqs. (3.1) and (3.2)):

$$\nabla \cdot \underline{u} = 0, \tag{5.41}$$

$$\rho\left(\frac{\partial \underline{u}}{\partial t} + \underline{u}\cdot\nabla\underline{u}\right) = -\nabla p + \mu\nabla^2\underline{u}, \tag{5.42}$$

To obtain the time-dependent flow fields in the alveolated duct during rhythmic motion, the conservation equations of mass, Eq. (5.41), and momentum, Eq. (5.42), are solved numerically on a moving grid using

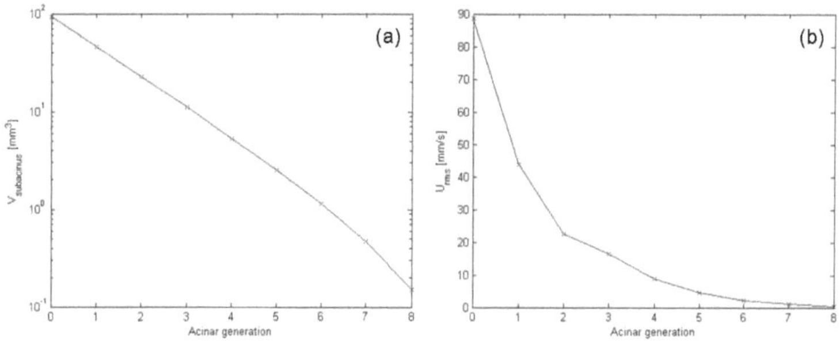

Figure 5.4: (a) Logarithmic plot of subacinar volume, $V_{subacinus}$, as a function of acinar generation z'. (b) RMS airflow velocity, U_{rms}, for the simple alveolated duct model.

a commercial finite-volume based program with fully implicit time marching techniques under isothermal conditions (CFX 5.7-1, ANSYS, INC. Canonsburg, PA, USA). Mesh displacement is achieved by implementing the displacement function described in Eq. (5.5) for each length scale of the geometrical model. The fluid flow equations are discretized with respect to the computational space coordinates with the implementation of the appropriate boundary conditions. All variables, including velocity components and pressure, are located at the centroids of the control volumes. The no-slip condition was invoked along the duct and alveolar walls such that in the case of moving walls, the fluid matched the wall velocity at the fluid-wall interface. Volume elements consisting of prisms are employed along the duct and alveolus walls to obtain an accurately fitted grid and to improve resolution of the flow at the wall for rhythmic breathing motion (see Fig. 5.2). Additionally, simulations were performed to ensure that the flow solutions are grid independent and converged, by performing a mesh refinement study and increasing the number of volume elements by 30% above that which was eventually used. For each simple alveolated duct at generation z', an unstructured mesh was generated using a hybrid mesh made of prisms, tetra- and hexahedron volume elements. Particular care was taken to accurately mesh the alveolar region to yield an accurate description of the flows fields near and inside an alveolus. For proximal generations of the acinus (generation 1–3), typical grids comprised of approximately 150'000 volume elements, while for distal acinar generations, grids consisted of 50'000 to 80'000 control volumes. To achieve sufficiently accurate results such that changes in resulting ductal flow Reynolds numbers, Re, were within $< 5\%$ upon further time step refinement, a time step of $\Delta t = T/200$ was eventually implemented.

The distal boundary at the duct outlet was defined as a surface of constant pressure, whose value was arbitrarily set to 1 bar. The velocity profile on the distal boundary was laminar parabolic. To simulate oscillatory breathing flows in the acinar airways, the proximal boundary condition was defined at the duct inlet by specifying a sinusoidal time-dependent volume flow rate ($\dot{Q}_T$ from Eq. (5.29)) and correspondingly a time-dependent ductal velocity ($U(z't)$ from Eq. (5.34)) in the physiologically relevant range to achieve hydrodynamic similarity, by matching Reynolds, (RMS) Re, and (RMS) Womersley, Wo, numbers in the model to those in the pulmonary acinus (see section 5.8.1). In particular, breathing conditions are replicated to model sedentary tidal breathing of an average human adult such that $T = 3$ s, $C \approx 16.7\%$ and $\beta \approx 5.3\%$ (see Table 5.1). Under the flow conditions tested presently, $Re_{max} \approx 3$, where Re_{max} is the maximum Reynolds number which occurred at peak inspiration and expiration in acinar generation $z' = 0$. For such flow conditions, the effects of the velocity profile on the alveolar flow are expected to be negligible since the length of the circular channels on both sides of the model alveolus are much greater than the entrance length, L_e, to yield a fully developed flow. Indeed, for low-Reynolds number flows in ducts [235], the correlation:

$$\frac{L_e}{D_d} \approx \frac{0.6}{1 + 0.035Re} + 0.056Re \tag{5.43}$$

may be used (compare with Eq. (3.17)). It then takes approximately 0.6 diameters for a non-inertial creeping flow to change from a uniform into a parabolic profile. Similarly for channel flows in the range $0.01 \leq Re \leq 5$, such as in microfluidic devices, the entrance length is approximately given by $L_e/D_d \approx 0.5$ [85, 213]. Therefore, the entrance length in an alveolar duct is expected to be smaller than the duct diameter and the influence of velocity profiles on the alveolar flow may be disregarded. These results are further confirmed from the magnitude and profile of the flow field at the duct entrance obtained from our simulations (see Fig. 5.8(a)).

To check and validate the computational methods presently used, several cases of relevant alveolar flows were computed and compared with numerical solutions available in the literature. As an initial validation, we computed the flow patterns without wall displacement (results are shown in section 5.8.2). The two-dimensional cross-sections of the flow patterns we obtained are in good agreement with previous results obtained for two-dimensional alveolar flows without wall motion (see Fig. 2 in [270] and Fig. 4 in [267]) as well as with streamline patterns obtained for flows inside spherical cavities, induced by a shear flow passing over their opening (see Fig. 4 in [195]). In a second step, we computed the flow patterns associated with alveolar and ductal wall displacement (see section 5.8.3). Cross-sections of the three-dimensional flow patterns we obtained compare very well with results obtained from recent studies on two-dimensional alveolar flow patterns [97, 270]. Hence, results obtained using our geometrical model for both static wall and wall displacement boundary conditions appear to confirm the validity of our computational scheme.

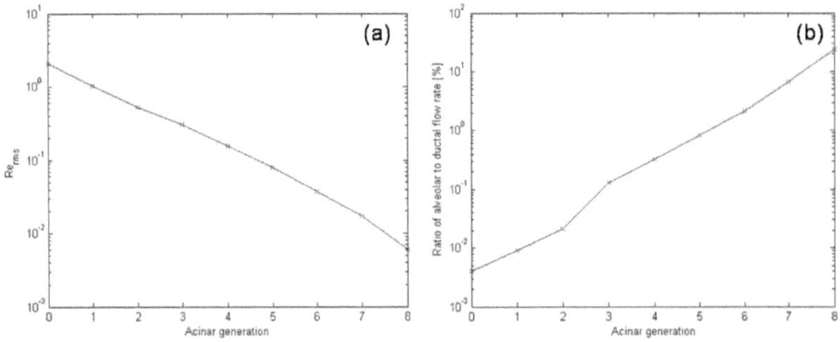

Figure 5.5: (a) Reynolds number as a function of acinar generation for the simple alveolated duct model. (b) Corresponding values of the ratio of alveolar to ductal flow ratio $\dot{Q}_a/\dot{Q}_T$.

5.8 Results and Discussion

5.8.1 Governing Parameters

The acinar flows may be characterized at each generation z' using dimensionless parameters including the ductal flow Reynolds number, Re, the Womersley number, Wo, which for oscillatory flows expresses the ratio of unsteady inertial to viscous forces (see Eq. (3.11)). Both non-dimensional parameters defined above are time-dependent due to the rhythmic motion of the model. A more representative result is then given by time averaged values of Reynolds and Womersley numbers with $\overline{U}(z') = 2/T \int_0^{T/2} U(z',t)\,dt$, where $U(z',t)$ is given in Eq. (5.34), and $\overline{D}_d(z') = 1/T \int_0^T D_d(z,t)\,dt$, such that $\overline{Re}(z') = \overline{U}\overline{D}_d/\nu$ and $\overline{Wo}(z') = \overline{D}_d\sqrt{f/\nu}$. Figure 5.5(a) illustrates a plot of $\overline{Re}$ as a function of acinar generation z'. Values of $\overline{Wo}$ range from 0.143 to 0.083 along the acinar generations. Results obtained for both Reynolds and Womersley numbers compare well with reference values noted for human sedentary breathing conditions [187] as well as with values employed in previous two-dimensional alveolar flow simulations [97,270].

As shall be seen in the results which follow, the three-dimensional alveolar flow patterns during cyclic wall motion may be characterized by a dimensionless parameter first introduced by Tsuda *et al.* [267]. This parameter is defined as the ratio of the alveolar, $\dot{Q}_a$ (see Eq. (5.25)), to ductal flow rate, $\dot{Q}_T$ (see Eq. (5.29)), and is analytically defined as:

$$\frac{\dot{Q}_a}{\dot{Q}_T} = \frac{\frac{9\pi^2}{4}\frac{\beta}{2}f{r_a}^3\left(1+\frac{\beta}{2}+\frac{\beta}{2}\sin\left(2\pi f t-\frac{\pi}{2}\right)\right)^2\cos\left(2\pi f t-\frac{\pi}{2}\right)}{\dot{Q}_{d,eq}+\eta\dot{Q}_A}, \tag{5.44}$$

$$= \frac{V_a(z')}{V_{subacinus}(z')}. \tag{5.45}$$

The ratio $\dot{Q}_a/\dot{Q}_T$ is then computed at each generation z' and plotted in Fig. 5.5(b). One may note that the resulting expression for $\dot{Q}_a/\dot{Q}_T$ is purely based on geometrical configuration and independent of parameters relating to breathing kinematics such as β and f. This result may be also understood by looking at the ratio of the alveolar to ductal volume inhaled over a complete inspiration phase expressed as:

$$\frac{\int_0^{T/2}\dot{Q}_a dt}{\int_0^{T/2}\dot{Q}_T dt} = \frac{C\cdot V_a\,|_{t=0}}{C\cdot(V_{d,t}+\eta\cdot V_A)\,|_{t=0}} = \left.\frac{V_a}{V_{subacinus}}\right|_{t=0}. \tag{5.46}$$

The ratio expressed in Eq. (5.46) depends solely on parameters describing the model geometry at $t=0$ and equals the aveolar to ductal flow rate ratio, $\dot{Q}_a/\dot{Q}_T$, when both alveolus and duct expand and contract self-similarly in phase. Otherwise, this observation does not hold true. This result has also been suggested by Haber *et al.* [89]. Therefore, each simple alveolated duct model describing an acinar generation z' is associated with a characteristic value for the ratio, $\dot{Q}_a/\dot{Q}_T$, which increases with generation depth, as seen in Fig. 5.5(b). As a final remark, one may note again that for an alveolar duct made of periodically spaced identical alveoli, similar flow patterns are to be expected within each alveolus of the duct, as $\dot{Q}_a/\dot{Q}_T$ is geometrically defined and remains constant for identical alveoli. Nevertheless, the implications of a multiple-alveolated ducts, which lie beyond the scope of the present investigation, are indeed relevant for aerosol transport and deposition as shown by Henry *et al.* in two-dimensional alveolated ducts [97]. We will consider the effect of multiple-alveolated ducts on particle deposition in the subsequent chapter, using a space-filling model of the pulmonary acinar tree (see chapter 6).

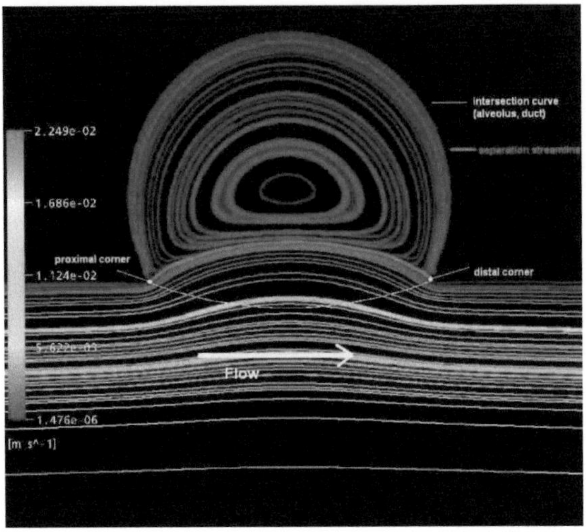

Figure 5.6: Cross-sectional view of alveolus and duct mid-plane, parallel to streamwise flow direction, illustrating streamlines with velocity field magnitude obtained in a rigid-wall ($\dot{Q}_a/\dot{Q}_T = 0$) alveolus of acinar generation $z' = 1$ ($Re = 0.47$). Color bar on left denotes velocity magnitude along streamlines, in [m/s]. The red line illustrates qualitatively the separation between the slow recirculating flow within the alveolus and the more rapid ductal flow. The line spanning from the proximal to distal corner denotes the intersection curve between the alveolus opening ring and the alveolar duct.

5.8.2 Flow Patterns in a Rigid Alveolus

We first present results obtained for the flow patterns in a rigid three-dimensional alveolus ($\dot{Q}_a/\dot{Q}_T = 0$). Although this scenario does not capture the real flow phenomena during rhythmical breathing motion, it is nonetheless essential to understand the influence of the ductal flow on the alveolar flow and subsequently compare static flow phenomenon with wall displacement one. Figure 5.6 presents streamlines with corresponding velocity magnitudes obtained for an alveolus of acinar generation $z' = 1$, where the flow is depicted from left to right at $Re = 0.47$. In the rigid case, convection in the duct induces a shear flow across the alveolus opening, thus generating a recirculation region filling the entire alveolar cavity. For illustration purpose and a better understanding, we introduce a separation line which connects the proximal and distal corners of the alveolus (see red line depicted in Fig. 5.6). This line qualitatively separates the ductal flow from the recirculating region in the alveolus, thus dividing the flow field into two distinct regions, where no fluid element from the duct crosses into the recirculating region. In reality, the ductal and alveolar regions of the flow may be viewed as separated by a three-dimensional surface rather than a line. Note however that the alveolus deflects a small portion of the ductal flow into its opening but the recirculating region prevents the ductal flow from encountering the alveolar wall. Thus for zero displacement ($\dot{Q}_a/\dot{Q}_T = 0$), convective exchange between the duct and the alveolus is prohibited. While the fluid in the alveolus recirculates very slowly, the fluid in the duct convects relatively quickly downstream, such that $\overline{U}_a/\overline{U} \ll 1$, where $\overline{U}_a = 2/T \int_0^{T/2} \dot{Q}_a/A_a\,dt$, A_a is the cross-sectional alveolus opening area, and $\overline{U} = 2/T \int_0^{T/2} U(z',t)dt$, with $U(z',t)$ given in Eq. (5.34).

The present simulation result is in good agreement with earlier findings obtained for shear flows across rigid spherical cavities, which exhibit creeping flow detachment inside the cavity [195, 260, 267, 270]. In particular, our simulation results (Fig. 5.6) illustrate two interesting qualitative flow features: (i) the recirculation region is essentially symmetrical inside the cavity, and (ii) the detachment zone does not fill entirely the cavity (the separation streamline resides within the alveolus, see Fig. 5.6). Similar experimental observations have been made in low-Reynolds number flows through sinusoidally constricted tubes [132], where, under creeping motion (i.e. $Re \ll 1$), cavity geometries exhibiting a large ratio of the duct radius to cavity opening diameter (i.e. approaching 1) give persistent rise to a detachment zone exhibiting symmetry. In the present simulation, this ratio yields $(D_d(z'=1)/2)/(2r_a(z'=1)\sin\alpha) \approx 1.08$, qualitatively consistent with Leneweit & Auerbach's experiments [132]. Hence, for a rigid alveolus, flow inside the cavity exhibits well defined flow separation and recirculatory motion characteristic of low-Reynolds cavity flows.

5.8.3 Alveolar Flow Patterns under Moving Walls

We consider again the alveolated duct of generation $z' = 1$ and implement periodic wall motion ($\dot{Q}_a/\dot{Q}_T = 0.009\%$). Figure 5.7 illustrates the resulting streamlines obtained at peak expiration for $Re = 1.46$. Al-

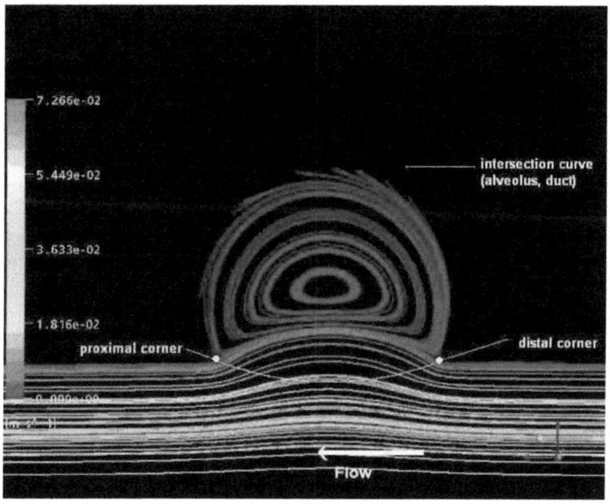

Figure 5.7: Cross-sectional view of alveolus and duct mid-plane, parallel to streamwise flow direction, illustrating streamlines with velocity field magnitude obtained at peak expiration at acinar generation $z' = 1$ ($Re = 1.46$, $\dot{Q}_a/\dot{Q}_T = 0.009\%$). Color bar on left denotes velocity magnitude along streamlines, in [m/s]. The line spanning from the proximal to distal corner denotes the intersection curve between the alveolus opening ring and the alveolar duct.

though the ratio of the two flow rates remains almost negligible, the alveolar flow topology is nevertheless now fundamentally different from the rigid-wall case (compare resulting alveolar flow topology at the alveolar wall in Figs. 5.6 and 5.7). The shear flow arising from the duct continues to dominate largely alveolar flow phenomena and one observes, similarly to the rigid wall case, a large recirculation region inside the alveolus. However, the rhythmic wall motion induces a new effect. As seen in Fig. 5.7 during wall contraction, a small portion of the flow now originates from and travels along the alveolar walls before entering the duct from the proximal side of the alveolar opening. Earlier two-dimensional simulations have shown that flow patterns at expiration are nearly identical to those at inspiration but in the opposite direction [270]. Wall expansion creates a radial flow originating from the proximal corner of the alveolus, which wraps around the recirculating region, and is directed towards the alveolar wall. Thus, the fundamental difference compared to the rigid alveolus case is that net convective transport from the duct into the alveolus now exists for $\dot{Q}_a/\dot{Q}_T > 0$. Fluid particles travel during inspiration from the duct into the alveolus along its wall and back from the alveolar wall into the duct during expiration. Although convective exchange now occurs between the duct and the alveolus, the velocity of the flow entering the alveolus remains very small relative to the flow in the duct such that $\overline{U}_a/\overline{U} = 0.04\%$.

As mentioned earlier, the ratio $\dot{Q}_a/\dot{Q}_T$ is entirely determined by geometrical parameters (see Eqs. (5.44) and (5.46)) and increases with acinar generation z' (see Fig. 5.5). For an alveolus located deeper in the acinar tree, the relative importance of wall induced radial flow to recirculating flow increases with larger $\dot{Q}_a/\dot{Q}_T$. Figure 5.8 illustrates alveolar streamlines with corresponding velocity magnitudes obtained at generation $z' = 5$ ($\dot{Q}_a/\dot{Q}_d = 0.819\%$), at peak inspiration ($Re = 0.112$). A larger portion of the flow is now radially flowing from the alveolar wall to the proximal corner of the alveolus. Note that the recirculating region has not only diminished in size but has also shifted to the proximal corner of the alveolus. Figure 5.9 illustrates the instantaneous flow patterns obtained during expansion and contraction over a breathing cycle at generation $z' = 5$. The resulting flow patterns remain essentially unchanged throughout a breathing cycle, regardless of the instantaneous Re number, with the recirculation region remaining on the proximal side of the alveolus. Such findings are in agreement with results obtained by Tsuda *et al.* for 2D simulations [270]. Although, intuitively one could perhaps expect that during exhalation the flow patterns inside the alveolus be "flipped" such that the recirculating region were to be located on the distal side of geometry, one must realize that during exhalation alveolar walls are contracting rather than expanding. Hence, during exhalation, the direction of the flow is reversed such that the flow is qualitatively "unwrapping."

One should note that although an increased portion of the ductal shear flow is deflected into the alveolar opening, alveolar and ductal flows remain largely isolated from each other (see Fig. 5.8(a)). Convective transport arises from the proximal corner and largely fills the alveolar space but the entire flow in the cavity remains very slow such that $\overline{U}_a/\overline{U} = 0.689\%$. Furthermore, the presence of the alveolus, which deflects a portion of the flow into its space, reduces locally the velocity of the flow in the region of the duct lying beneath it. Looking at Fig. 5.8(b), the recirculating region exhibits a complex flow structure specific to the three-dimensional nature of the problem. The recirculation zone in the cavity is formed by two characteristic flow structures which appear to be slightly twisted and symmetrical with respect to the plane cutting through the alveolar mid-plane along the streamwise flow direction. These results confirm earlier findings for 3D alveolar flow simulations [89] and suggest that in order to describe accurately alveolar flow patterns, one cannot neglect the three-dimensional nature of the real geometry.

For the simple alveolated duct models investigated here, the transition to alveolar flow phenomena entirely dominated by radial flows was found to occur at generation $z' = 6$, where $\dot{Q}_a/\dot{Q}_T = 2.14\%$. Under

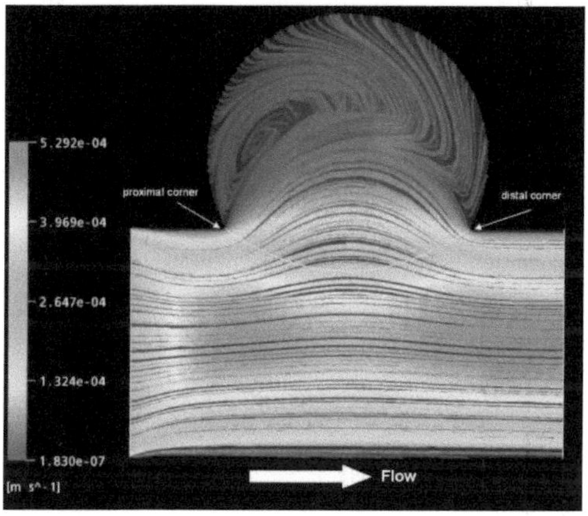

(a)

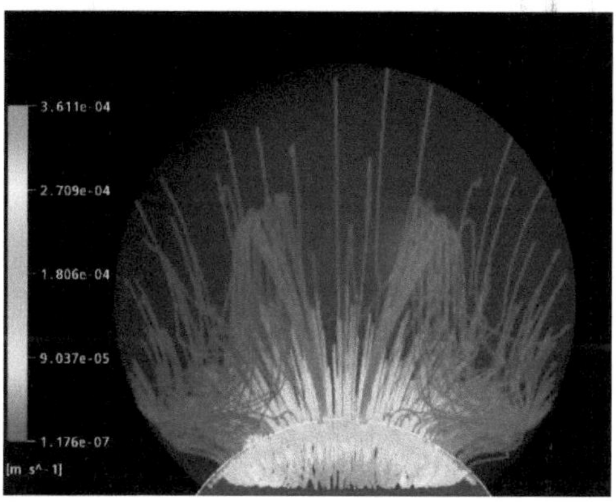

(b)

Figure 5.8: Illustration of instantaneous alveolar streamlines with velocity field magnitude obtained at peak inspiration at acinar generation $z' = 5$ ($Re = 0.112$, $\dot{Q}_a/\dot{Q}_T = 0.82\%$). Color bar on left denotes velocity magnitude along streamlines, in [m/s]. (a) Cross-sectional view of alveolus and duct mid-plane in streamwise flow direction: note the slower recirculating flow within the alveolus compared to that flowing through the duct; the line spanning from the proximal to distal corner denotes the intersection curve between the alveolus opening ring and the alveolar duct. (b) Projection of streamlines with corresponding velocity magnitude in 3D space onto cross-sectional view of alveolus in spanwise direction.

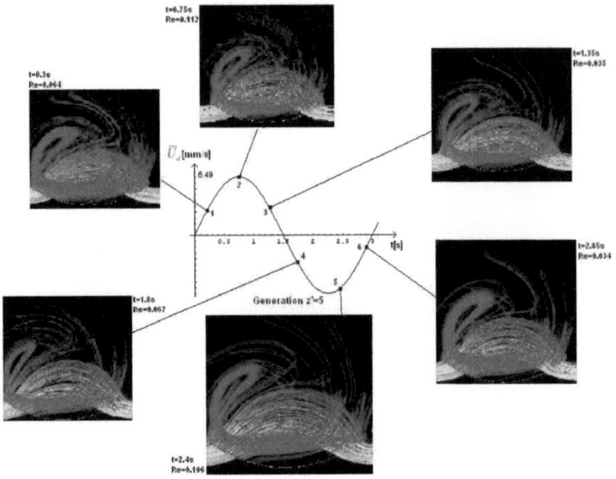

Figure 5.9: Recirculation streamlines within alveolus, obtained from the projection in 3D space onto alveolus mid-plane in streamwise flow direction, and illustrating different instantaneous breathing times, over a complete breathing cycle at generation $z' = 5$ ($\dot{Q}_a/\dot{Q}_T = 0.82\%$). Each subfigure is annotated with the instantaneous breathing time (in [s]) and the ductal Reynolds number, Re. Note that the location of the recirculation region remains essentially unchanged over the entire cycle along the proximal side of the alveolus. Resulting streamlines compare well with instantaneous alveolar flow patterns obtained in previous 2D simulations (Fig. 6 in [270]).

moving wall boundary conditions for geometrical configurations with $\dot{Q}_a/\dot{Q}_T > 2.14\%$, the alveolar flow is then purely radial as illustrated in Fig. 5.10 in the last acinar generation, $z' = 8$ ($\dot{Q}_a/\dot{Q}_T = 24.25\%$), but the flow continues to enter and exit through the proximal side of the alveolus, similar to our observation in more proximal acinar generations. Once wall motion comes to dominate flow phenomena within an alveolus relative to the induced shear flow across the alveolar opening, it is precisely the alveolar wall velocity that sets the scale of the fluid velocities inside the alveolus, following the no-slip condition. A scale of the radial wall velocity may then be given by taking directly the derivative of Eq. (5.5) with respect to time, t, where a suitable length scale corresponds to the initial radius of the alveolus, r_a, at $t = 0$, such that $u_w = r_a f \beta \pi \cdot \cos(2\pi f t - \pi/2)$. Although the geometrical ratio, $\dot{Q}_a/\dot{Q}_T$, largely dominates alveolar flow phenomena and dictates the resulting alveolar flow patterns based on acinar generation depth, it may be foreseen that for sufficiently large physiological breathing parameters f and β, the radial wall velocity, u_w, will be large enough such that alveolar velocity scales are effectively dominated by radial flows and therefore independent of acinar generation depth.

Past generation $z' = 6$, the radial flows now fill entirely the alveolus such that convection effectively transports flow from the duct to the alveolar wall. Nevertheless, the alveolar velocity field remains much slower than that in the duct with $\overline{U}_a/\overline{U} = 9.09\%$. One may note that the ratio, $\overline{U}_a/\overline{U}$, increases with generation similarly to $\dot{Q}_a/\dot{Q}_T$, keeping in mind that the ductal flow rate, $\dot{Q}_d$, is strongly decelerated at each deeper generation as a consequence of applying mass conservation at each bifurcating airway. In summary, for the present tidal breathing simulations, alveolar flow patterns are predominantly governed by the ratio, $\dot{Q}_a/\dot{Q}_T$, a geometrically defined quantity. Physiologically, this result implies that alveolar flow patterns are uniquely determined by the location of an alveolus along the acinar tree, while the magnitude of the flow velocities is, however, dependent on the breathing conditions, β and f. It is suspected that local differences in alveolar flow topologies along the acinar tree may influence the local kinematics and deposition of inhaled aerosol particles as suggested in previous simulations [89, 97]. Moreover, under the breathing conditions tested here, alveolar flow patterns remain at all acinar generations essentially time-independent, which results from the low Womersley numbers, $Wo < 1$, implying quasi-steady flow conditions.

5.9 Conclusions

We have simulated three-dimensional low Reynolds number alveolar flows at each generation of the human pulmonary acinus, using moving wall boundary conditions to replicate lung expansion and contraction during sedentary tidal breathing. Alveolar flows may be highly complex, with flow structures pertinent to the three-dimensional nature of the problem and driven by the inherent motion of the walls during rhythmical breathing. However, velocity magnitudes within alveoli remain very slow relative to ductal flows travelling through the acinar airways. Alveolar flow patterns are largely time-independent and governed by their geometrical configuration which relates to the location of the alveoli along the acinar tree. For alveoli located in the proximal acinar generations, flows are dominated by recirculation patterns. In the deeper acinar generations, flows become largely radial due to rhythmic wall motion and increasing alveolar dimensions, while the recirculation region gradually decreases in the distal region until it eventually vanishes.

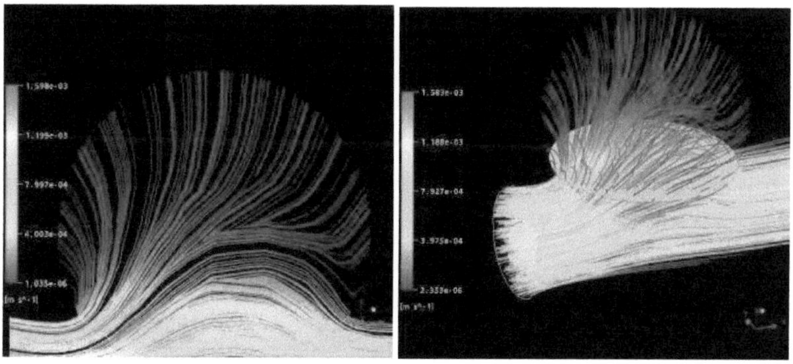

(a) (b)

Figure 5.10: Illustration of instantaneous alveolar streamlines with velocity field magnitude obtained at acinar generation $z' = 8$ during inspiration with $Re = 0.008$ and $\dot{Q}_a/\dot{Q}_T = 24.25\%$. Color bar on left denotes velocity magnitude along streamlines, in [m/s]. (a) Cross-sectional view of alveolar mid-plane in streamwise flow direction (flow is from left to right). (b) Corresponding view of alveolar radial streamlines and ductal streamlines in 3D space.

Chapter 6

Flow Phenomena and Sedimentation in a Space-Filling Pulmonary Acinar Tree

The inhalation of micron-sized aerosols into the lung's acinar region may be recognized as a possible health risk or a therapeutic tool. In an effort to develop a deeper understanding of the mechanisms responsible for acinar deposition, we have numerically simulated the transport of non-diffusing fine inhaled particles (1 and 3 μm in diameter) in two acinar models of varying complexity: (i) a simple alveolated duct (see chapter 5) and (ii) a novel space-filling, asymmetrical acinar branching tree following the description of lung structure by Fung [71]. Detailed particle trajectories and deposition efficiencies, as well as acinar flow structures, were investigated under different orientations of gravity, for tidal breathing motion in an average human adult. Trajectories and deposition efficiencies inside the alveolated duct are strongly related to gravity orientation. While the motion of larger particles (3 μm) is relatively insensitive to convective flows compared to the role of gravitational sedimentation, finer 1 μm aerosols may exhibit, in contrast, complex kinematics influenced by the coupling between (i) flow reversal due to oscillatory breathing, (ii) local alveolar flow structure, (iii) initial location of a particle at injection, and (iv) streamline crossing due to gravity. These combined mechanisms may lead to irreversible twisting and undulating trajectories in the alveolus, over multiple breathing cycles. The extension of our study to a space-filling acinar tree was well suited to investigate the influence of bulk kinematic interaction between ductal flows and alveolar flows on aerosol transport. We found the existence of intricate trajectories of fine 1 μm aerosols spanning over the entire acinar airway network, which cannot be captured by simple alveolar models. In contrast, heavier 3 μm aerosols yield trajectories characteristic of gravitational sedimentation, analogous to those observed in the simple alveolated duct. For both particle sizes, however, particle inhalation yields highly non-uniform deposition. While larger particles deposit within a single inhalation phase, finer 1 μm particles exhibit much longer residence times over multiple breathing cycles. With the on-going development of more realistic models of the pulmonary acinus, we hope to capture some of the complex mechanisms leading to acinar deposition of inhaled aerosols. Such models may lead to a better understanding towards the optimization of pulmonary drug delivery to target specific regions of the lung, such as the acinus.

6.1 Introduction

Under normal circumstances, only small aerosol particles (typically ≤ 5 μm) penetrate into the distal region of the lung (i.e. pulmonary acinus) without being deposited in the nasopharynx or conducting airways [163]. Because these particles are too large to undergo significant Brownian diffusion and too light to be substantially affected by inertia, their fate may be mainly determined by the balance between aerodynamic and gravitational (sedimentation) forces [100]. However, since these particles carry far more mass than sub-micron particles (< 1 μm), aerosols in the micron-size range play an important role in a variety of physiological processes. Carcinogenic materials, coal dust and bacteria amongst other may enter the lung in aerosolized form and cause parenchymal disease as a consequence of environmental and occupational exposure [287]. Alternatively, aerosolized drugs containing bronchodilators, surfactant, or genes are ubiquitous in the treatment of pulmonary diseases such as asthma, chronic obstructive diseases, cystic fibrosis and infant or acute respiratory distress syndrome (RDS) [10, 135, 159, 264]. In particular, for aerosol delivery to infants, findings from in vitro studies using nebulizers recommend the use of fine particles (< 3 μm) for increased lung deposition [115, 225], and breath-holding remains a widely advocated practice to enhance acinar lung deposition of pharmaceutical aerosols by augmenting the time for deposition through sedimentation [59, 66]. Hence, whether the inhalation of aerosols is recognized as a possible health risk or a therapeutic tool, a comprehensive knowledge of deposition mechanisms of inhaled micron-sized particles in the distal regions of the lung is fundamental.

Due to the sub-millimeter dimensions, accessibility and complexity of the pulmonary acinus, alveolar flow characteristics and particle deposition mechanisms remain, however, difficult to assess directly. Thus, the understanding of such flows and their influence on aerosol transport and deposition has been significantly contributed by numerical simulations. Commonly, acinar airways have been modelled using simple alveolated duct structures, such as cylindrical channels mounted with spherical or toroidal cavities, both in two- [47, 97, 268, 270] and three-dimensional [87–89] simulations. In particular, Tsuda *et al.* [268] demonstrated in a two-dimensional (2D) alveolated duct that the geometrical structure of the alveolar duct itself has an important role for gravitational sedimentation, and gravitational cross-streamline motion may depend on the coupled effects of curvature of gas streamlines and duct orientation relative to gravity. More recently, Haber *et al.* [89] showed for a hemispherical alveolus with its opening plane located normal to the gravity field that alveolar wall motion is crucial in determining aerosol deposition inside the alveolus. In addition, fine particles (i.e. 1 μm) are particularly sensitive to the detailed alveolar flow structure (e.g. recirculating flow), as they undergo gravity-induced convective mixing and deposition. Clearly, simple geometric models of the pulmonary acinus have provided insightful knowledge on the complex nature of local alveolar flow structure and its influence on the deposition of inhaled aerosols inside model alveoli. However, computational investigations have generally looked at aerosol kinematics in generic isolated alveolar ducts, or in a single alveolus, rather than in networks of acinar airways forming a multi-generation branching tree, more representative of realistic anatomical properties. Hence, an acinar model capturing these latter features would be particularly well-suited to study bulk kinematic interaction between ductal flows in branching networks and local alveolar flows, and the associated aerosol behavior resulting in such a tree structure during breathing motion. Moreover, existing studies modelling alveolar flows have not accounted for the densely-packed, space-filling nature of the distal regions of the lung [138, 152, 201, 211].

In our previous study (see chapter 5), we investigated convective flow phenomena in three-dimensional (3D) models of simple alveolated duct structures, detailing the nature of alveolar flow topology in relation to acinar generation depth. In an effort to extend our recent contribution and develop more realistic models of the pulmonary acinus to study specifically the transport and deposition of non-diffusing fine particles as well as acinar flow phenomena, we have developed a space-filling, asymmetrical branching model of a sub-acinar region following the original description of lung structure by Fung [71, 72]. Detailed computational fluid dynamics (CFD) simulations, under moving wall boundary conditions mimicking breathing motion, are presented for quiescent tidal breathing in an average human adult. Specifically, settling trajectories and deposition sites of fine inhaled micron-sized particles (1 and 3 μm) are illustrated for different orientations of the acinar tree with respect to gravity, and detailed alveolar flow fields are presented. Findings for the space-filling acinar tree are compared with results obtained concurrently for sedimenting aerosol particles in the recently developed simple alveolated duct geometry (chapter 5). In particular, deposition efficiencies of inhaled particles are measured both in the simple alveolated duct and in the space-filling geometry to investigate the influence of gravity orientation and assess particle residence times inside the acinar airspace prior to wall deposition. With the modularity of the present space-filling acinar model, future investigations may be foreseen including the transport and deposition of diffusing sub-micron particles, the influence of heterogeneous ventilation [2], the role of inter-alveolar communication (i.e. pores of Kohn [12]), or alternatively the influence of modifying the dimensions and structure of the space-filling geometry itself.

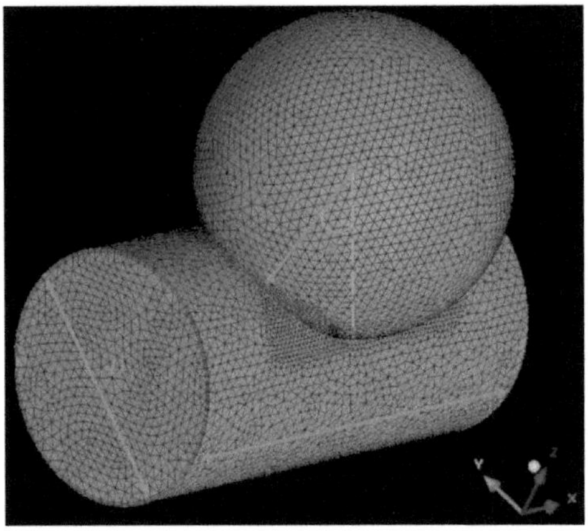

Figure 6.1: Computational mesh of the simple alveolated duct structure at the 5th acinar generation. The alveolus radius is given by r_a, the airway duct diameter and the length are, respectively, D_d and l_d. The alveolus half-opening angle is denoted by α.

6.2 Model Geometry

6.2.1 Simple Alveolated Duct

The alveolated duct follows the description reported in detail in section 5.3. Briefly, the duct is modelled as a cylindrical shell with open ends, defined by a length, $l_d = 0.556$ mm, and a diameter, $D_d = 0.286$ mm. The alveolus itself is modelled by a spherical cap connected to the duct, located at the center of the duct (Fig 6.1). The spherical cap is described by a radius, $r_a = 0.18$ mm, and an opening half angle, $\alpha = 60^o$, defining the arc of the alveolus opening. The angle, α, is assumed time-independent under self-similar breathing motion [97, 270]. Note, however, that all geometrical length scales vary with time due to breathing motion (see section 5.2). The anatomical dimensions of the alveolated duct follow morphometric measurements of the pulmonary acinus [90, 284], such that the alveolated duct corresponds approximately to the 5th generation of the human pulmonary acinar tree. Our choice to study particle sedimentation at this specific acinar generation, rather than at another generation, stems from our recent results (see chapter 5), where complex recirculating alveolar flow structures are encountered at this particular generation. Such flows come in contrast with perhaps more trivial flow topologies encountered in the deeper acinar generations (i.e. alveolar sacs), where alveolar streamlines are found to be purely radial [97, 270]. Hence, as discussed recently by Haber et al. [89], alveoli exhibiting recirculating flows may potentially illustrate the complex coupling of gravitational settling and convective mechanisms responsible for transport and deposition of fine inhaled particles. Thus, the idealized geometrical model of a 5th acinar generation seems suitable to investigate detailed aerosol kinematics due to local alveolar flow structure.

6.2.2 Space-Filling Acinar Tree

Although there exists a history for the representation of alveoli figured as isolated spheres [158], it has been long recognized that, rather, pulmonary alveoli are densely-packed hollow polyhedra sharing common boundary walls (i.e. interalveolar septum) [138, 152, 201, 211], whose shape and structure are comparable to honeycombs [57, 145] or soap foams [281], and where the wall between two adjacent alveoli may be described as flat [254]. Our idealized computational geometry is based on the original description of the acinar ventilatory unit by Fung [71]. This model assumes that all alveoli are equal and space-filling and alveoli are ventilated as uniformly as possible. Of the existing geometries suggested for an alveolus, a suitable choice is the truncated octahedron (or 14-hedron) - a fourteen sided polyhedron with eight hexagonal and six square faces (Fig. 6.2), as first proposed by Dale *et al.* [38]. The main advantages of this alveolar geometry are that it is space-filling, enabling the assemblage of several of such polyhedra to form ducts without leaving any voids. Furthermore, it has the minimum surface area to volume ratio of all space-filling polyhedra, and the most common shapes for alveolar septa found in lung parenchyma are hexagons and rectangles [71]. Previously, the 14-hedron alveolar geometry has been employed in models of the mechanical behavior of lung parenchyma, using finite element methods [38, 51–53]. However, hitherto, this geometry has not yet been implemented for respiratory simulations of alveolar ventilation. In particular, a space-filling acinar branching tree is thought to be suitable to study bulk kinematic interaction between ductal flows and alveolar flows, and the associated aerosol behavior, while the simple alveolus model (see chapter 5) is rather aimed at capturing local alveolar flow structures and resulting aerosol kinematics within the cavity.

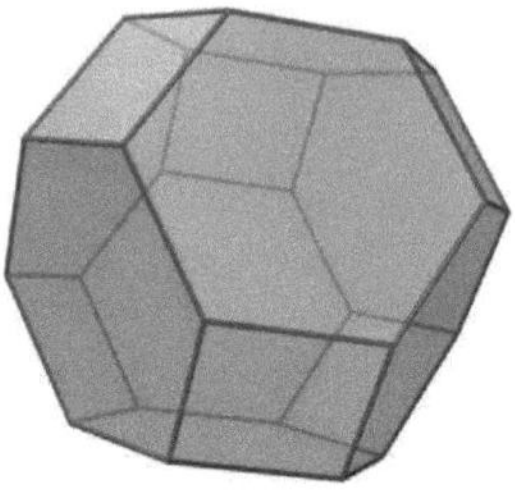

Figure 6.2: Model of a truncated octahedron (14-hedron) alveolus: a 14-sided polyhedron with 8 regular hexagonal faces, 6 regular square faces, 24 vertices and 36 edges.

We briefly describe the assembly of such polyhedra to form a 3D space-filling tree. Further details are given by Fung [71]. Every alveolus of the lung must be ventilated to the atmosphere; hence none can be a closed polyhedron. To vent a polyhedron, one or more of the walls must be removed. A 14-hedron surrounded by 14 identical polyhedra contacting and matching each of its faces will form a solid unit in space that resembles the 14-hedron in shape. Following Fung [71], we call this larger unit a polyhedron of order 2, whereas the original basic unit is termed a polyhedron of order 1. Now if all the walls of the polyhedron of order 1 lying at the center of a polyhedron of order 2 are removed, then all the alveoli surrounding it are ventilated. All remaining units have equal access to the center and the edges of the polyhedron of order 1 at the center become the mouths of the surrounding alveoli. In particular, an order-2 polyhedron can be connected and ventilated to other order-2 polyhedra to form alveolar ducts (Fig. 6.3). Figure 6.4 shows how order-2 polyhedra can be assembled to form a space-filling acinar ductal tree. The structure of the tree so obtained is a 3D version of the schematic acinar model constructed by Fung (Fig. 7B in [71]), which has remarkable resemblance with the anatomical description presented by Hansen *et al.* [93].

The space-filling geometry (Fig. 6.4) models in fact a sub-region of the pulmonary acinus (i.e. acinar airway generations 3–8 are modelled here, while a complete acinus would stretch approximately from generations 0 to 8 [90]). The model is dichotomous but exhibits asymmetry; with some of the acinar branches coming to an abrupt end past airway bifurcations (e.g. gen. 4 and 6, see Fig. 6.4). All alveoli are identical in size, independent of acinar generation. This property differs slightly from actual morphometrical measurements [90,281,284], where alveolar size increases slowly with acinar generation. Since alveolar ducts are modelled here by a series of basic 14-hedra, the length of any duct must be an integral multiple of the alveolar dimension of the 14-hedron. Hansen & Ampaya [92] measured linear regressions for ductal lengths where generations 1, 2, and 3 have approximately a length of 0.56 mm, generations 4 and 5 a length of 0.40 mm, and generations 6, 7, and 8 a length of 0.26 mm. Following Fung [71], we set Λ to 0.14 mm at total lung capacity (TLC) to match Hansen & Ampaya's measurements [92] (the alveolar dimension, Λ, is the hexagon- to hexagon-face distance in a 14-hedron alveolus). Thus, generation 3 has an effective length of $4\Lambda = 0.56$ mm, generations 4 and 5 a length of $3\Lambda = 0.42$ mm, and generations 6 and 7 a length of $2\Lambda = 0.28$ mm. The entire geometry consists of 190 14-hedra elements making up for a total acinar volume of ~ 0.2 mm^3 at functional residual capacity (FRC). Note that our model represents a mere $\sim 0.2\%$ of the average volume of an entire acinus ($\sim$ 187 mm^3) [90]. Finally, as a consequence of the space-filling assumption, generation 8 (i.e. alveolar sac) consists of a single alveolus, and bifurcation

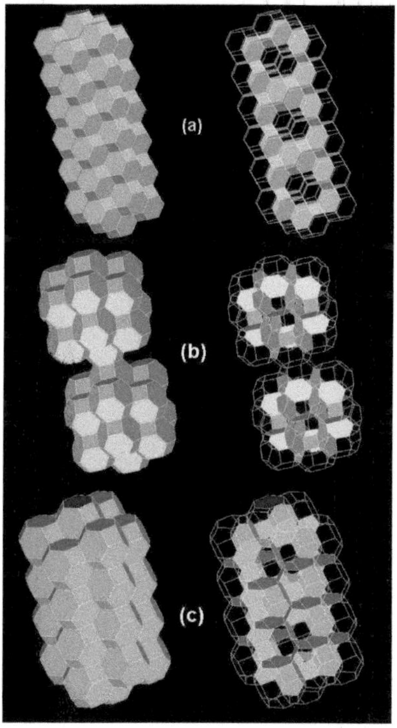

Figure 6.3: Three-dimensional models of alveolar ducts assembled using the order-2 polyhedron with fourteen 14-hedra surrounding 1 central 14-hedron, following Fung [71]. Left column illustrates outer alveolar walls and right column reveals the inner walls. (a) Alveolar duct corresponds to generation 3 of the ductal tree (Fig. 6.4); (b) Two order-2 polyhedra are distinguishable and constitute the ductal models for generations 4 and 5 of the ductal tree; (c) Model corresponds to generations 6 and 7 of the ductal tree.

opening angles between parent and daughter ducts are by definition a multiple of $\approx 70.5^o$.

6.3 Numerical Methods

The numerical methods follow closely that presented earlier in section 5.7. In particular, breathing kinematics are described in detail in section 5.2 where quiet tidal breathing in an average human adult is replicated ($T = 3$ s, $C \approx 16.7\%$ and $\beta \approx 5.3\%$, see Table 5.1).

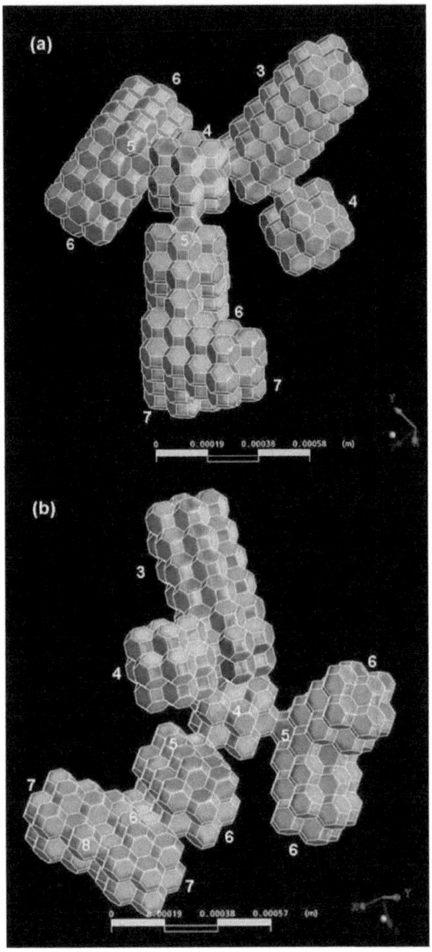

Figure 6.4: Example of assembling order-2 polyhedra into an alveolar ductal tree, following Fig. 7B of Fung [71]. Two three-dimensional views ((a) and (b)) of the same geometry are illustrated here with corresponding acinar airway generation numbers. The entrance inlet for airflow is visible on the proximal side of generation 3 in (a). Scale of model is shown in [m].

6.3.1 Governing Equations of Fluid Motion

In sub-millimeter acinar airspaces, the Mach number (ratio of fluid to sound speed) is very small, and changes in air density caused by molecular diffusion of oxygen and carbon-dioxide across alveolar walls are negligible, such that flow is effectively incompressible [47]. Therefore, the equations of motion (conservation of mass and momentum) of the fluid (i.e. air) are governed by the unsteady, incompressible Navier-Stokes equations (see section 3.2 as well as Eqs. (5.41) and (5.42)):

$$\nabla \cdot \underline{u} = 0, \tag{6.1}$$

$$\rho \left(\frac{\partial \underline{u}}{\partial t} + \underline{u} \cdot \nabla \underline{u} \right) = -\nabla p + \mu \nabla^2 \underline{u}. \tag{6.2}$$

In the above equations, laminar flow conditions are assumed [47]. To obtain the time-dependent flow field, the conservation equations of mass, Eq. (6.1), and momentum, Eq. (6.2), are solved numerically on a moving grid using a commercial finite-volume based program with fully implicit marching techniques under isothermal conditions (CFX-11, Ansys Inc., Canonsburg PA, USA). The fluid flow equations are discretized with respect to the computational space coordinates, and all variables, including velocity components and pressure are located at the centroids of the control volumes. In the present study, respiratory flows are generated from the wall motion induced during rhythmical breathing by implementing the length scale displacement function described in Eq. (5.5) and the appropriate boundary conditions. The no-slip condition is invoked along all acinar walls, such that the air matches the wall velocity at the solid-fluid interface. For the space-filling acinar tree, airflow is entirely induced through wall motion of the geometry such that the boundary at the entrance of the space-filling geometry is defined as a surface of constant pressure, whose value is arbitrarily set to 1 bar. Following our recent study (see chapter 5), the distal boundary of the simple alveolated duct is defined as a surface of constant pressure (1 bar), while the proximal boundary at the duct inlet is defined by specifying a sinusoidal time-dependent mass flow-rate. Under the flow conditions tested for the simple alveolated duct, effects of velocity profile on the alveolar flow may be disregarded since the entrance length to yield fully-developed flow is much smaller than the length of the cylindrical channel on both sides of the alveolus (see section 5.7). For both geometries, hydrodynamic similarity was achieved by matching root mean square (rms) Reynolds, $Re = UD/\nu$ (ratio of inertial to viscous forces), and Womersley numbers, $Wo = D\sqrt{f/\nu}$ (ratio of unsteady inertial forces to viscous forces), to physiologically relevant values, where U is taken as the uniform ductal flow velocity.

An unstructured mesh was generated for the space-filling tree, using a hybrid mesh made of tetra- and hexahedron. Particular care was taken to accurately mesh the alveolar region near walls to yield an accurate description of the flow field near and inside alveoli. Simulations were performed to ensure that flow solutions were grid independent and converged, by performing a mesh refinement study, such that approximately 1.4 million volume elements were eventually used for the space-filling geometry. Similarly, for the simple alveolated duct, a total of approximately 500'000 volume elements were employed. Based on the chosen mesh size for each geometry, transient solutions at any time step, Δt, were ensured such that the (RMS) Courant number, $Co = \Delta t u/\Delta x$, relating the ratio of a time step, Δt, to the cell residence time, $\Delta x/u$, where Δx is the cell element size, yielded consistently $Co < 0.1$, following Ferziger & Peric [64]. To guarantee this condition, a normalized time step in the range $\Delta t/T \approx 1.6 \times 10^{-4}$ to 3.3×10^{-3} was eventually implemented, depending on the computational geometry (i.e. simple alveolus or space-filling tree). Finally, residuals measuring the imbalance on conservation equations were monitored to stay within a specified tolerance value of $\leq 10^{-5}$.

6.3.2 Particle Motion

The differential equation governing the motion of a spherical particle subjected to the gravity field, $\underline{g}$, is given by (see equivalent Eq. (4.1)):

$$m_p \frac{d\underline{u}_p}{dt} = \underline{F}_D + \underline{F}_B, \tag{6.3}$$

where $\underline{u}_p$ is the particle velocity vector, m_p is the particle mass of a sphere and the term on the left-hand side of Eq. (6.3) is a summation of all the forces acting on a particle expressed in terms of the particle acceleration. Note that the equation above is assumed for flows where the particle density is much greater than the fluid density. Furthermore, numerical simulations are "one-way coupled", such that particles are assumed not to influence the continuous-phase flow. Rather, aerosol particles are passively introduced in the fluid [89, 268]. The viscous drag force, $\underline{F}_D$, over the particle surface follows Stokes law:

$$\underline{F}_D = \frac{1}{8}\pi\rho_f {d_p}^2 C_D |\underline{u}_f - \underline{u}_p|(\underline{u}_f - \underline{u}_p), \tag{6.4}$$

where d_p is the particle diameter, and subscripts f and p differentiate between fluid and particle properties, respectively. The drag coefficient, C_D, for flow past a spherical particle is computed from the widely used correlation of Schiller & Neumann [219]:

$$C_d = \frac{24}{Re_p}\left(1 + 0.15{Re_p}^{0.687}\right), \tag{6.5}$$

where Re_p denotes the particle Reynolds number and C_d reduces effectively to $24/Re_p$ for $Re_p \ll 1$ (i.e. Stokes law, see Eq. (4.3) and Appendix B). For a spherical particle, the buoyancy force, $\underline{F}_B$, due to gravity is then:

$$\underline{F}_B = \frac{1}{6}\pi {d_p}^3(\rho_p - \rho_f)\underline{g}. \tag{6.6}$$

Following the analysis of Haber *et al.* [89] for gravitational sedimentation of aerosols in a hemispherical alveolus under oscillatory breathing conditions, Eq. (6.3) may be rewritten in non-dimensional form:

$$\frac{{d_p}^2\rho_p\omega}{18\mu_f}\frac{d^2\underline{x}'_p}{dt'^2} = \frac{{d_p}^2\rho_p g}{9\mu_f D\omega}\underline{g} + \frac{d\underline{x}'_p}{dt'}, \tag{6.7}$$

where $t' = \omega t$ is the dimensionless time and $\underline{x}'_p = \underline{x}_p/R = 2\underline{x}_p/D$ is the dimensionless particle position. The angular breathing frequency is $\omega = 2\pi/T$ and $D = 2R$ represents a characteristic length scale of the acinar geometry (i.e. alveolar dimension). For inhaled pharmaceutical aerosols where $\rho_p \gg \rho_f$ densities of compounds are typically near that of water [66]. Specifically, we are concerned with non-diffusing fine particles in the range 1–3 μm in diameter such that the maximum Stokes number, Stk, which determines the magnitude of the left-hand side term of Eq. (6.7) is (compare with Eq. (4.9)):

$$Stk = \frac{{d_p}^2\rho_p\omega}{18\mu_f} \approx 6\times10^{-5}, \tag{6.8}$$

whereas the gravity number, H, is of the order of:

$$H = \frac{{d_p}^2\rho_p g}{9\mu_f D\omega} \approx 0.1 - 2.5\,. \tag{6.9}$$

Therefore, the role of particle inertial effects leading to impaction is negligible relative to the significance of gravitational sedimentation. Note that following Kojic & Tsuda's notation [121], the gravity number may be expressed as:

$$H = \frac{1}{P_d} = \frac{T}{T_s} = \frac{u_t}{R\omega}, \tag{6.10}$$

where P_d is the particle sedimentation parameter, and H may be interpreted as the ratio between the oscillatory flow time, T (i.e. breathing period), and the characteristic gravitational sedimentation time, $T_s = R/u_t$, where the terminal sedimentation velocity, u_t, was given earlier in Eq. (4.5):

$$u_t = \frac{\rho_p g {d_p}^2}{18\mu_f}. \tag{6.11}$$

Computationally, a bolus of particles, uniformly distributed over the inlet cross-section, is injected at the beginning of the inhalation phase ($t = 0$), between the first and second time step. Particle displacement, $\underline{x}_p$, is calculated using a forward Euler integration scheme of the particle velocity, $\underline{u}_p$, over the time step, Δt, defined as:

$$\underline{x}_p^n = \underline{x}_p^o + \underline{u}_p^o \Delta t, \tag{6.12}$$

where the superscripts o and n refer to old and new values, respectively. During forward integration, the particle velocity calculated at the start of the time step, Δt, is assumed to prevail over the entire time step. At the end of a time step, the new particle velocity, $\underline{u}_p$, is calculated using the analytical solution to Eq. (6.3):

$$\underline{u}_p = \underline{u}_p + (\underline{u}_p^o - \underline{u}_f)e^{\frac{-\Delta t}{\tau}} + \tau \underline{F}_B \left(1 - e^{\frac{-\Delta t}{\tau}}\right), \tag{6.13}$$

where the parameter τ is defined as:

$$\tau = \frac{4 d_p \rho_p}{3 \rho_f C_D} |\underline{u}_f - \underline{u}_p|. \tag{6.14}$$

The validity and accuracy of our computational schemes for particles subject to a gravity field in small acinar airways were verified with a test case for gravitational deposition of particles in horizontal laminar pipe flow (see Appendix D). We open a short parenthesis noting that for a dense bolus (i.e. high number concentrations) introduced in small airways, where $d_p/D \approx 1\%$, particles may indeed influence the continuous-phase flow. Amongst several possible effects, settling velocities, u_t, would be lower than that predicted by Eq. (6.11), as particles travel in each other's wakes (i.e. "hindered settling") [35, 54]. However, such effects remain beyond the scope of the present study and a one-way coupling approach is adopted.

6.4 Results and Discussion

6.4.1 Aerosol Kinematics in the Simple Alveolated Duct

We investigated gravitational sedimentation for three distinctive orientations of the alveolar duct with respect to gravity (cases (i) to (iii) in Fig. 6.5). Simulations were conducted for fine inhaled particles of 1 ($P_d = 4.06$) and 3 μm ($P_d = 0.45$) diameter. A detailed description of the alveolar flow topology at the 5th acinar generation of the pulmonary acinus illustrating a characteristic recirculating flow structure (rms $Re = 0.07$, rms $Wo = 0.1$) was given in section 5.8.3 (see chapter 5) and is illustrated in Fig. 5.8. For low Womersley numbers ($Wo < 1$), resulting flow patterns remain essentially unchanged throughout the breathing cycle (i.e. the recirculation region remains on the proximal side of the alveolus) such that the basic flow characteristics are rather insensitive to global Re effects [97, 270]. For each simulation, a bolus consisting of a total of 1'000 particles was injected uniformly across the duct inlet. Simulations were conducted until particles either deposited on walls or left the computational domain. Results for the deposition efficiency, $n(t)/N$ (as introduced in Appendix D), are illustrated in Fig. 6.5 and depend

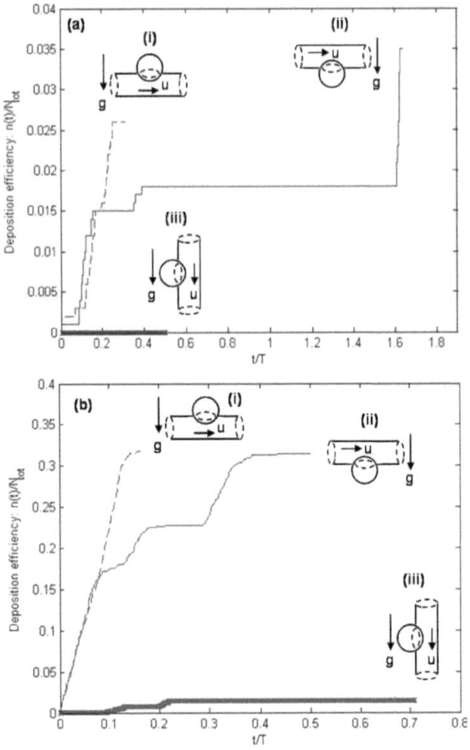

Figure 6.5: Influence of gravity orientation (cases (i)-(iii)) on deposition efficiency, $n(t)/N$, as a function of normalized time, t/T, for (a) 1 and (b) 3 μm diameter particles in the simple alveolated duct model (see section 6.2.1).

strongly on both the particle sedimentation parameter, P_d, and the specific orientation of the alveolated duct with respect to gravity. We detail results obtained for cases (i) through (iii) in what follows.

Gravity Orientation: Case (i)

Case (i) illustrated in Fig. 6.5(a) and (b) corresponds to an alveolus opening facing upwards relative to the gravity orientation. Here the ductal flow orientation is normal to the gravity direction. Particle trajectories and deposition sites are illustrated in Figs. 6.6 and 6.7, respectively for 1 and 3 μm diameter particles. These two cases are qualitatively similar to gravitational sedimentation occurring for laminar horizontal pipe flow (see Appendix D). Indeed, a qualitative inspection of resulting deposition sites reveals that particles settle along the bottom of the duct (Figs.6.6 and 6.7). This may be quantitatively observed in

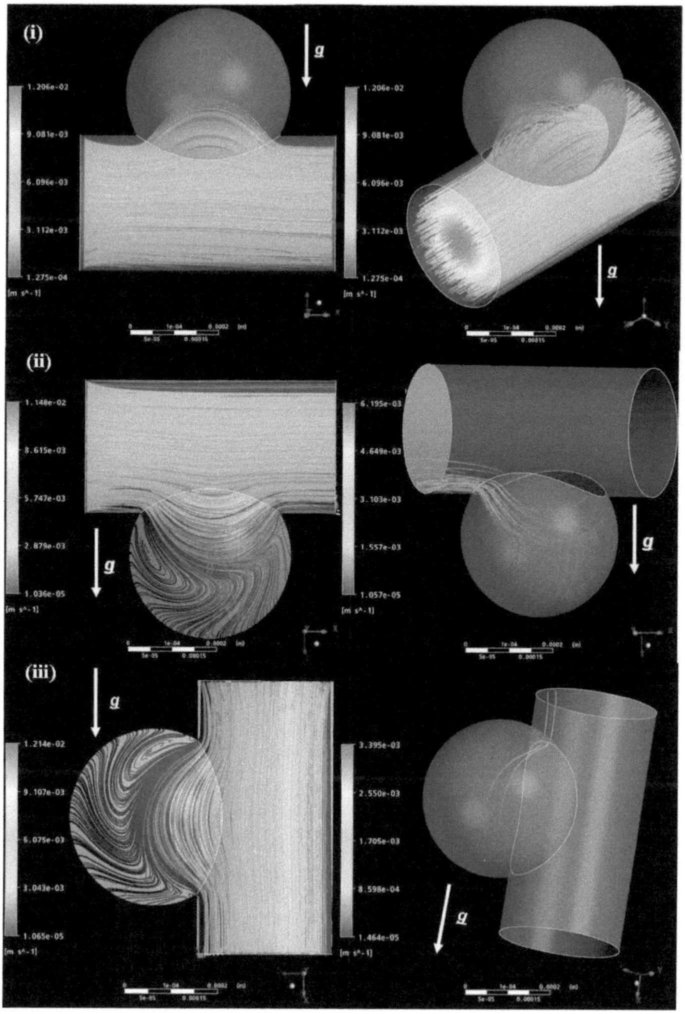

Figure 6.6: 1 μm particle trajectories, with velocity magnitude along trajectories (scale in m/s). (i)-(iii) (left and right column) correspond to cases (i)-(iii) in Fig. 6.5(a). (i) Deposition occurs only on the bottom of the duct. (ii) All particle trajectories are shown with alveolar flow pattern illustrated in the background (left). Trajectories are shown for deposited particles only (right). Note the complex trajectories inside the alveolus. (iii) All particle trajectories are shown with alveolar flow pattern in the background (left). Trajectories are shown for deposited particles only (right).

Fig. 6.5(a) and (b), where deposition efficiency curves follow closely the trend of the curve illustrating sedimentation in a horizontal pipe (see Fig. D.3 in Appendix D). In particular, deposition occurs intuitively faster for the larger aerosols (3 μm) over a similar breathing time, t/T, since P_d is approximately an order of magnitude smaller than for 1 μm particles. However, since the alveolated duct here is very short, the curves (Fig. 6.5(a) and (b)) stop abruptly when the particles have exited the computational domain at the duct outlet, during the inhalation phase.

It is interesting to note that streamline crossing is operating relatively strongly for the larger 3 μm aerosols (Fig. 6.7), such that particle trajectories are only slightly disturbed by the presence of the alveolar opening. Indeed, particles illustrate only a small bulge in their trajectories in the region near the alveolus opening. In contrast, the smaller aerosols (1 μm) follow closely the ductal streamlines (Fig. 6.6) since streamline crossing due to sedimentation occurs at a much slower rate (terminal sedimentation velocity follows $u_t \propto {d_p}^2$). Consequently, particles get deflected well into the alveolar opening region. However, under the present configuration, 1 μm aerosols do not get trapped inside the alveolar cavity, but remain rather along trajectories following the separation streamline between the alveolar and ductal flow as defined earlier (see results in section 5.8 of chapter 5). Therefore, no deposition occurs inside the alveolar cavity.

Gravity Orientation: Case (ii)

The configuration illustrated for case (ii) (Fig. 6.5) bears resemblance with the simple hemispherical alveolus model investigated previously by Haber *et al.* [89]. Particle trajectories and deposition sites are illustrated in Figs. 6.6 and 6.7 for 1 and 3 μm, respectively. As we have now been familiarized with deposition patterns along the ductal segment of the alveolated geometry (see Appendix D and case (i) above), we now concentrate on describing in more detail particle trajectories near and within the alveolar cavity. Looking at Fig. 6.7, the motion of 3 μm particles is largely unaffected by the convective alveolar flow structure. Indeed, resulting trajectories exhibit a nearly perfect vertical sedimenting path once particles have crossed the ductal-alveolar streamline separation. In particular, when particles cross into the alveolar cavity, they are no longer influenced by axial flow motion and their terminal sedimentation velocity, $u_t \approx 265$ μm/s, is much larger than the local alveolar flow velocity (i.e. at peak inspiration, $t = T/4$, flow velocity inside the cavity is on the order of < 10 μm/s, see results of section 5.8). Thus, deposition of particles inside the alveolus occurs rapidly and all particles entering the cavity are ultimately deposited within the end of the first inhalation phase (Fig. 6.5(b)). Based on such findings, one can intuitively expect that for larger particles (> 3 μm) for case (ii) configuration, aerosol kinematics in the alveolus will follow a similar trend while alveolar deposition will occur even faster.

In contrast, however, for the smaller non-diffusing aerosols (1 μm), kinematics differ substantially. While the bulk of particles within the duct follow closely the axial flow (i.e. streamline crossing operates very slowly), particles residing along streamlines deflected into the alveolar opening may be locally subjected to complex kinematics (Fig. 6.6, case (ii)). In particular, particles which have the tendency to enter the region where they may potentially be deflected into the alveolus space must all originate from ductal streamlines located on the bottom outer edges of the inlet opening, where velocities are relatively weak (due to the parabolic profile resulting from no-slip conditions at the wall). Since flow magnitudes in proximity of the wall are relatively small, particles do not have the time to travel beyond the alveolar opening towards the duct outlet within the end of the first inhalation phase. Simultaneously, near flow reversal at $t \approx T/2$, the velocity field within the computational space approaches zero everywhere. Therefore, over

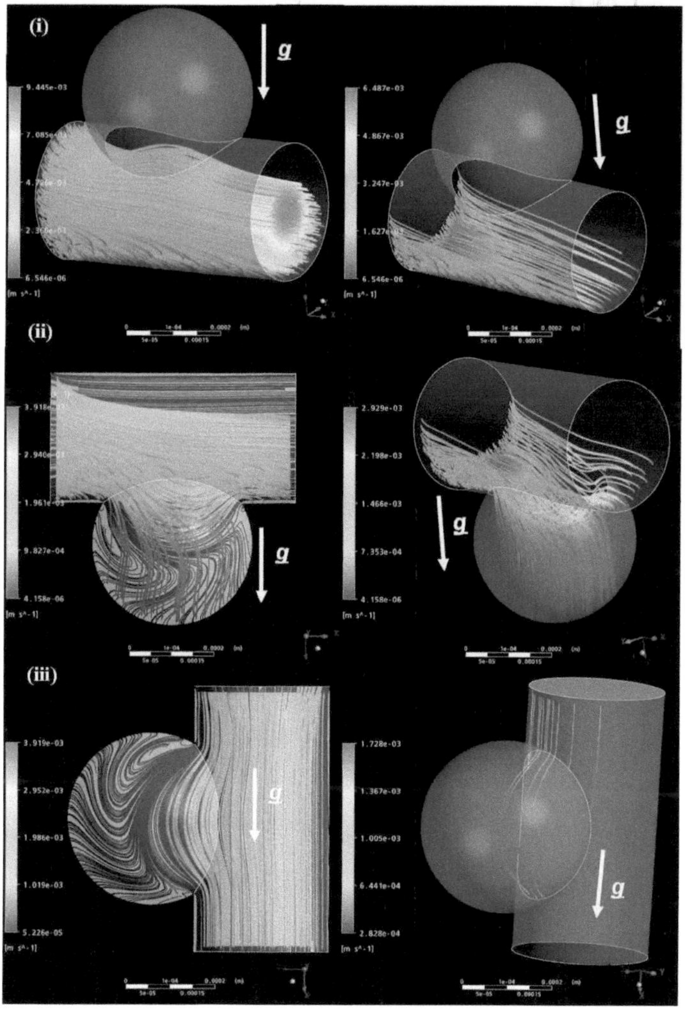

Figure 6.7: $3\ \mu$m particle trajectories, with velocity magnitude along trajectories (in m/s). (i)-(iii) (left and right column) correspond to cases (i)-(iii) in Fig. 6.5(b). (i) Deposition occurs only on bottom of the duct. Trajectories are shown for deposited particles only (right). (ii) All trajectories are shown with alveolar flow pattern illustrated in background (left). Trajectories are shown for deposited particles (right). (iii) All trajectories are shown with alveolar flow pattern in background (left). Trajectories are shown for deposited particles only (right). Deposition occurs around the opening ring.

a short period of time particles are essentially only subjected to their own weight during which a small degree of streamline crossing may operate. On the onset of the exhalation phase, particles will then begin to be convected back towards the duct inlet but simultaneously they are now located slightly deeper within the alveolar cavity. At their new location, particles are now subjected to the slow but complex alveolar flow structure. Therefore, such fine particles will exhibit a slow sedimentation process, which results from the combination of flow reversal leading to a swinging motion and the local topology of the alveolar flow. The resulting trajectories are thus complex and intrinsically three-dimensional, illustrating twisting motion (Fig. 6.6) similar to earlier findings by Haber *et al.* [89]. When aerosols eventually approach the alveolar walls, streamlines are then nearly radial, and particle trajectories describe a slightly undulating yet largely vertical sedimentation fall.

For such non-diffusing micron particles in case (ii) configuration, alveolar deposition becomes a slow process (see Fig. 6.5(a)), where particle residence times inside the alveolus are relatively long (i.e. no alveolar deposition occurs between the end of the first inhalation phase, $t/T \approx 1/2$, and the end of the second inhalation phase at $t/T \approx 3/2$). Deposition at the alveolar wall concludes only at the onset of the second exhalation phase ($t > 3T/2$), with a sudden jump along the deposition efficiency curve.

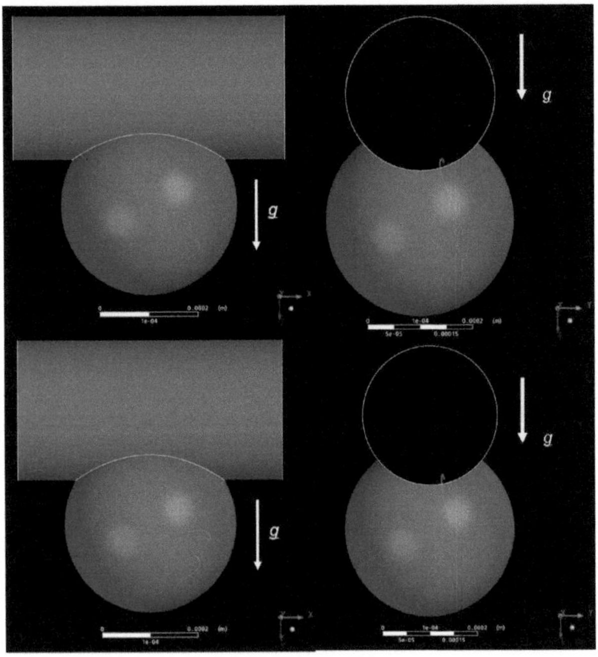

Figure 6.8: Example of two trajectories of 1 μm diameter particles originating close one from another at the duct inlet, for case (ii) configuration (left column: side view; right column: front view). Particles are highly sensitive to initial conditions and local alveolar flow structure, leading to unique irreversible trajectories.

Furthermore, for such fine aerosols, kinematics are highly sensitive to initial conditions, pertinent to their starting location across the inlet cross-section at the onset of inhalation ($t = 0$). Each trajectory is irreversible, unique and strongly influenced by the local alveolar flow structure, as illustrated in Fig. 6.8 and similarly discussed in previous 2D studies [268].

Gravity Orientation: Case (iii)

Case (iii) illustrated in Fig. 6.5(a) and (b) corresponds to the configuration where the gravity vector points parallel to the duct and in the direction of the inhalation flow. For both aerosol sizes (1 and 3 μm), the bulk of particles is transported parallel to the ductal flow and leaves intuitively the computational domain. Therefore, no deposition occurs along the ductal walls, since gravity is parallel to the duct orientation and no streamline crossing may arise in the duct in this configuration. However, interesting aerosol kinematics may arise for particles transported near the alveolar opening. Specifically, for the larger aerosols (3 μm), what appears to be gravitational settling effects may be observed at the proximal and distal side of the alveolar ring (Fig. 6.7, case (iii)). Such kinematics may develop from the specific combination of a particle's own weight acting in the same direction as the ductal flow, ultimately resulting in minor streamline crossing relative to the curved flow streamlines at the alveolar entrance. Indeed, the present findings suggest that the relatively heavier particles cannot follow flawlessly the curved ductal flow at the alveolar opening and may therefore deposit around the alveolar ring. However, deposition efficiency remains very low (see Fig. 6.5(b)).

For smaller aerosols (1 μm) transported into the region within the alveolar opening, gravitational sedimentation is not expected to play a significant role as the particle's weight is 27 times smaller here than for the larger 3 μm one ($m_p \propto {d_p}^3$). Since such fine aerosols have consequently a much slower terminal sedimentation velocity, u_t, the local alveolar flow structure can potentially influence aerosol kinematics, similar to findings for case (ii). This may be observed in Fig. 6.6 (bottom row, right column), where two particles have been effectively deflected into the alveolar cavity. In particular, their kinematics illustrate complex directional changes at the end of the inhalation phase, when flow reversal occurs. Here, trajectories show again evidence of three-dimensionality with slight twisting motion, although these features are less pronounced than in case (ii) for 1 μm particles (see Fig. 6.6, middle row, right column). This configuration illustrates once more that fine 1 μm particles are indeed sensitive to the detailed alveolar flow structure. However, as illustrated for case (iii) in Fig. 6.5(a) and (b), very few particles in fact enter the alveolus and deposit at the wall, due to the specific orientation of the geometry with respect to gravity. Therefore deposition efficiency remains very low (Fig. 6.5(a)).

Although the above results (cases (i) through (iii)) are pertinent to a rather simple and generic acinar geometry, they illustrate nevertheless important features relevant for particle transport and alveolar deposition as noted in previous studies [88, 89, 268]: 1) the structure of the alveolated duct, 2) wall motion due to breathing, 3) the orientation of gravity, as well as 4) the initial location of particles at $t = 0$. Our results suggest that aerosol trajectories and alveolar deposition are strongly dependent on the geometrical orientation of the duct and alveolus with respect to gravity. In particular, if particles are somewhat large, where sedimentation is expected to play a significant role (i.e. smaller P_d), our findings show that kinematics in the alveolus may then be fairly trivial and result largely from vertical settling trajectories, which are not affected by the local alveolar flow structure. In contrast, however, for finer non-diffusing micron-sized particles (i.e. 1 μm), aerosol kinematics may illustrate complex motion under the condition that particles cross the ductal-alveolar streamline separation barrier and enter the alveolar cavity. From

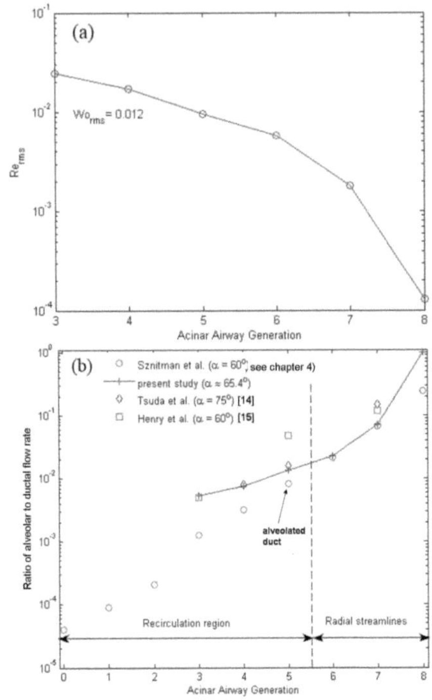

Figure 6.9: (a) Profile of (RMS) Re number vs. acinar generation (RMS Wo number is indicated and constant over all generations). (b) Ratio of alveolar to ductal flow rate in the space-filling tree vs. acinar generation (continuous line). Values are compared to previous investigations of alveolar flows (see details in text) and the simple alveolated duct model is indicated with an arrow.

that point onwards, the coupling of recirculating alveolar flow patterns with flow reversal due to oscillatory breathing motion and slight streamline crossing due to sedimentation give rise to intricate irreversible trajectories, illustrating 3D twisting and undulating motion leading ultimately to alveolar wall deposition over long residence times ($t > T$).

6.4.2 Flow Phenomena in Space-Filling Acinar Airway Tree

In the space-filling geometry, airflow ventilates the entire network of acinar ducts, while flow velocities gradually decrease with acinar depth, as a consequence of mass conservation applied progressively along airway bifurcations. Quantitatively, this is well captured by the cascade of values taken by (RMS) Re (see Fig. 6.9(a)), measured at each airway generation by following the longitudinal path length starting from the inlet (generation 3) until the alveolar sac (generation 8). During rhythmical wall motion, alveolar

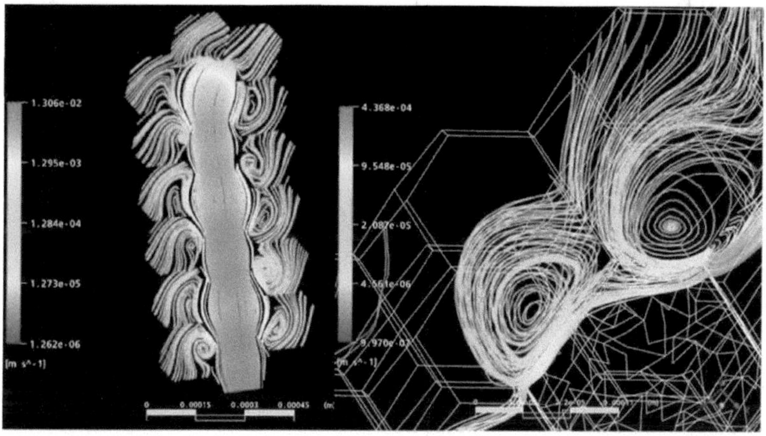

Figure 6.10: Left: 2D cross-sectional streamlines with velocity field magnitude obtained parallel to streamwise flow direction in generation 3 of the space-filling tree. Note the slower flow within alveoli compared to within the duct (scale is logarithmic in m/s). Right: Close-up of 3D recirculating flow patterns observed in alveoli located in generation 3.

flow topology may substantially differ according to acinar location along the airway tree. In the more proximal generations (i.e. gen. 3–5), flows are generally characterized by the existence of alveolar recirculation patterns (Fig. 6.10), as seen in the simple alveolated duct (see section 6.4.1). In particular, flows inside the cavities recirculate slowly and may exhibit the formation of open streamlines that spiral into singular points (Fig. 6.10, right), a property known to exist in 3D cavity flows while absent from 2D motions [239, 266]. In contrast, however, in the deeper acinar generations (i.e. gen 6–8), or conversely past asymmetrical bifurcations leading prematurely to an airway end (i.e. gen. 4 and 6), flow fields are generally characterized by radial streamlines (Fig. 6.11).

Qualitatively, along the acinar tree, alveolar flows may be understood as follows. In proximal acinar generations, only a small portion of the ductal fluid enters individual alveolar airspaces, while the bulk of the flow is carried towards deeper generations to feed more distal alveoli. The relatively strong ductal flows in the proximal acinar generations create a relatively strong shear layer over the alveolar mouth openings. These in turn generate flow separation and ultimately a recirculation region with the cavities, similar to classic low-Reynolds shear-driven cavity flows [101, 239, 260]. It is the relative strength of each driving mechanism (i.e. shear layer vs. wall motion) which ultimately governs the resulting alveolar flow topology, as noted previously [97, 270]. As one travels towards regions where the strength of the ductal flow decreases, consequently, recirculation regions will disappear and fluid fills alveolar cavities with a radial-like motion (see section 5.8.3 and Tsuda *et al.* [268]).

Along the longitudinal path length from generation 3 to 8, alveolar flow phenomena along the acinar tree may be captured by investigating values for the ratio of the alveolar to ductal flow rate, $\dot{Q}_a/\dot{Q}_T$ (Fig. 6.9(b)), a parameter originally introduced by Tsuda *et al.* [268]). For self-similar breathing motion, this ratio is a purely geometrical parameter independent of breathing pattern and flow conditions (see

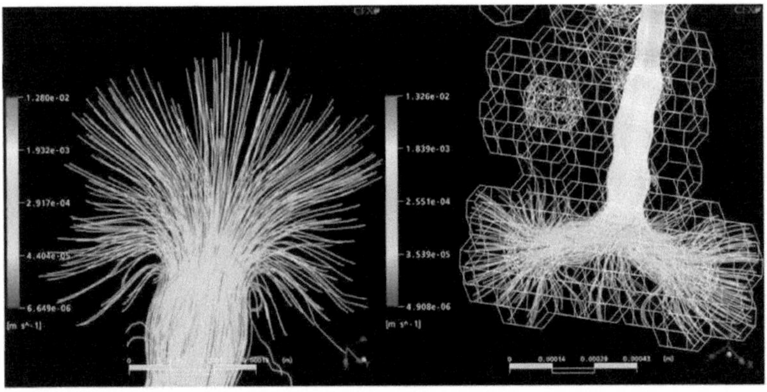

Figure 6.11: 3D view of instantaneous radial streamlines, with velocity magnitude in m/s (logarithmic scale) at airway generation 4 (left) and 7/8 (right).

Appendix B). Results suggest that low values of $\dot{Q}_a/\dot{Q}_T$ are associated with recirculating cavity flows, while past a certain threshold value, $\dot{Q}_a/\dot{Q}_T$ describes radial flow in alveoli, where the ductal flow is too weak to induce recirculation motion. As a general observation, if the space-filling model were symmetrical, values of $\dot{Q}_a/\dot{Q}_T$ would be associated as well with the exact location of an alveolus along the tree, as suggested earlier in chapter 5 (see section 5.8). However, due to asymmetry along the branches in the model, more representative of realistic anatomical features [71, 92, 93], a given acinar generation may be described by different values of $\dot{Q}_a/\dot{Q}_T$, depending on which daughter branch at a bifurcation one follows. Indeed, radial streamlines may be found in rather proximal generations of the space-filling tree (see Fig. 6.11, left). Note that following the space-filling assumption, $\dot{Q}_a/\dot{Q}_T$=1 at generation 8 (i.e. alveolar sac), since the alveolus and duct may not be distinguished between one another.

Values of $\dot{Q}_a/\dot{Q}_T$ reported here are consistent with previous findings [97,270], as illustrated in Fig. 6.9(b). Note that the present study is the only one to date to report values of $\dot{Q}_a/\dot{Q}_T$ in a multi-generation acinar tree (marked as a continuous line in Fig. 6.9(b)), while past studies have looked at in isolated alveolated ducts or single alveoli represented as spherical cavities (scatter points in Fig. 6.9(b)), rather than in polyhedra-shaped alveoli, sharing common boundaries (i.e. interalveolar septum). Such geometrical differences, as well as variations in the alveolar opening half-angle (see α in Fig. 6.9(b)), may influence locally the flow topology, as suggested previously [268]. One consequence is the dependence of the threshold value beyond which recirculating flows disappear entirely. In the present space-filling tree, this threshold value was found approximately at $\dot{Q}_a/\dot{Q}_T \approx 0.02$, in comparison with $\dot{Q}_a/\dot{Q}_T \approx 0.05$ [268], 0.01 [270], and ~ 0.021 (see earlier results for the simple alveolated duct in section 5.8) from previous studies. Such values correspond approximately to the passage between the 5th and 6th acinar airway generation (Fig. 6.9(b)). Despite small discrepancies in the threshold values found, these remain nevertheless very similar, suggesting indeed that the ratio $\dot{Q}_a/\dot{Q}_T$ is an appropriate parameter to describe alveolar flows, as proposed originally by Tsuda *et al.* [268]. Furthermore, alveoli represent, irrespective of variations in the geometrical assumptions, a biological example of complex low-Reynolds boundary-driven cavity flows. Indeed, the overall flow phenomenon results principally from the coupling between expansion/contraction wall motion and a low-Re shear driven cavity flow, rather than from the intrinsic details of the cavity geometry. Note finally that within the space-filling tree, $\dot{Q}_a/\dot{Q}_T = 0.53\%$ at generation 3 (Fig. 6.9(b)). Along the space-filling tree, this value is closest to the one investigated in the single alveolus of section 6.4.1 ($\dot{Q}_a/\dot{Q}_T = 0.82\%$). Locally then, resulting alveolar flows are indeed similar (compare Figs 5.8 and 6.10).

6.4.3 Aerosol Transport and Deposition in Space-Filling Tree

The transport of 1 and 3 μm particles was investigated for two distinct orientations of the space-filling acinar tree with respect to gravity. The first orientation, i.e. configuration (a), corresponds to the case where the gravity vector was chosen orthogonal to the inlet entrance at generation 3 (i.e. gravity vector points in the same direction as the ductal flow during inhalation). Configuration (b) illustrates the case where the gravity vector was tangential to the cross-sectional surface at the entrance inlet (i.e. gravity is orthogonal to the ductal flow in generation 3). In particular, gravity points along the entrance into the 4th acinar generation which terminates abruptly without further bifurcations (see Fig. 6.12(a)). For each simulation, a bolus consisting of a total of 5'000 particles was injected at $t = 0$ uniformly across the inlet cross-section.

Gravity Orientation: Configuration (a)

Figure 6.12(a) illustrates a general view of 1 μm particle trajectories in the space-filling tree. A first qualitative inspection of trajectories shows that particles are transported mainly along the branching alveolar ducts and reach relatively deep into the acinar tree. However, aerosols do not enter homogeneously into individual alveolar cavities. In particular, at generation 3, where $\dot{Q}_a/\dot{Q}_T$ is relatively strong, the bulk of particles is convected axially along the duct such that aerosols do not deposit within the alveolar cavities at that acinar generation. This phenomenon resembles closely to results obtained in case (iii) for the simple alveolated duct model (see section 6.4.1). In particular, one recognizes the wavy trajectory deflections occurring near the alveolar entrances (Fig. 6.12), as characterized earlier in the single alveolus model (Fig. 6.6). This may be observed as well for 3 μm particles under the same configuration (a) (see Fig. 6.12(b)). Here, the simple alveolus model in case (iii) gives useful insight into the general transport of aerosols occurring through generation 3 of the space-filling tree for this configuration.

It is interesting to note that qualitatively, 1 μm particles reach not only deeper into the acinar tree but they also seem to be transported more homogeneously along the different generations of acinar ducts, in comparison with 3 μm particles (compare Fig. 6.12 and (b)). This may be attributed to the fact that 1 μm particles are less influenced by transport mechanisms due to gravitational sedimentation and hence act to some extent more as passive tracers of the ductal flow, illustrating closely the flow distribution along the network of acinar branches. This property may be observed for example past the bifurcation at generation 3 (Fig. 6.12(a)), where a portion of 1 μm particles follow the ductal flow and are convected into the short duct at generation 4. Comparing with trajectories obtained for 3 μm particles (Fig. 6.13), aerosols which enter the short duct at generation 4 do not follow the convective flow into the bulk of the airspace but rather illustrate streamline crossing leading to short vertical sedimentation paths which come quickly into contact with alveolar walls near the entrance of generation 4.

Although trajectories within generation 3 are relatively similar for 1 and 3 μm particles (i.e. resembling case (iii) for the simple alveolated duct), the bifurcation leading to the daughter branches of generation

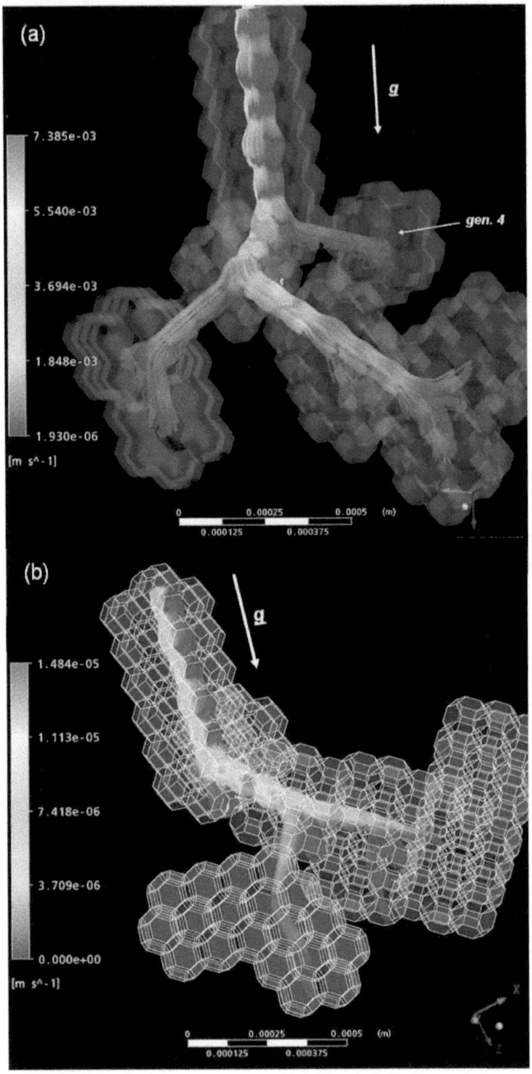

Figure 6.12: General view of trajectories of (a) 1 and (b) 3 μm diameter particles in the space-filling acinar tree with velocity magnitude along trajectories (scale in m/s). Geometrical orientation with respect to gravity corresponds to configuration (a) (see section 6.4.3).

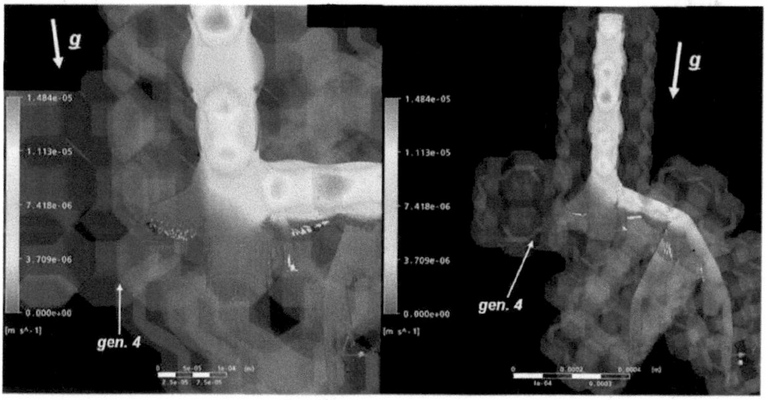

Figure 6.13: Detail of sedimenting $3\ \mu$m diameter particle trajectories with velocity magnitude (scale in m/s). Left: Close-up of trajectories at the bifurcation of generation 3. Right: Alternative view of sedimenting trajectories.

4 marks the onset where particle trajectories differ substantially between lighter and heavier aerosols. Indeed, for the heavier $3\ \mu$m aerosols, particles illustrate well gravitational sedimentation trajectories (Fig. 6.13), as early as the first bifurcation from parent generation 3 to daughter generation 4, where particles do not follow the bifurcating flow but settle straight into the alveolus beneath them (see detail in Fig. 6.13, left). In the deeper acinar generations where the ductal flow magnitude decreases, trajectories are largely vertical and particles enter alveoli residing along their straight path. Consequently, deposition is a highly localized phenomenon, since heavy particles can only enter into alveoli where the alveolar cavity openings are facing downwards with respect to the gravity orientation. Moreover, the local alveolar flow structure cannot influence particle transport of $3\ \mu$m particles, as observed for case (ii) in the simple alveolated duct. For even heavier particles ($> 3\ \mu$m) in configuration (a), aerosol trajectories are expected to follow a similar trend, where the role of gravitational sedimentation will become even more significant.

For smaller $1\ \mu$m particles, we have found evidence of aerosols illustrating complex 3D swinging and undulating motions within the entire space-filling geometry. Figure 6.14 illustrates examples of such distinct trajectories encountered, with residence times plotted along the particle trajectories. It is interesting to note that these fine aerosols may be swept along long distances, deep into the acinus, without depositing, before flow reversal occurs during which particles cross streamlines due to their own weight and end up along different ductal flow streamlines, which initiate new trajectories. During the exhalation phase, particles may then be convected back towards proximal generations. However, due to gravity this process is irreversible and particles may either be swung for a number of cycles before deposition, or they may possibly be ejected out of the computational domain if they are located along ductal streamlines with sufficient velocity (e.g. Fig. 6.14, bottom row). In the proximity of and within alveolar cavities, particles may then illustrate similar trajectories to the ones observed in the simple alveolated duct for cases (ii) and (iii) (Fig. 6.7). The simple alveolated duct model illustrated the importance of flow reversal, in particular in case (ii), in the transport and deposition of fine particles (i.e. $1\ \mu$m). Here, flow reversal is even more so relevant in the space-filling geometry, where intricate trajectories span over the entire

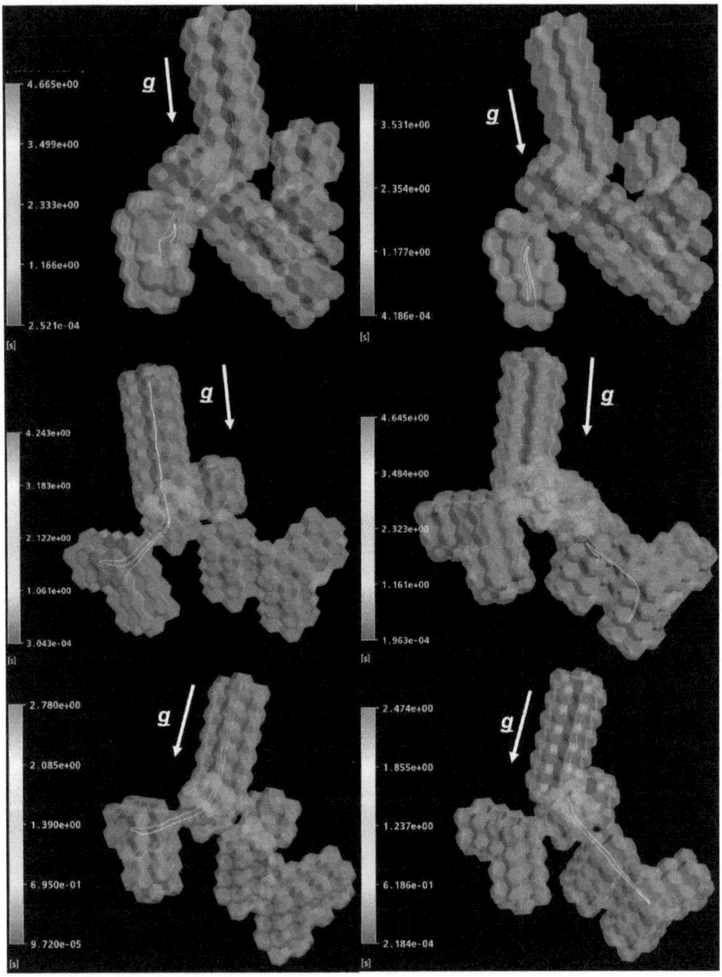

Figure 6.14: Examples of distinct $1\ \mu$m particle trajectories for configuration (a). Color code corresponds to particle residence time along trajectory (scale in seconds). Bottom row illustrates examples of particles leaving the computational domain during first exhalation phase.

network of space-filling airways. Such kinematics cannot, of course, be captured by simple models of isolated cavities or alveolated ducts [88, 89, 268], illustrating again the relevance of investigating aerosol transport in networks of acinar airways. Hence, results for configuration (a) suggest that fine aerosols (i.e. $1\ \mu$m) are strongly influenced by convective acinar respiratory flows (in particular ductal flows) as well as by flow reversal due to rhythmic breathing coupled with slight streamline crossing effects due to sedimentation, such that particles may be swept back and forth through large regions of the acinar tree before ultimately depositing. These mechanisms give rise to relatively long residence times ($t > T$) within the geometry (see Fig. 6.14).

Gravity Orientation: Configuration (b)

We now turn our attention to configuration (b) for 1 and $3\ \mu$m particles, respectively. Figure 6.15(b) illustrates trajectories for the heavier $3\ \mu$m particles. Here, the orientation of gravity plays a decisive role in determining actual deposition sites of individual particles. In particular, these heavier aerosols are dominated by relatively strong sedimentation mechanisms such that deposition sites are confined within alveoli located along the bottom-side of generation 3. Consequently, the entire network of more distal alveoli remains void. Aerosols illustrate here trajectories which are somewhat analogous to the superposition of deposition occurring under laminar horizontal pipe flow (see Appendix D, Fig. D.4) with deposition observed for case (ii) in the simple alveolated duct (Fig. 6.7). For even heavier particles ($> 3\ \mu$m) under configuration (b), we expect a similar deposition trend to occur such that particles will be entirely confined within generation 3 of the tree and exhibit even shorter axial motion. Comparing with results obtained for $3\ \mu$m particles in configuration (a), our findings suggest that the orientation of gravity does indeed play an essential role in determining the deposition pattern for relatively heavier particles, whose transport is largely determined by gravitational sedimentation.

For finer aerosols (i.e. $1\ \mu$m), a qualitative inspection of Fig. 6.15(a) seems to suggest at first that trajectories appear to be widely similar to those obtained in configuration (a), where particles are convected along all acinar branches of the tree (compare with Fig. 6.13(a)). In particular, a detailed inspection of some trajectories (Fig. 6.16) illustrates analogous sets of intricate particle motion, as described earlier in configuration (a), where the coupling of convective mechanisms with slight gravitational sedimentation and flow reversal results in aerosols travelling first deep along one region of the acinar model but depositing in another, after exhibiting long residence times in the airspace. However, as noted earlier, deposition sites for these fine particles are not homogeneously distributed, with many alveolar cavities remaining void, suggesting again that deposition may be a highly localized phenomenon. Although configurations (a) and (b) yield qualitatively similar transport of fine particles (i.e. $> 1\ \mu$m), it is interesting to note that the orientation of gravity gives rise, nevertheless, to slight variations in trajectories despite the relatively weak influence of the sedimentation process (in comparison with $\geq 3\ \mu$m particles). In particular, we have located aerosols which deposit in the smaller airspace branch at generation 4 (see examples of trajectories terminating in generation 4, Fig. 6.16 top row and Fig. 6.17), after very long residence times ($t > 3T$). Indeed, the orientation of gravity favors slightly the entrance of a portion of particles into this region of the tree. Since velocities are very weak in this particular region, particles exhibit irreversible trajectories which are very slow and cannot exit back out into other airway branches, since gravity opposes such motion. This situation is somewhat analogous to kinematics occurring in the alveolated duct for case (ii), since the airspace along the shorter duct at generation 4 may be seen as one large alveolus leading to swinging and sedimentation as seen in the simple alveolus.

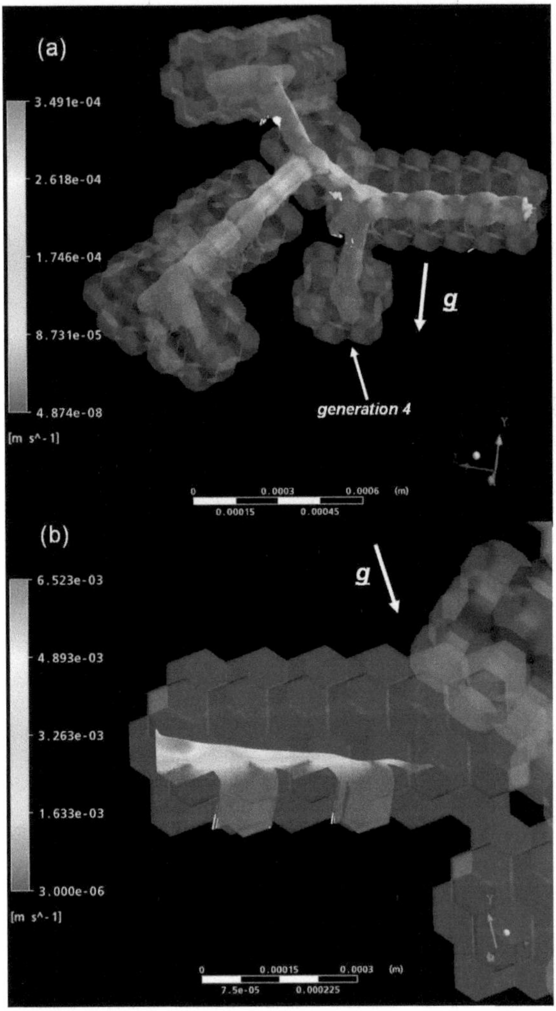

Figure 6.15: General view of trajectories of (a) 1 and (b) 3 μm diameter particles in the space-filling acinar tree with velocity magnitude along trajectories (scale in m/s). Geometrical orientation with respect to gravity corresponds to configuration (b) (see section 6.4.3).

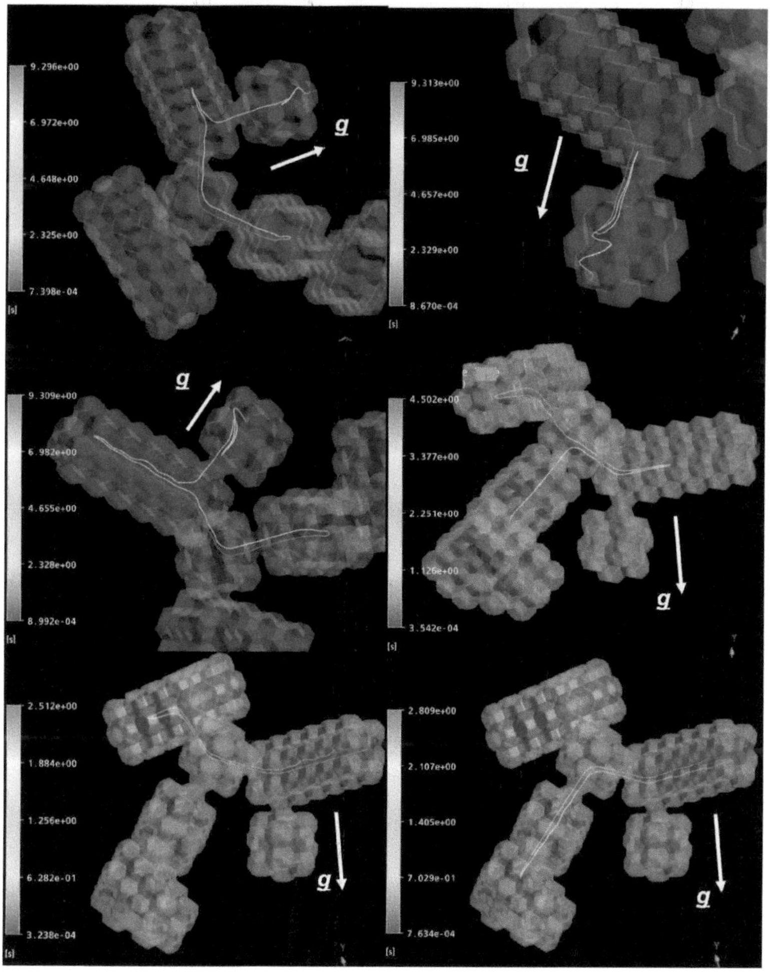

Figure 6.16: Examples of distinct 1 μm particle trajectories for configuration (b). Color code corresponds to particle residence time along trajectory (scale in seconds). Top row illustrates examples of particles which settle in the shorter branch of generation 4, due to the specific orientation of gravity. Bottom row illustrates examples of particles leaving the computational domain during first exhalation phase.

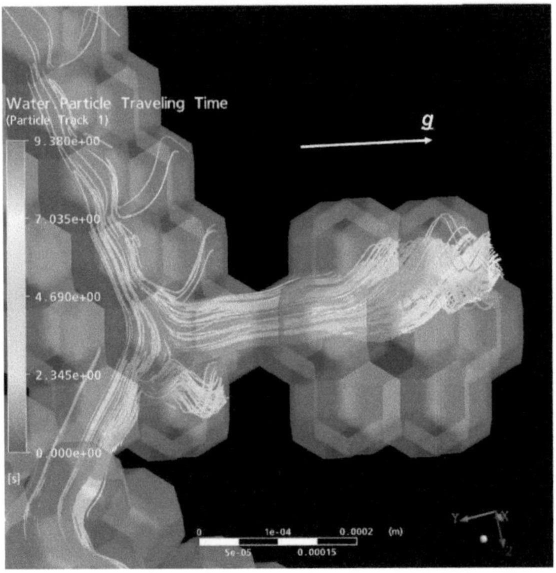

Figure 6.17: Detail of particle trajectories inside generation 4, in configuration (b) (see section 6.4.3). Scale corresponds to particle residence time in seconds. Particles entering generation 4 exhibit very long residence times ($t > 3T$) before depositing due to the specific orientation of gravity.

Deposition Efficiency in the Space-Filling Acinar Tree

Figure 6.18 illustrates the deposition efficiencies, $n(t)/N$, obtained for 1 and 3 μm diameter particles, respectively, for sedentary tidal breathing in configurations (a) and (b). For heavier particles, $n(t)/N$ reaches unity within the end of the first inhalation phase (all particles are deposited), although intuitively, configuration (b) yields slightly quicker deposition since particles need to sedimentate over shorter distances to reach the nearest alveolar wall. It is interesting to note that while actual deposition patterns (where particles deposit along the tree) differ strongly between each configuration (compare Figs. 6.12(b) and 6.15(b)), profiles of the two efficiency curves illustrate, however, surprisingly similar behaviors. This preliminary result seems to suggest that for relatively heavier particles, deposition efficiency is influenced perhaps more by the gravitational sedimentation mechanism itself rather than the actual orientation of the geometry with respect to the gravity field. Indeed, for both configurations, 3 μm particles are characterized by the same sedimentation parameter, $P_d = 4.06$ (or alternatively the same gravity number $H = 1/P_d$). These findings contrast sharply with deposition profiles of 3 μm particles observed in the simple alveolated duct which vary strongly with the orientation of gravity (see Fig. 6.5(b)). The differences noted between the simple alveolated duct and the space-filling model may perhaps be due to the fact that the combination of a large number (i.e. 190 14-hedra) of identical but differently oriented alveoli assembled into a space-filling geometry could give rise to global isotropy with respect to gravity orientation, when considering deposition efficiency of particles whose transport is dominated by sedimentation (i.e. the role of convective flow is much weaker).

For finer aerosols (i.e. $1\ \mu$m), residence times of particles in the acinar airspace are substantially longer (up to 3 times longer than for $3\ \mu$m particles), and efficiency curves in both configurations yield $n(t)/N \approx$ 0.9–0.95, since a small portion of the particles have exited the computational domain during the first exhalation phase, as described earlier (e.g. bottom rows of Figs. 6.14 and 6.16 for configuration (a) and (b), respectively). In particular, over the interval, $0 < t < 1.5T$, the deposition efficiency curves share again comparable profiles until efficiencies reach $n(t)/N \approx 0.8$. However, beyond $t > 1.5T$, the curves begin to diverge such that for configuration (b) deposition terminates after $t > 3T$, while in configuration (a) deposition terminates at approximately $t \approx$ 1.6–1.7T. The sharp difference noted in configuration (b) for $t > 1.5T$, may be attributed to the portion of particles which has entered the small airspace region at generation 4 (as discussed earlier in section 6.4.3). In configuration (b), the specific orientation of gravity favors the entrance of a small fraction of aerosols into generation 4's shorter branch (Figs. 6.16 and 6.17). Such particles ultimately settle after very long residence times, > 9 s, since the local ductal flow in this short branch is very slow (as a consequence of mass conservation) and fine particles are sensitive to flow reversal coupled with small but significant sedimentation effects. Hence, for lighter $1\ \mu$m particles whose transport is governed by complex mechanisms independent of gravity such as convective ductal and alveolar flow structures as well as flow reversal due to oscillatory breathing, it is likely that the precise orientation of gravity may be responsible for the small differences observed in deposition sites as well as deposition efficiencies.

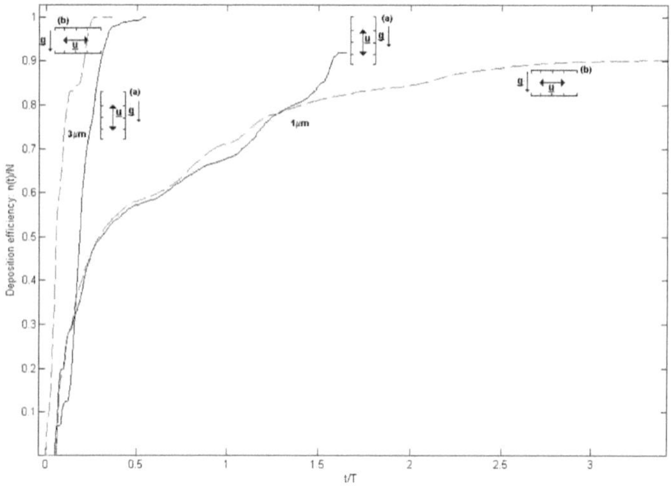

Figure 6.18: Deposition efficiency, $n(t)/T$, in the space-filling geometry as a function of normalized time, t/T, for $3\ \mu$m (curves on the left) and $1\ \mu$m diameter particles (curves on the right) under configuration (a) and (b) (see text for details). Schematic corresponds to the orientation of acinar generation 3 with respect to gravity.

6.5 Conclusions

We have investigated, using CFD methods, the transport of non-diffusing micron-sized (1 and $3\ \mu$m) inhaled particles in models of the pulmonary acinus, under rhythmic breathing motion. Two acinar geometries of varying complexity were constructed: (i) a previously introduced simple alveolated duct (see chapter 5) following morphometric measurements [90] and (ii) a novel space-filling acinar tree following the description of lung structure by Fung [71]. Detailed particle trajectories and deposition efficiencies, as well as acinar flow structures, were investigated under different geometrical orientations with respect to gravity, for tidal breathing in an average human adult.

The simple alveolated duct model was aimed at capturing the detailed motion of aerosol particles locally within an alveolus and simultaneously identifying the role of individual transport mechanisms for lung deposition. Our findings illustrate that resulting trajectories inside the alveolus, as well as deposition efficiencies, are strongly tied to the geometrical orientation of the model with respect to gravity. While the motion of larger particles ($3\ \mu$m) is relatively insensitive to convective flow structures compared to the determining role of gravitational sedimentation leading to straight vertical trajectories inside the alveolus, finer aerosols ($1\ \mu$m) may exhibit, in contrast, complex kinematics. In particular, the precise motion of such fine aerosols is influenced by the coupling between (i) flow reversal effects due to oscillatory breathing, (ii) the local convective alveolar flow structure, (iii) initial conditions relating to the location of a particle at injection, as well as (iv) small but significant sedimentation mechanisms leading to effective streamline crossing. These combined mechanisms may lead to highly 3D particle trajectories observed within the alveolus, exhibiting irreversible twisting and undulating motions over long residence times ($t > T$).

The extension of our study to a space-filling acinar tree model was well suited to investigate the influence of bulk kinematic interaction between ductal flows and alveolar flows on aerosol behavior. Although there exist a number of analogies between local particle trajectories observed in the simple alveolated duct and the space-filling model, the latter and more complex acinar geometry illustrates the existence of intricate trajectories of fine $1\ \mu$m aerosols which span over the entire network of space-filling airways due to flow reversal, and cannot be captured by simple models of isolated cavities or alveolated ducts. In contrast, heavier $3\ \mu$m aerosols yield trajectories characteristic of gravitational sedimentation, largely insensitive to local acinar flow structures. For both lighter ($1\ \mu$m) and heavier ($3\ \mu$m) aerosols, however, individual particle trajectories yield a highly non-uniform distribution of deposition sites, leaving many individual alveoli and entire regions of the acinar geometry void. Such findings may give further insight for inhalation therapy, where targeting the delivery of aerosols to different regions of the lung is desired for localized treatments [9]. Moreover, while larger particles deposit within a single inhalation phase, fine $1\ \mu$m particles exhibit long residence times during which they are suspended in the bulk of the acinar space. Such findings suggest that multiple breathing cycles may be needed for deposition to finalize. With the development of more realistic CFD models of the acinar structure of the lung, it is our hope to capture and explain some of the complex mechanisms leading to local acinar deposition of inhaled aerosols. Such numerical models may lead in the future to a better understanding of the physical requirements which need to be considered for the optimization of pulmonary drug delivery to target specific regions of the lung [218].

Chapter 7

Reconstruction of Alveolar Airspaces from X-ray Tomographic Microscopy

A deeper knowledge of the three-dimensional (3D) structure of the pulmonary acinus has direct applications in studies on acinar fluid dynamics and aerosol kinematics. Until present, limitations in the spatial resolution of lung imaging techniques have largely prevented the possible 3D reconstruction of acinar structures. Moreover, acinar flow simulations have been often based on simple geometrical models inspired by morphometrical studies. In the present investigation, high-resolution, synchrotron-based X-ray Tomographic Microscopy (XTM) images of the pulmonary acinus of a mouse are used to reconstruct 3D alveolar airspaces, corresponding to terminal alveolar sacs. After fitting a computational mesh to the reconstructed geometries, transient respiratory simulations are conducted under moving wall boundary conditions to simulate rhythmic lung motion during sedentary tidal breathing. The resulting alveolar flow patterns in the alveolar sacs are governed by creeping radial motion and are fundamentally time-independent, confirming findings from previous studies using geometrical models. Whether respiration is modelled as self-similar or exhibits a small degree of geometric hysteresis, the general flow topology remains largely insensitive to shape complexity but, rather, is driven by the basic wall motion induced in the alveolar cavities. Convective flow patterns obtained presently therefore suggest that the possible existence of chaotic acinar flows may rather be confined to the more proximal generations of the acinar tree, where recirculating flows are found to exist. The feasibility of the present CFD simulations using reconstructed 3D XTM geometries opens the path towards future, more realistic aerosol kinematics and deposition studies in the pulmonary acinus.

7.1 Introduction

Relatively few quantitative data exist describing the 3D geometry of the respiratory region of the lung (i.e. pulmonary acinus). As interest in the fate of inhaled substances in the airways increases, whether the lung may be considered as a target (inhalation aerosols) or an unfortunate recipient (e.g. airborne contaminants and pollutants) of inhaled particles, the lack of 3D information on the acinar structure becomes more and more critical if we hope, one day, to predict accurately, and perhaps even locally target, the deposition of inhaled substances in a given individual. Traditionally, acinar airway morphometry has been studied using measurements of mammalian-lung cast models [15, 90, 224] or alternatively, acinar geometry has been described using serial histological section techniques [92, 93, 184]. Historically, the introduction of three-dimensional reconstructions of alveolar geometries was first brought from serial histological sections [155, 255], but due to technical limitations, reconstruction schemes have been restricted to only but a few alveoli [155]. However, with the recent introduction of new imaging techniques, such as computed tomography (CT) [17, 151], anatomically-based realistic 3D models of the lung have become more widespread. While this important advancement has led towards the measurement and reconstruction of the 3D structure of the bronchial tree and the small airways [4, 183, 202, 216, 233, 293], the successful reconstruction and visualization of the acinar region has been largely prohibited due to limitations in the spatial resolution offered using standard micro-CT techniques. An alternative to this barrier has been recently implemented with the use of synchrotron-based radiation CT, although this technique still remains exclusive due to the few facilities available worldwide. Synchrotrons constitute a type of cyclic particle accelerator in which the magnetic field and the electric field are carefully synchronized with the travelling particle beam, and are mostly used for producing high-intensity X-ray beams. This technique has opened the path towards high-resolution visualization and 3D reconstruction of small airways and alveoli [110, 234] with spatial resolutions capable of reaching from < 15 μm down to < 1 μm. In particular, synchrotron-based imaging of the acinus may have a strong appeal for aerosol transport and deposition studies in anatomically-based 3D geometries using computational fluid dynamics (CFD) methods. Therefore, the objective of the present study is twofold: to reconstruct 3D alveolar airspaces from high-resolution synchrotron-based imaging of the lung; and implement physiologically realistic simulations of respiratory flows in the reconstructed acinar geometries to study acinar flows and in a later step aerosol kinematics.

The pursuit towards an anatomically realistic description of the 3D structure of the pulmonary acinus has important and direct applications in studies on fluid dynamics and particle deposition in the lungs. The motivation for such investigations has risen, amongst other, from the increased interest in targeted pulmonary drug delivery in which the site of deposition of the particles may be a key factor in the success or failure of the treatment [129]. In particular, the numerical study of alveolar flows has significant relevance for aerosol kinematics and acinar deposition of inhaled fine particles [87–89, 267, 268], and simulations have offered explanations for the existence of experimentally observed convective aerosol mixing in the pulmonary acinus [41, 99, 208]. While respiratory simulations of airflow and particle transport have recently been performed in a realistic 3D upper bronchial tree based on CT imaging [261, 276], flows in the pulmonary acinus have remained usually more difficult to assess due to the sub-millimeter dimensions, the accessibility of the region and the lack of 3D imaging data. Hence, the measurement and simulation of alveolar flow phenomena in such region continues to present challenging problems.

Until present, insight into acinar flows has been brought on the one hand by experimental flow visualization studies using in-vitro [29, 116, 265, 271] and in-vivo [272] setups, but has been largely driven by numerical computations. These simulations have often made use of simple alveolated duct structures inspired by morphometrical studies from measurements of human airway casts [90, 281]. Commonly, the acinar airways have been modelled using alveolated channels, where central cylindrical ducts were mounted with spherical cavities, both in 2D [47, 61, 97, 267, 268, 270] and 3D [87–89] simulations. While such geometries have remained relatively simple, previous numerical simulations have given better insight into the complex nature of acinar flows, such as the relevance of rhythmical boundary wall motion [47, 270], the existence of chaotic behavior due to both alveolar flow recirculation [97, 270], and flow asynchrony at airway bifurcations [87, 89, 271], likely generated by a small degree of geometric hysteresis in the expanding and contracting lung [157]. Hence, alveolar flows can be substantially more complex than previously thought, due to the unique alveolated duct structures and their time dependent motion. However, an exact understanding of acinar fluid dynamics and realistic kinematics and deposition of aerosols calls, most likely, for the use of anatomically based three-dimensional alveolar geometries in respiratory flow simulations.

In the present investigation, we make use of high-resolution imaging data ($1.4\ \mu$m $\times$ $1.4\ \mu$m $\times$ $1.4\ \mu$m voxels) of the pulmonary acinus of a mouse obtained from synchrotron-based X-ray Tomographic Microscopy (XTM) to reconstruct 3D geometries of terminal alveolar airspaces, corresponding to alveolar sacs. A computational mesh is then generated for the reconstructed airspaces before performing CFD simulations of small-scale respiratory flows to simulate physiologically realistic rhythmical breathing. Flow results are discussed and compared with the existing literature. Furthermore, we study the feasibility and limitations in the reconstruction of 3D alveolar geometries from current XTM technology. Finally, we discuss the promising relevance and potential impact for future aerosol deposition studies using CFD simulations with 3D reconstructed alveolar geometries.

7.2 Methods

7.2.1 Animal Preparation and Data Acquisition

Lungs of 129/SV mice were prepared according to Schittny *et al.* [222] at postnatal day 10. Briefly, the airspace was filled with 2.5% glutaraldehyde in 0.03 M potassium-phosphate buffer (pH 7.4, 370 mOsm) at a constant pressure of 20 cm water column. At this pressure, the lung reaches roughly its mid-respiratory volume. In order to prevent a recoiling of the lung, the pressure was maintained during fixation (minimum of 2 h). Samples were postfixed in 0.1 M sodium cacodylate (pH 7.4, 340 mOsm), containing 1% OsO_4, and stained en bloc with 0.5% uranyl acetate in 0.05 M maleate buffer. After dehydration in a graded series of ethanol, the samples were embedded in Epon 812 [221]. Handling of the animals before and during the experiments, as well as the experiments themselves, were approved and supervised by the Swiss Agency for the Environment, Forests and Landscape and the Veterinary Service of the Canton of Bern.

The samples were shaped down to a rod of a diameter of 1.3 mm on a watchmaker's lathe and glued into a hole of 1.6 mm at the top of a rod like sample holder. Special care was taken such that the samples were mounted perpendicularly to the surface of the sample holder in order to fit exactly into the window of the camera.

The samples were scanned at a X-ray wavelength of 1 Angstrom (monochromatic X-ray beam corresponding to an energy of 12.398 keV; DE/E = 0.014%) at the micro-tomography station of the Materials Science beamline at the Swiss Light Source (SLS) of the Paul-Scherrer-Institut (Villigen, Switzerland) [253]. After penetration of the sample, X-rays were converted into visible light by a thin Ce-doped YAG scintillator screen (Crismatec Saint-Gobain, Nemours, France). Projection images were further magnified by diffraction limited microscope optics and finally digitized by a high-resolution CCD camera (Photonic Science Ltd., East Sussex, UK) [253]. For the tissue samples, the optical magnification was set to $10\times$ and on-chip binning was selected to improve the signal to noise ratio, resulting in isotropic voxels of $1.43\ \mu$m^3 for the reconstructed images. 1001 projections were acquired along with dark and periodic flat field images for each sample. Data were post-processed and rearranged into flat field corrected sinograms online. Reconstruction of the volume of interest was performed on a 16-node Linux PC

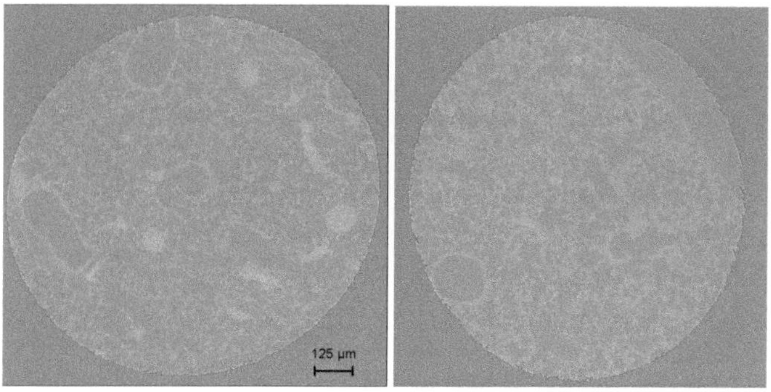

(a) (b)

Figure 7.1: Illustration of typical XTM image slices with a spatial planar resolution of $1.4\ \mu$m $\times$ $1.4\ \mu$m $\times$ $1.4\ \mu$m obtained from the pulmonary acinus of a 10 days old mouse. Scale is given in the bottom right of (a). Ductal cross-sections of small airways are visible (e.g. bottom left of (b)), while the outer edge of the lung parenchyma is visible along the upper right region of (b).

farm (Pentium 4, 2.8 GHz, 512 MB RAM) using highly optimized filtered back-projection routines. Typical XTM planar slice images obtained from the pulmonary acinus of a 10 days old mouse are illustrated in Fig. 7.1.

7.2.2 Three-Dimensional Reconstruction

As the focus of our study is concerned with the reconstruction of 3D alveolar airspaces towards respiratory CFD simulations, computational costs will increase drastically with large geometries and computational mesh sizes. Consequently, for simulations to remain computationally converging while reasonably affordable, simulations of respiratory flows in complete multi-generation pulmonary acinar branching trees remain currently unfeasible, in particular due to limitations in the reconstruction schemes (as will be discussed). For such reason, the three-dimensional reconstruction of acinar airspaces was restricted, for the time being, to sub-regions extracted from entire XTM image stacks. Image segmentation (separation of lung tissue from airspace) and three-dimensional surface rendering were obtained separately using both a commercial software (Imaris, Bitplane AG, Zrich, Switzerland) and an in-house developed software based on a MATLAB platform (MATLAB 7.0.4, The Mathworks, Inc, MA USA). Both methods delivered similar 3D reconstructed geometries, while the in-house developed software enabled greater flexibility to investigate possible optimization schemes during the reconstruction steps. A flow chart of the general image processing steps is given in Fig. 7.2.

Successful reconstructions of acinar airspaces were typically obtained for XTM data (approximately 100 pixels $\times$ 100 pixels $\times$ 100 slices) extracted near the outer edges of the lung parenchyma in the XTM image slices (Fig. 7.1(b)). These locations generally coincided with the more distal regions of the pulmonary

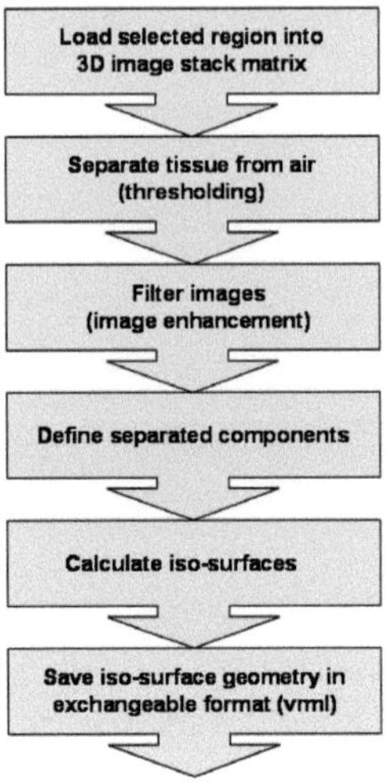

Figure 7.2: Flow chart illustrating image processing algorithm steps implemented for the three-dimensional reconstruction of alveolar airspaces.

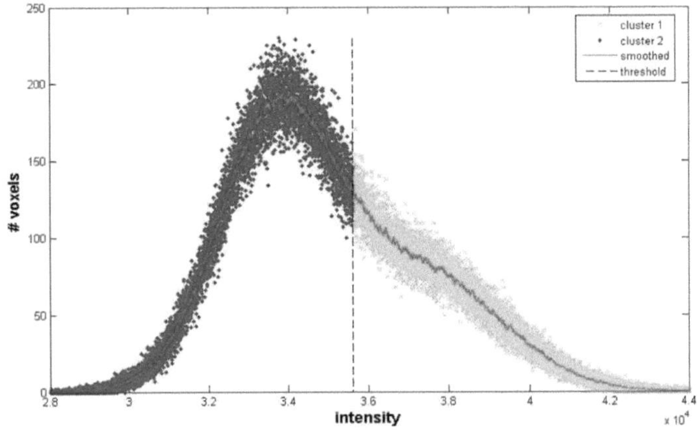

Figure 7.3: Histogram of the intensity values of an image stack example extracted from the original XTM data for a 10 days old mouse. The threshold value separating air (cluster 1) from lung tissue (cluster 2) was calculated by taking the mean of the resulting centers obtained from a 2-means clustering algorithm.

acinus, where terminal alveolar airspaces (i.e. alveolar sacs) were thought to be found. Separation of lung tissue from air (for flow simulation purposes, we are interested in reconstructing airspaces rather than alveolar wall septa) was obtained using a thresholding technique applied on the intensity values of the voxels. High intensity values corresponded to lung tissue and lower ones were attributed to air. Since there are only two different materials present, namely air and lung tissue, the problem was reduced to finding a single threshold value over the entire image stack. However, looking at a characteristic intensity histogram of an XTM image stack (Fig. 7.3), it becomes clear that the intensity distribution is not purely bimodal, but rather, air and tissue exhibit imperfect contrast and their intensity ranges overlap significantly, such that two distinct intensity peaks are not discernible. Therefore, setting a single threshold value will always amount to a trade-off between having too thick alveolar walls and correspondingly creating a loss of airspace, versus setting a threshold value too high and risking to create artifacts such as holes in the alveolar walls. To optimize separation of lung tissue from air, a balance was chosen between direct visual thresholding and an iterative K-means clustering algorithm [232], which minimizes the sum of point-to-centroid distances, summed over K clusters (in the present case, $K = 2$). The mean of the resulting two cluster centers was calculated and used as an initial threshold value (Fig. 7.3) and further correction, if needed, was then implemented by visual thresholding.

The presence of intrinsic noise in the original XTM raw data could potentially jeopardize the successful 3D geometry reconstruction. To obtain meaningful reconstructed geometries and avoid the generation of artifacts inside airspaces (scatter voxels due to noise could be wrongfully attributed with tissue because of their relatively high intensity values), an elimination of noise through the use of digital filters was sought. Accordingly, a median filter (with adjustable $N \times N$ window size) was applied to each image slice [114]. The advantages of this filter were its simplicity and that it is reasonably edge-preserving. Figure 7.4(a) and (b) illustrate a pair of an original XTM image and its corresponding filtered version. Median filtering yields satisfactory results, although small drawbacks in edge-preserving filtering techniques such as edge smoothing were unavoidable. Within the image stack, the next step consisted in distinguishing individual components and shapes of airspaces (i.e. segmentation). To accomplish this step, an iterative algorithm was applied over the image stack which assigned one component to each voxel. For each voxel attributed

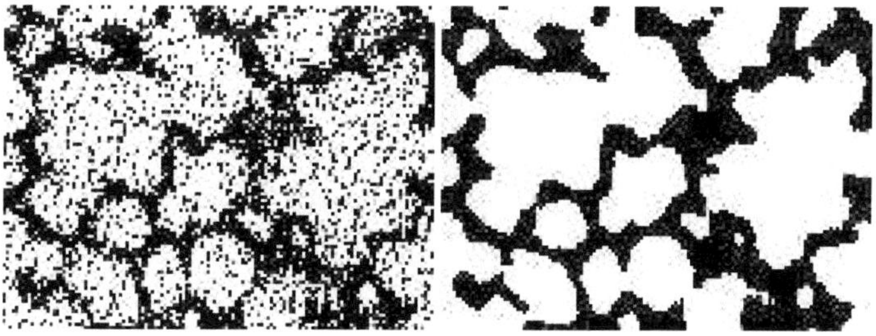

(a) (b)

Figure 7.4: (a) Extracted region of a thresholded XTM raw image illustrating the presence of noise compared with (b) the resulting image after applying a 5×5 window median filter. Note that applying a median filter smoothens slightly the edges (alveolar walls).

with air, the neighboring, previously visited voxels were checked for voxels also attributed with air. If an air-voxel was found in this neighborhood, the current voxel was assigned the same component number as the neighboring air-voxel, thus added to the component corresponding to this number. If no such air-voxel was found in the previously visited neighborhood, the current voxel was assigned with the next free component number. The procedure for the separation of components is schematically illustrated in Fig. 7.5. Finally, to generate three-dimensional geometries, iso-surfaces were constructed. For a three-dimensional matrix representing an image stack, a surface within the volume that had the same value at each vertex (referred to as the iso-value) was calculated. Optionally, the image stack matrix was first smoothed to reduce abrupt changes between neighboring polygon normals of the calculated polygonal iso-surfaces. On the outer borders, where iso-surfaces were cut by the bounding box spanned by the size of the image stack, so called isocaps were defined to form closed bodies together with the iso-surfaces. Finally, the mesh formed by the calculated iso-surfaces was stored in an exchangeable format compatible with the flow solver software.

7.3 Breathing Kinematics

The breathing kinematics described here follow closely the methodology described earlier in section 5.2. To accommodate for both self-similar lung expansion [3, 80, 83] and wall motion exhibiting characteristics of geometric hysteresis [157], our reconstructed alveolar airspace geometries are designed to expand and contract in a simple sinusoidal manner, with a breathing period T (see Eq. (5.5)). Any length scale, $L(t)$, in the geometry is then described by the kinematic displacement function:

$$L(t) = L_0 \left[1 + \frac{\beta}{2} + \frac{\beta}{2} \sin\left(2\pi f t - \frac{\pi}{2} + \alpha(\underline{x}, t) \right) \right] = L_0 \cdot \lambda(\underline{x}, t). \tag{7.1}$$

The equation above is essentially identical to Eq. (5.5). However, an additional term is now included. Namely, the function, $\alpha(\underline{x}, t)$, defines the time- and spatially-dependent phase shift to mimic geometrical

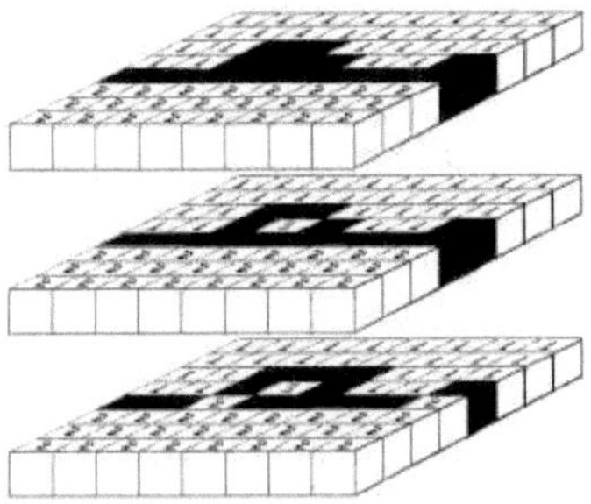

Figure 7.5: Schematic illustration of an image stack with all voxels of separated air components (in white) assigned with the number of the component they belong to.

hysteresis during rhythmical breathing (see below). Physiological breathing conditions are replicated to model approximately tidal breathing of a mouse [13, 194, 223], such that $T = 0.4$ s and $C \approx 19\%$ (see section 5.2).

Kinematics of Self-Similarity

Let us consider the self-similar wall motion of a simple geometry, whose time-dependent volume is given by $V(t) = CR^3(t)$, where $R(t)$ is the length scale of the geometry and C is chosen here as a constant (for a sphere, $R(t)$ is the radius and $C = 4\pi/3$). Rewriting the volume, $V(t)$, in Cartesian coordinates such that $R(t) = (x^2(t) + y^2(t) + z^2(t))^{1/2}$, the volume may then be expressed as:

$$V(t) \propto \left[(x_0\lambda_x(t))^2 + (y_0\lambda_y(t))^2 + (z_0\lambda_z(t))^2\right]^{3/2}, \tag{7.2}$$

where the subscript 0 denotes the coordinates at time $t = 0$ and $\lambda_x(t)$, $\lambda_y(t)$ and $\lambda_z(t)$ are time-dependent cyclic length scaling functions, not necessarily equal to one another. Similarly, the total surface area, $S(t)$, may be expressed as:

$$S(t) \propto \left[(x_0\lambda_x(t))^2 + (y_0\lambda_y(t))^2 + (z_0\lambda_z(t))^2\right]. \tag{7.3}$$

Following Miki *et al.* [157], the geometric hystersis curve may be formally described by the function $S(t)/V(t) = f(V(t))$. Using the two equations above, and dropping the variable t for clarity, yields the ratio:

$$\frac{S}{V} \propto \left[(x_0\lambda_x)^2 + (y_0\lambda_y)^2 + (z_0\lambda_z)^2\right]^{-1/2}. \tag{7.4}$$

Substituting for $V(t)$ into the above yields $S/V \propto V^{-1/3}$ (for a sphere, $S/V = KV^{-1/3}$ with $K = 3/(3/(4\pi))^{1/3}$). This result suggests that if breathing is defined by cyclic length scaling functions solely

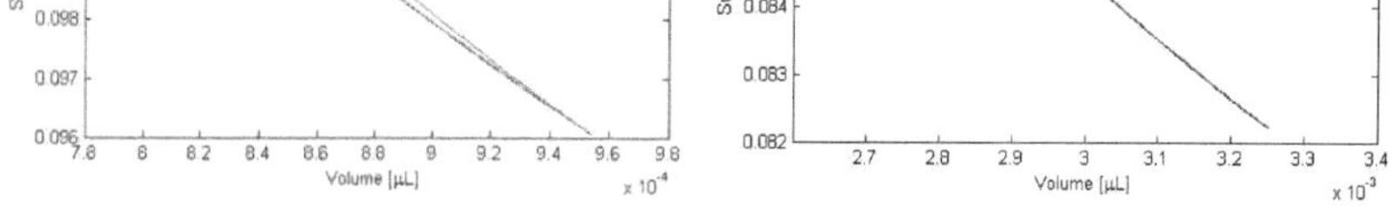

(a) (b)

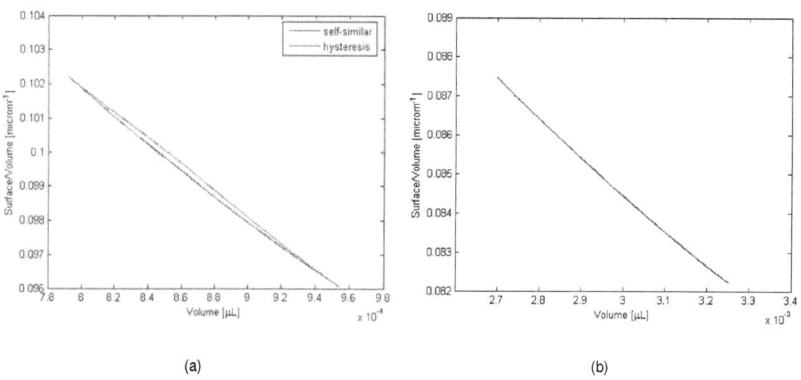

Figure 7.6: Plot of function $S(t)/V(t) = f(V(t))$ exhibiting no hysteresis, for self-similar cases in geometry (a) I and (b) II, between inspiration and expiration. For geometry I, implementing a phase shift, α, in the kinematic wall motion over the expiration phase effectively generates a degree of geometric hysteresis ($\approx 10^o$).

dependant on time, t, geometric hysteresis cannot be kinematically achieved. Any point within the volume, or at its boundary, retraces during expiration, the same path traced during inspiration. Therefore, a time-dependent kinematic scaling function (and not spatially dependent) will result exclusively in self-similar motion. Furthermore, during inspiration, as the volume V increases, the function S/V must be monotonically decreasing, following $S/V \propto V^{-1/3}$ (see Fig. 7.6(b)).

Kinematics of Geometric Hysteresis

Based on the above result for self-similarity, we now introduce both a temporal and spatial dependency in the wall motion. While the possibilities to create cyclic wall kinematic displacement functions exhibiting a degree of geometrical hysteresis are vast, we will restrict our simple displacement model to fulfill the following considerations: 1) the actual variation of lung volume with respect to time is not perfectly sinusoidal but rather slightly asymmetrical. While the inspiration phase resembles closely a sinusoidal function, the expiration curve, in contrast, has a steeper (negative) gradient during its initial phase [193]. 2) The amount of geometric hysteresis observed experimentally lies approximately around 10° [157,271]. 3) The total volume at the beginning and the end of each breathing cycle must be equal, $V(t=0) = V(t=T)$. 4) The wall displacement function should avoid any spatial as well as temporal discontinuities. Indeed, spatial discontinuities may lead to angular edges or even holes in the alveolar walls, while temporal discontinuities will create abrupt jumps in the alveolar wall displacements. 5) Finally, the displacement function should be able to run over cumulative breathing cycles, namely $t = nT$, where $n = 1, 2, ..., \infty$.

To fulfill the above conditions in a simple manner, the phase shift, introduced in Eq. (7.1), is described as follows:

$$\alpha(\underline{x}, t) = g(t) \cdot h(t) \cdot \alpha'(\underline{x}). \tag{7.5}$$

The phase shift, $\alpha(\underline{x}, t)$, is constructed of two parts: a temporal component, $g(t) \cdot h(t)$, and a spatial component $\alpha'(\underline{x})$. To model the asymmetry during respiration, we first assume that the inspiration phase is sinusoidal and self-similar, such that $\alpha(\underline{x}, t) = 0$ over the interval $nT \leq t \leq (T/2 + nT)$ with $n = 0, 1, 2, ..., \infty$. To fulfill the asymmetry condition, we make use of the Heaviside step function (also known as "unit step function") expressed as [1]:

$$g(t) = \begin{cases} 0, & \sin(2\pi f t - \pi) < 0, \\ 1, & \sin(2\pi f t - \pi) > 0. \end{cases} \tag{7.6}$$

Therefore, the function yields $g(t) = 0$ over the interval $nT \leq t \leq (T/2 + nT)$ and $g(t) = 1$ over the interval $(T/2 + nT) \leq t \leq (T + nT)$. The function $h(t)$ is responsible for eliminating the discontinuity generated at the transition between inspiration and expiration, occurring at the jump between values of 0 and 1 of the step function $g(t)$, and is defined as:

$$h(t) = \frac{1}{2} + \frac{1}{2} \sin\left(4\pi f t - \frac{\pi}{2}\right). \tag{7.7}$$

An illustration of the temporal component, $g(t) \cdot h(t)$, of $\alpha(\underline{x}, t)$ is shown in Fig. 7.7, over two breathing cycles. In the work of Miki *et al.* [157], a precise description of the local alveolar wall motion is not available but rather, macroscopic geometric hysteresis is observed. Therefore, geometric hysteresis may be kinematically modelled in various ways. For analytical simplicity, we impose a spatial component, $\alpha'(\underline{x})$, solely dependent on one direction, namely x, and thus make use of the y–z symmetry plane in the reconstructed XTM alveolar airspaces (see results in section 7.4). While reducing the analytical complexity of the phase shift, $\alpha(\underline{x},t)$, the spatial component, $\alpha'(\underline{x})$, assures, nevertheless, the kinematic existence of geometric hysteresis.

Pragmatically, the spatial component, $\alpha'(\underline{x})$, is implemented such that along the centerline of the geometry at $x = 0$, the wall displacement during expiration is phase shifted relative to the outer regions of the geometry, $x = \pm x_{max}$, where x_{max} is the maximal distance from the origin in the x-direction. Furthermore, for simplicity, we assume that the spatial component, $\alpha'(\underline{x})$, takes a simple linear form such that:

$$\alpha'(x) = \alpha_{max} + \frac{\alpha_{max}}{|x_{max}|} - step(x)\frac{2\alpha_{max}}{|x_{max}|}, \tag{7.8}$$

where α_{max} is the maximal phase shift and $step(x)$ is a Heaviside step function. Therefore, the maximal phase shift, α_{max}, is located at $x = 0$ and will occur at $t = n \cdot 3T/4$, through the implementation of $g(t) \cdot h(t)$, which corresponds to the maximum expiratory velocity. The minimal phase shift at location $x = \pm x_{max}$ for any time t is given by $\alpha(x = \pm x_{max}, t) = 0$. A representation of the phase shift, $\alpha(\underline{x},t)$ (Eq. (7.5)), obtained through the multiplication of Eqs. (7.6), (7.7), and (7.8), is illustrated in Fig. 7.8 at inspiration and at expiration time $t = 3T/4$, with $\alpha_{max} = \pi/9$. Thus, at any time, t, during expiration, the function $\alpha(\underline{x},t)$ has the shape of a triangular saw tooth whose peak at $x = 0$ varies between 0 and α_{max} over the interval $t = (T/2 + nT) \leq t \leq (T + nT)$. On average then, the phase shift obtained is on the order of 10°, as suggested by Miki *et al.* [157]. An illustration of the resulting geometric hysteresis, formally represented by values of the ratio S/V plotted with respect to V over the breathing cycle, is given in Fig. 7.6(a).

7.3.1 Numerical Methods

The numerical methods follow closely the description given in section 5.7 for the simple alveolated duct model. At the entrance of the reconstructed alveolar airspaces (see Fig. 7.9), an additional duct was

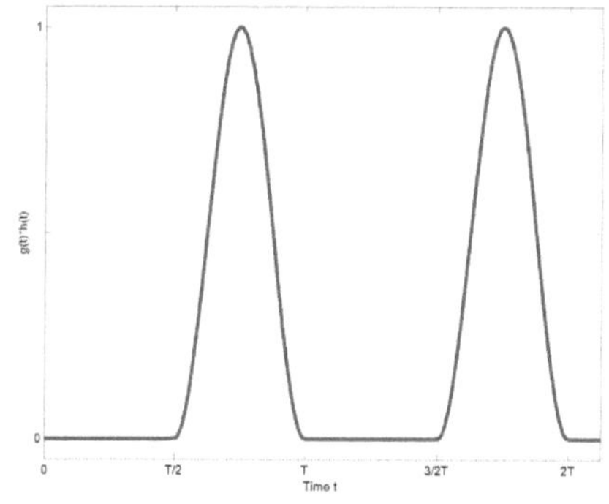

Figure 7.7: Time-dependent component of the phase shift, α, obtained through the multiplicative function, $g(t) \cdot h(t)$, of Eqs. (7.6) and (7.7).

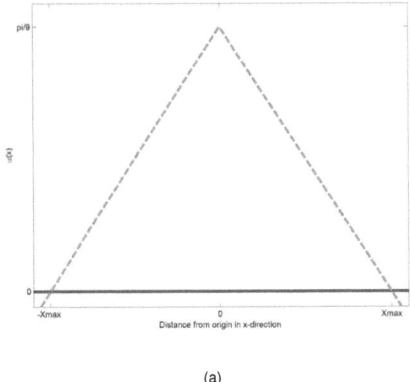

(a)

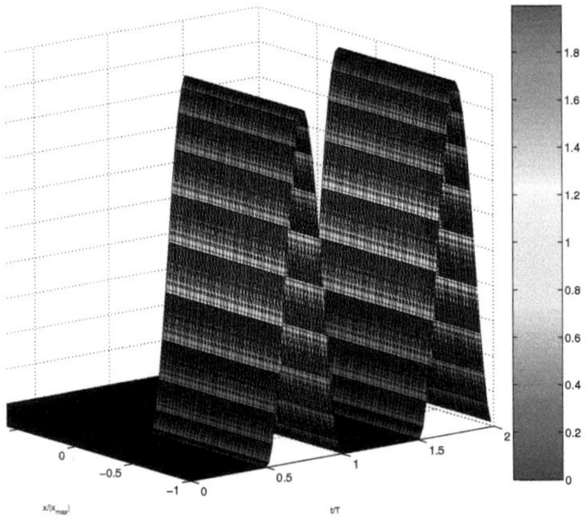

(b)

Figure 7.8: (a) Representation of the phase shift, α, illustrated during inspiration (full line) and at time $t = 3T/4$ (dashed line), which corresponds to maximal expiratory flow. (b) Phase shift, α, as a function of time, t, and spatial location x. Color bar indicates non-dimensional α.

added to guarantee that the effects of the velocity profile on the alveolar flow were negligible. In particular, for low-Reynolds flows in ducts [235], the entrance length, L_e, to achieve fully developed flow was given in Eq. (5.43). Following these considerations, the entrance ducts of the reconstructed airspaces were conservatively designed with $L \geq D$, where L is the length of the entrance duct (thus, $L > L_e$), and the original dimensions of the alveolar airspace opening are approximately $D \approx 55 - 60$ μm (the duct cross-section is not perfectly circular, see Fig. 7.9). Therefore, the entrance length of the duct feeding the flow into the alveolar airspace guaranteed that the influence of the velocity profiles on the flow within the airspace were negligible (see results in section 7.4).

For each alveolar sac geometry (see results in section 7.4), an unstructured hybrid mesh was generated consisting of prisms and tetrahedron volume elements. The first alveolar sac geometry (geometry I, Fig. 7.11 (b)) consisted of approximately 280'000 volume elements, corresponding to an initial volume at $t = 0$ of approximately 0.8×10^{-3} μl, while the larger alveolar sac (geometry II, Fig. 7.11 (c)) consisted of approximately 600'000 volume elements for an initial volume of approximately 2.7×10^{-3} μl. For rhythmic wall motion, displacement gradients near the wall called for an accurately fitted grid in the direction perpendicular to the wall to avoid unfavorable velocity angles between velocity vectors and vectors normal to the cell surfaces. Therefore, volume elements consisting of layers of prisms were employed to improve the resolution of the flow in the vicinity of the wall (Fig. 7.9). Simulations were performed to ensure that the flow solutions were grid independent and converged, by performing a mesh refinement study. For this, we increased the density of volume elements in a specified alveolus (see bottom right region of Fig 7.11 (b)) by approximately 200% above the value which was eventually used. Since the reconstructed alveolar sac geometries employed are symmetrical along the y–z plane (see results in section 7.4), resulting flows were compared between the more densely meshed alveolus and the benchmark one. No noticeable changes were observed between the symmetrical alveolar flows, for the computational mesh eventually used. Furthermore, to achieve sufficiently accurate results such that changes in the resulting entrance flow Reynolds number were within $< 5\%$ upon further time step refinement, a time step of $\Delta t = 0.05T = 0.002$ s was eventually implemented.

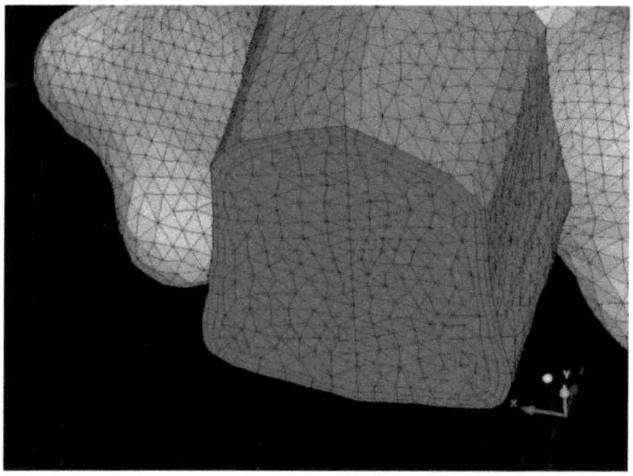

Figure 7.9: Close-up of the entrance duct for the alveolar airspace geometry I (Fig. 7.11 (b)) illustrating the use of three prism layers near the wall (here shown at the duct entrance) for improved near wall flow resolution.

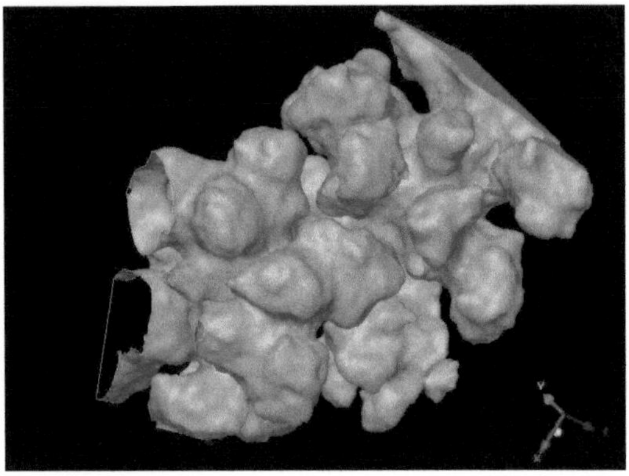

Figure 7.10: Three-dimensional alveolar airspaces reconstructed from X-ray tomographic microscopy (XTM). Typical alveolar diameters for the 10 days old mouse, as obtained from counting voxels and multiplying values with the spatial scale (1.4 μm), range between 15 μm and 40 μm. Alveolar airspaces consist of cavities with complex geometries, which outer surfaces are composed of polygonal planes.

7.4 Results

7.4.1 3D Alveolar Geometries

A typical example of a reconstructed terminal alveolar airspace is shown in Fig. 7.10. While the reconstruction steps yield recognizable alveolar structures, an adequate and bounded flow domain must be determined for respiratory CFD simulation purposes. To achieve this, we sought to minimize any distortion in the reconstructed geometries and preserve at best the geometry in its original configuration. However, the 3D reconstruction of a complete multi-generation pulmonary acinar airspace branching tree remained beyond the current capabilities. This was a direct consequence of the first restriction imposed through the extraction of a subset from the original XTM stack largely intended to limit the computational costs for flow simulation. Furthermore, the search for an optimal threshold value for air-tissue separation, as well as the presence of intrinsic noise in the raw data and the subsequent smoothing steps, slightly influenced the topology of the reconstructed geometry. Finally, the low contrast in the raw XTM images acted largely as an additional barrier to the possible reconstruction of an entirely connected acinar airspace branching tree.

With such restrictions in mind, we limited the scope of the study, for the present time, to respiratory flow simulations in reconstructed terminal alveolar airspaces (i.e. alveolar sacs), as schematically shown in Fig. 7.11(a). We reconstructed two distinct alveolar sac geometries of variable size and complexity (geometry I is slightly smaller than geometry II, see section 7.3.1), as illustrated in Figs. 7.11(b) and (c). These geometries consisted of clusters of alveolar airspaces obtained directly from the three-dimensional XTM reconstruction, as shown in the example of Fig. 7.10. Nevertheless, these geometries originally exhibited artificial planes near the domain boundaries, resulting from the combination of the 3D reconstruction steps, the separation of air volumes, and the presence of the exterior bounding box. To

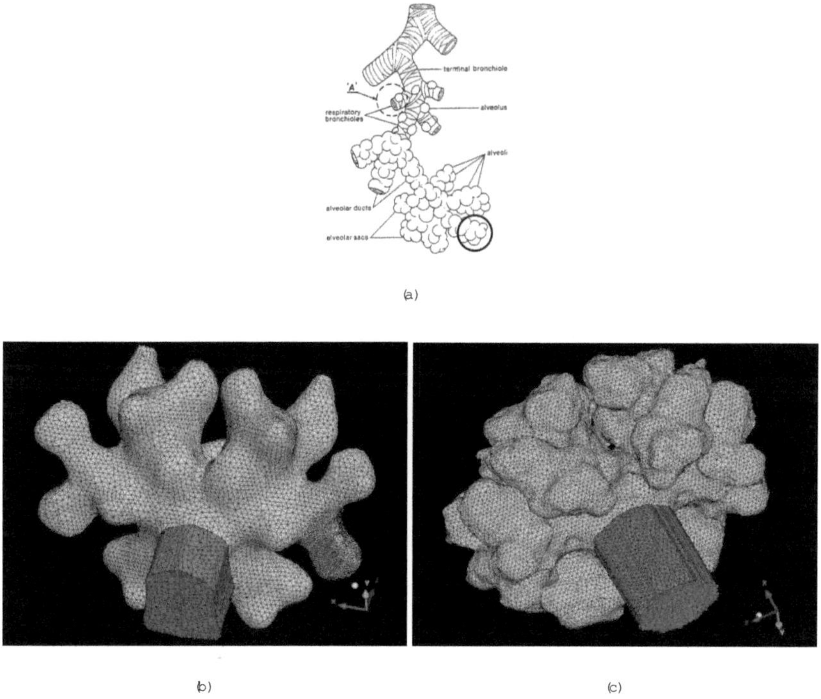

Figure 7.11: (a) Schematic representation of the pulmonary acinus as depicted in [88], with the location of an alveolar sac identified (circle). Resulting meshes for the reconstructed three-dimensional alveolar sacs are illustrated for (b) geometry I and (c) II. Both geometries are characterized by the existence of symmetry planes and the presence of a short entrance duct feeding the alveolar space (shown in a distinct color). Geometry I is composed of approximately 280'000 volume elements and geometry II, approximately 600'000 elements. Note in the right side region of Geometry I (b) the densely meshed alveolus employed for the mesh refinement study.

solve this problem, the alveolar geometries were mirrored about such planes and connected along the mirrored surfaces to obtain a fully bounded flow domain. This way, airflow into and out of the alveolar space could be generated entirely through respiratory wall motion without prescribing any additional flow assumptions. To provide an airflow passage with the external environment, a short duct was added to allow fluid to be fed into the reconstructed alveolar airspace (Figs. 7.9 and 7.11 (b) and (c)). A surface from the original opening in the alveolar sac geometries was extruded and connected to the entrance of the domain (details on duct design with respect to flow considerations are given in section 7.3.1).

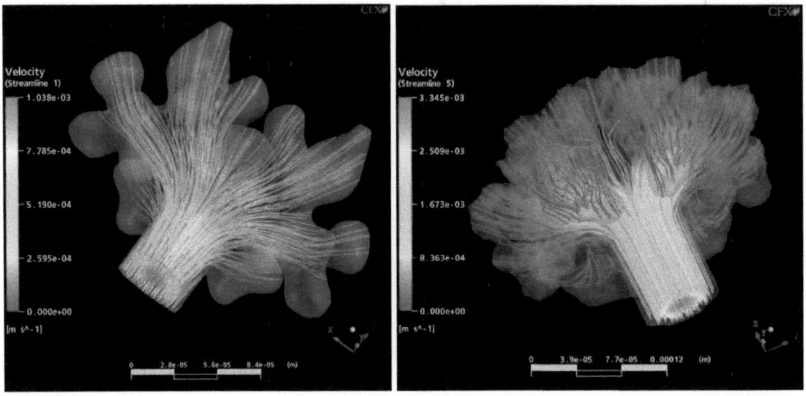

(a) (b)

Figure 7.12: Illustration of instantaneous alveolar stream lines with velocity field magnitude in three-dimensional space, obtained at peak inspiration ($t = 0.1$ s) in alveolar sac geometries (a) I and (b) II. Color bar on left denotes velocity magnitude in [m/s].

7.4.2 Flow Patterns

Alveolar flow patterns were first computed under self-similar breathing conditions for both alveolar sac geometries I (Fig. 7.11 (b)) and II (Fig. 7.11 (c)). The resulting three-dimensional stream lines with corresponding velocity magnitudes are illustrated at peak inspiration ($t = 0.1$ s) in Figs. 7.12 (a) and (b), for each geometry, respectively. The resulting flow topology in both alveolar sacs is highly similar, despite variations in the complexity of the geometries. Namely, stream lines are essentially radial, filling individual alveoli. Indeed, rhythmic wall expansion generates stream lines originating from the duct opening and reaching to the alveolar walls, as fluid is dragged into the cavities by creating a negative pressure gradient through wall displacement. Hence, flow at the duct entrance rapidly exhibits a fully developed parabolic profile, and entrance effects due to velocity profiles are avoided. Following conservation of mass, the velocity along stream lines within the alveolar cavities sharply decreases as the fluid travels further into the alveolar sac. The Reynolds numbers defined at the duct entrance yield a mean value of $\overline{Re} \approx 0.001$ and $\overline{Re} \approx 0.0035$, for geometry I and II respectively, as illustrated in Fig 7.13 (locally the flow reaches a maximum velocity at the duct entrance ranging from approximately 1 to 3.4 mm/s, for geometry I and II respectively). Under such flow conditions, alveolar flow in the last generation of the pulmonary acinus is governed by Stokes flow (see description in section 3.3.1), where inertial effects are negligible. The overall flow topology is driven predominantly by the basic rhythmical wall motion and to a much lesser extent, by the detailed alveolar geometry. As expected, self-similar wall motion does not exhibit characteristics of geometric hysteresis (Fig. 7.6 (b)). Wall reversibility induces a prescribed curve which follows $S/V \propto V^{-1/3}$, as described earlier in section 7.3.

Flow patterns were further examined at several different oscillation points (Fig 7.14). Regardless of

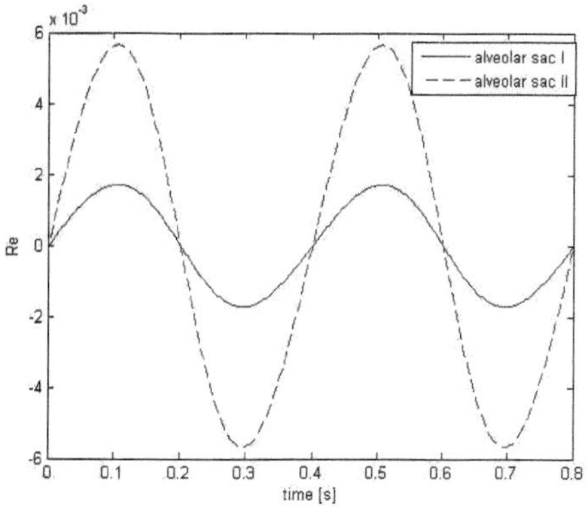

Figure 7.13: Time dependent Reynolds number, Re, defined at duct entrance, plotted over two breathing cycles for alveolar sac geometries I and II, respectively, under self-similar wall motion.

the instantaneous Re number that spanned from zero to a maximum of $Re \approx 0.002$ (geometry I) and $Re \approx 0.006$ (geometry II), the flow topology did not change appreciably throughout the breathing cycle, suggesting that the basic flow characteristics are insensitive to global Re effects. This follows from the small values of the Womersley numbers obtained, with $\overline{Wo} \approx 0.02$ for both geometries, suggesting that flow phenomenon in alveolar sacs is indeed quasi-steady. At flow reversal, when $\underline{u}(\underline{x}, t = 0.2s) \rightarrow 0$ over the entire domain under Stokes' flow conditions, slight alterations in the local flow patterns were suggested, in particular near the alveolar walls where closed streamlines were seen visible. For the alveolar sac (geometry I), we further examined the effects of imposing a phase shift, $\alpha(\underline{x}, t)$, during the expiration phase, on the flow patterns (Fig. 7.6 (a)). Although the sinusoidal volume change over time exhibits a degree of asymmetry (Fig. 7.16), with a steeper gradient in the expiratory phase [193], and correspondingly, an appreciable geometric hysteresis is kinematically generated in the S/V loop (Fig. 7.6 (a)), no noticeable differences were, however, noted in the resulting flow patterns. Therefore, whether geometric hysteresis was imposed or self-similarity was preserved over the entire breathing cycle, flow patterns at expiration remain largely identical to those at inspiration, for the low Reynolds boundary-driven cavity flows generated here.

7.5 Discussion

7.5.1 General Feasibility

With the present study, we have first shown that it is, in principle, not only feasible to reconstruct 3D alveolar airspaces but also to conduct small-scale acinar flow simulations with the use of anatomically based three-dimensional image reconstruction, provided that high spatial resolution imaging techniques are available. Here, XTM images were employed with a planar resolution of $1.4\ \mu m \times 1.4\ \mu m \times 1.4\ \mu m$.

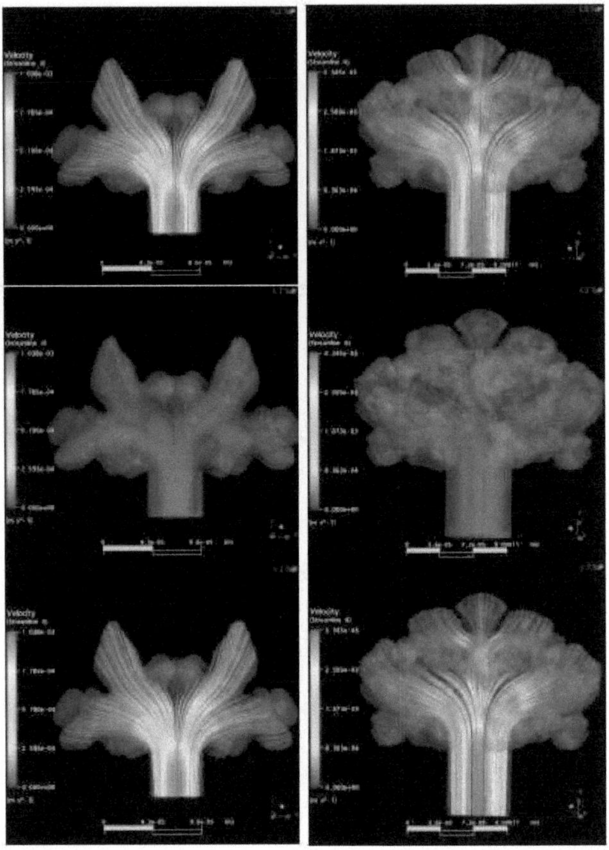

Figure 7.14: Two-dimensional stream lines with velocity field magnitude obtained along symmetry plane in alveolar sac geometry I (left column) and II (right column) for different oscillation points in the breathing cycle. Color bar on left denotes velocity magnitude in [m/s].

XTM offers a reliable technique which in fact yields possibly even lower spatial resolutions (< 1 μm) [253], and thus, may perhaps open the path towards even more structurally detailed reconstructed geometries. Furthermore, acinar flow simulations could now be foreseeable using reconstructed geometries from samples of human pulmonary acini instead. However, as mentioned earlier, two major barriers must be overcome to obtain in the future more reliable 3D alveolar geometries and hence acinar flow simulations. Intrinsic noise (Fig. 7.4) and low intensity contrast (Fig. 7.3) observed in the raw XTM images, combined with the standard reconstruction schemes, impede to a large extent the successful generation of a

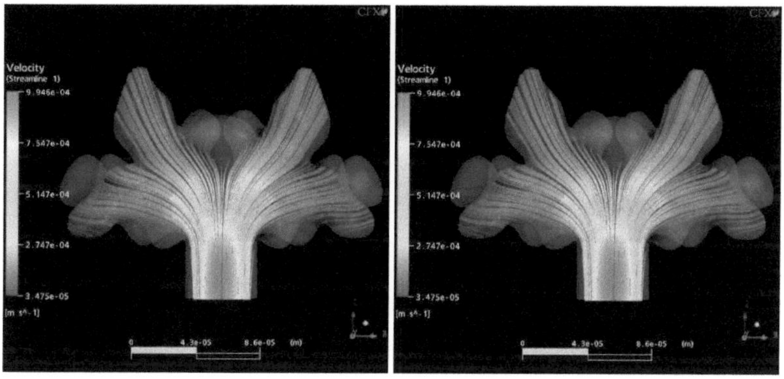

(a) (b)

Figure 7.15: Comparison between two-dimensional stream lines with velocity field magnitude obtained along symmetry plane in alveolar sac geometry I for the (a) self-similar wall expansion case and (b) the geometric hysteresis case, at peak expiration ($t = 0.3$ s). Color bar on left denotes velocity magnitude in [m/s].

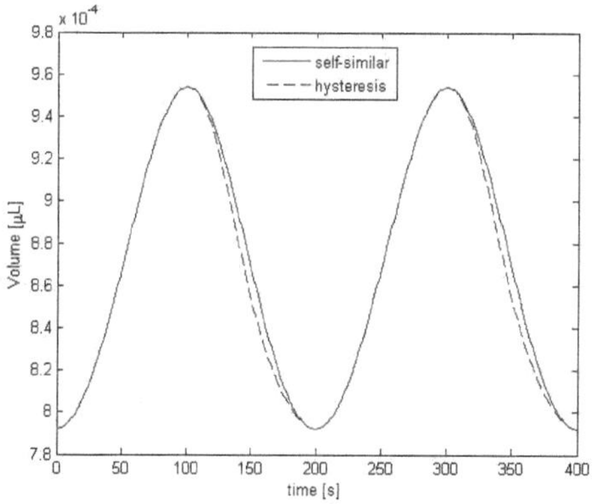

Figure 7.16: Evolution of total alveolar sac volume (geometry I) over 2 breathing cycles under self-similar wall motion (full line) and wall motion with geometric hysteresis (dashed line). Note the steeper (negative) gradient in the expiratory phase under geometric hysteresis.

complete multi-generation pulmonary acinar tree. Moreover, computational costs linked with increasing geometry and mesh sizes continue to represent a potential burden towards full-scale acinar flow simulations. Therefore, flow simulations have been limited, here, to sub-regions extracted from XTM image stacks, thought to coincide with the last generation of the acinar tree, namely the alveolar sacs. While this study remains a first step towards a wider use of anatomically based reconstructed acinar geometries in respiratory CFD simulations, our preliminary flow results deliver, nevertheless, some useful insights into alveolar fluid dynamics. Furthermore, they confirm results from earlier studies with geometrical alveolated duct models.

Before discussing our flow results in more detail, we open a short parenthesis on the actual reconstructed alveolar airspaces. It is perhaps interesting to note that the reconstructed 3D alveoli (Figs. 7.10 and 7.11 (b) and (c)) do not form tightly bounded space-filling foam-like structures [71,138,201] as one may typically expect (compare space-filling model of Fig. 6.4). This intuitively results from the fact that our reconstructed geometries are constituted of alveolar airspaces only. Indeed, the reconstruction of alveolar septum was disregarded for flow simulation purposes (see section 7.2.2). Therefore, individual alveolar airspaces cannot lie in direct contact with their neighbors due to the finite thickness of the alveolar septum separating each alveolar cavity. However, the relatively large distances qualitatively observed, separating individual alveoli, may arise from additional factors. During lung development [220], the alveolar septa of a mouse are relatively thicker at 10 days old than for an adult [18,210], yielding effectively a relative increase in the space separating each alveolar cavity. Furthermore, the global threshold value chosen during segmentation may slightly increase the alveolar wall thickness to avoid the generation of artificial holes in the alveolar septum.

Finally, one must consider the possibility of artificial changes in the tissue dimensions occurring with preparation. Indeed, the influence of fixing, dehydrating, and embedding agents may introduce some changes in dimensions of lung tissue structures from the fresh to the processed specimen. However, as shown in a previous study [283], shrinking of the specimen may be on the order of approximately 5%, which remains largely negligible. Consequently, we believe that the final shape of the reconstructed airspaces was not substantially influenced by the specimen preparation.

7.5.2 Flows in Alveolar Sacs

Flow topology in the deepest regions of the pulmonary acinus (i.e. alveolar sacs) is characterized by low-Reynolds boundary driven cavity flows, governed by creeping motion under quasi-steady conditions. In particular, flows in reconstructed alveolar sacs exhibit purely radial streamlines (Fig. 7.12 (a) and (b)). It is in fact the basic wall expansion/contraction motion, under low Re and Wo numbers flow conditions, which is the driving mechanism governing flow phenomenon at this scale, as suggested in previous studies [29,47,270] and shown earlier in the distal regions (i.e. generation 8 of the acinus) for the simple alveolated duct (see section 5.8.3). This is first intuitively understood by the fact that if no wall motion were generated, the existence of alveolar flows, and hence respiration, would be prohibited. Furthermore, subtle changes in wall motion, induced through kinematic phase shifts illustrating a small degree of geometric hysteresis, result in inconspicuous changes in flow patterns compared with the principal, self-similar mode of lung expansion (Fig. 7.15). Our results also show that flows in terminal alveolar airspaces is largely insensitive to the relative complexity in the alveolar geometries, as flow patterns remain essentially similar (i.e. radial) at all oscillation times for both alveolar sac geometries I and II. This observation is further confirmed with the use of simplified geometrical models as seen in

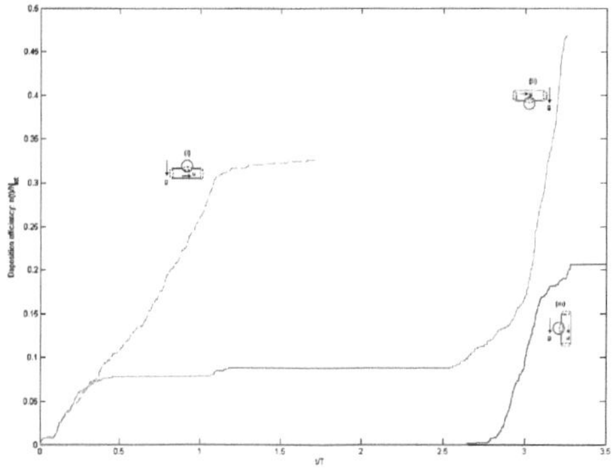

(a)

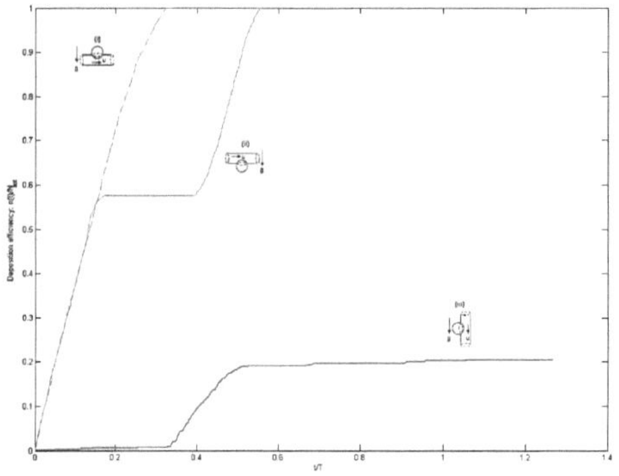

(b)

Figure 7.17: Influence of gravity orientation (cases (i)–(iii)) on deposition efficiency, $n(t)/N$, as a function of normalized time, t/T, for (a) 1 and (b) 3 μm diameter particles in the simple alveolated duct model at generation 8 of the pulmonary acinus.

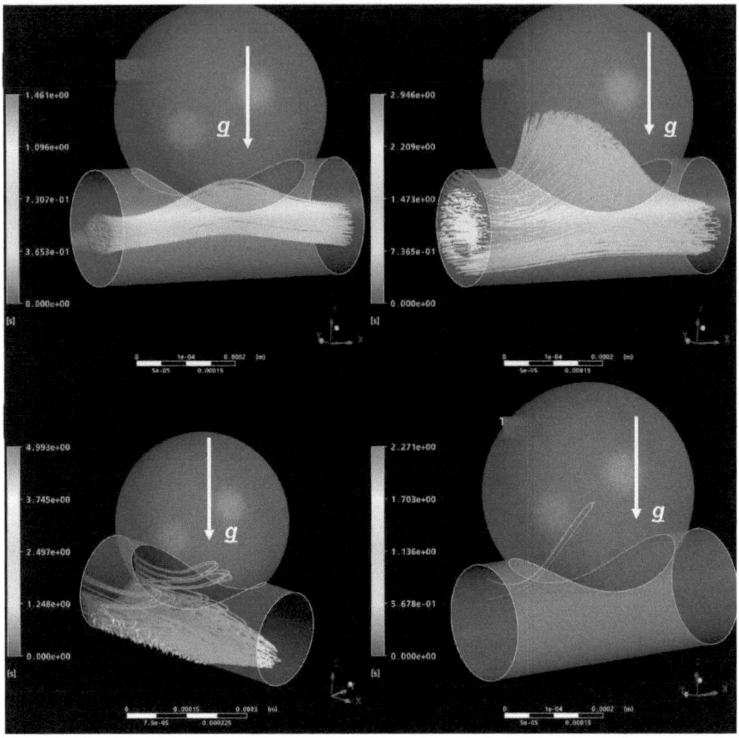

Figure 7.18: Examples of 1 μm particle trajectories for gravity orientation of case (i) depicted schematically in Fig. 7.17 (a), illustrating particle residence time in seconds. Top left: Particles convected out of the computational domain at distal end of duct. Top Right: Particles convected back out of the domain through the duct inlet within the end of the first inhalation phase. Bottom left: Examples of particles sedimenting at bottom of duct. Bottom right: Example of single particle trajectory entering and then exiting the alveolus.

chapter 5 (see Fig. 5.10 depicting flows in generation 8). Indeed, under physiologically relevant flow conditions in terminal acinar generations, radial alveolar flow patterns are well captured using simple spherical alveolar cavity models [47,97,270]. Our results obtained with reconstructed XTM geometries, therefore, point towards the relevance of acinar flow studies using simplified acinar structures. It is indeed the basic existence of wall motion in a cavity which characterizes the general alveolar flow topology at such low Reynolds numbers.

Based on our simulations, the existence of complex alveolar flows, described by the presence of recirculation regions with stagnation saddle points leading to chaotic flow behavior [87,270,272], seems to be confined to more proximal generations of the pulmonary acinar tree. For flow separation and recirculation regions to occur in alveolar cavities, the existence of a relatively strong shear flow arising in the alveolar

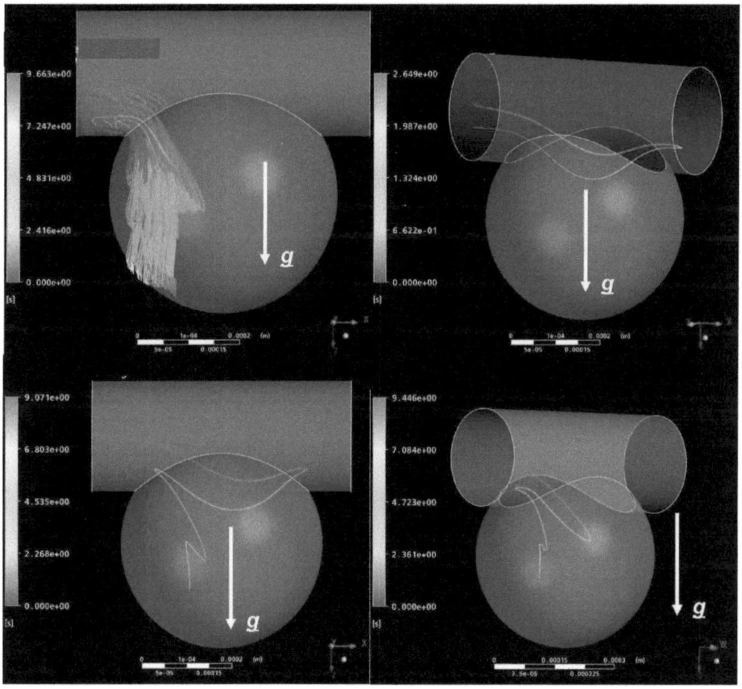

Figure 7.19: Examples of 1 μm particle trajectories for gravity orientation of case (ii) depicted schematically in Fig. 7.17 (a), illustrating particle residence time in seconds. Top left: Particles deposited inside the alveolus after long residence times ($t > 3T$). Top Right: Example of a particle convected back out of the domain through the duct inlet within the end of the first inhalation phase. Second and third rows: Examples of individual particles depositing within the alveolus.

duct and passing over an alveolar opening is required. Such ductal flows are relatively stronger in more proximal regions of the acinar tree, since they feed the entire network of distal airways and alveoli located downstream. This is well captured in the relatively low values of the ratio, $\dot{Q}_a/\dot{Q}_T$, describing acinar flows in geometrical models of alveolar ducts located in proximal generations (see sections 5.8.1 and 6.4.2). In contrast, flow topology in the deeper acinar generations is characterized by the prevalence of radial flows induced by wall expansion captured in relatively larger values of the ratio. In particular, alveoli located in alveolar sacs do not cover per se a duct, but rather, they form a closed end chamber. Therefore, ductal shear flow cannot exist there due to the specific spatial configuration of the deepest acinar region.

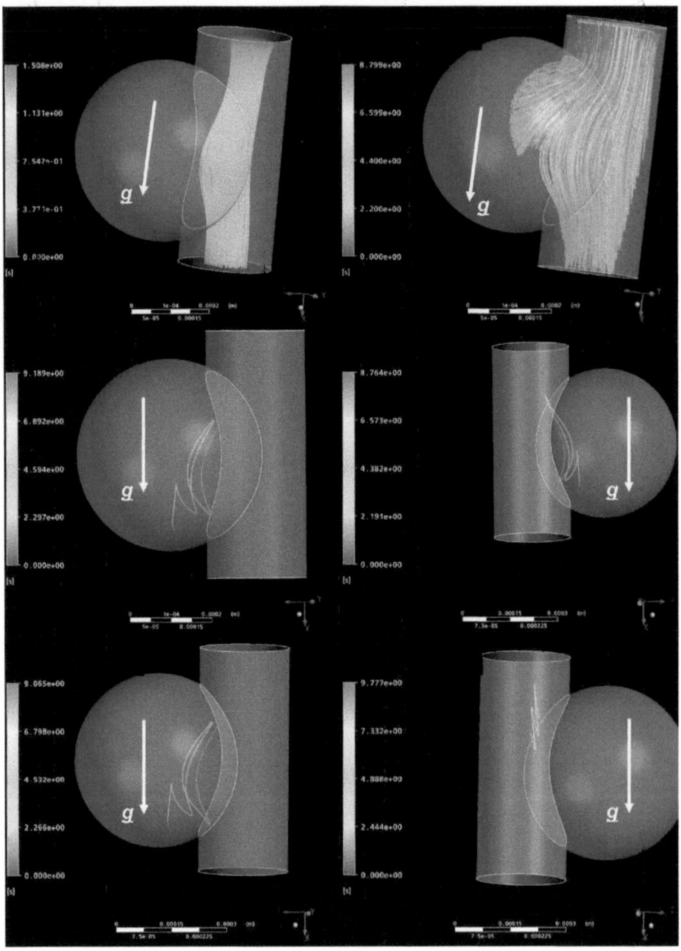

Figure 7.20: Examples of 1 μm particle trajectories for gravity orientation of case (iii) depicted schematically in Fig. 7.17 (a), illustrating particle residence time in seconds. Top left: Particles convected out of the domain through the duct outlet. Top Right: Particles convected back out of the domain through the duct inlet. Bottom left and right: Examples of individual particles sedimenting within the alveolus.

7.6 Deposition in a Simple Alveolated Duct: Generation 8

As discussed earlier, our results for flow patterns obtained in reconstructed XTM alveolar sacs (see Fig. 7.12 and section 7.4.2) illustrate strong similarities with flow patterns obtained in generation 8 of the simple alveolated duct model (compare with Fig. 5.10 from section 5.8.3). Namely, flows are radial and governed by the wall motion of the alveolar walls. For this reason, we have investigated the transport and deposition, under different orientations of gravity, of 1 and 3 μm inhaled particles in the simple alveolated duct model (see chapter 5) at generation 8 of the pulmonary acinus (dimensions are given in Table 5.2). Numerical methods are detailed in section 6.3 and the theory for particle motion is given explicitly in section 6.3.2. Here, the mesh of the alveolated duct model at generation 8 is made up of approximately 700'000 unstructured (tetra- and hexahedron-) volume elements and flow conditions at the duct inlet ($\overline{Re} = 0.005$) were derived earlier in section 5.5 for quiet tidal breathing. For both particle sizes (1 and 3 μm), three different orientations of gravity with respect to the duct geometry were investigated, as discussed in detail in chapter 6 (cases (i) through (iii)) for the simple alveolate duct of generation 5 (see section 6.4.1). We describe briefly the resulting aerosol kinematics including deposition efficiencies in what follows.

Aerosol Kinematics: 1 μm Particles

Although the flow topology resulting within the alveolus of generation 8 (see Fig. 5.10 of chapter 5) is fundamentally different from the one observed in generation 5 (see Fig. 5.8), aerosol kinematics of 1 μm particles seen in generation 8 preserve many features described earlier for generation 5. In particular, independent of the orientation of gravity considered, fine 1 μm aerosols are subject to the influence of the local alveolar flow structure. Again, the precise motion of these aerosols is mainly influenced by the coupling between flow reversal effects due to oscillatory breathing, the local convective alveolar flow structure, and small but significant sedimentation mechanisms leading to effective streamline crossing. These combined mechanisms may yield again examples of 3D particle trajectories exhibiting irreversible twisting and undulating motions, with characteristic oscillating paths observed earlier for instance in case (ii) of generation 5 (Fig. 6.6). However, since the ductal flow is considerably weaker in generation 8 of the acinus compared to the one resulting in generation 5, fine aerosols may illustrate much longer residence times in the bulk of the acinar airspace ($t \sim 3T$, see Fig. 7.17 (a)), specifically in cases (ii) and (iii). These comparatively slower acinar flows in generation 8 yield enough time to obtain higher deposition efficiencies ($n(t)/N \sim 0.2$–0.5, depending on the case considered), since airflow does not convect particles out of the domain as quickly as in generation 5.

Looking at each gravity orientation case individually, we see that case (i) of generation 8 illustrates a deposition efficiency curve profile qualitatively analogous to the one seen both in laminar horizontal pipe flow (see Appendix D) and in generation 5 (Fig. 6.5 (a)). This observation results from the fine particles which deposit on the walls of the duct, rather than inside the alveolus. In contrast, however, the deposition efficiencies obtained are higher in case (i) of generation 8 ($n(t)/N \approx 0.3$). However, they are reached over much longer respiratory times ($t > T$). Figure 7.18 illustrates examples of individual particle trajectories obtained in generation 8 for case (i). While a large portion of particles is convected through the duct outlet, fine aerosols which are radially transported into the alveolar cavity during the inhalation phase follow a nearly reversible trajectory back out (although a small amount of streamline crossing due to gravity does operate, in particular at times approaching flow reversal). Hence, deposition

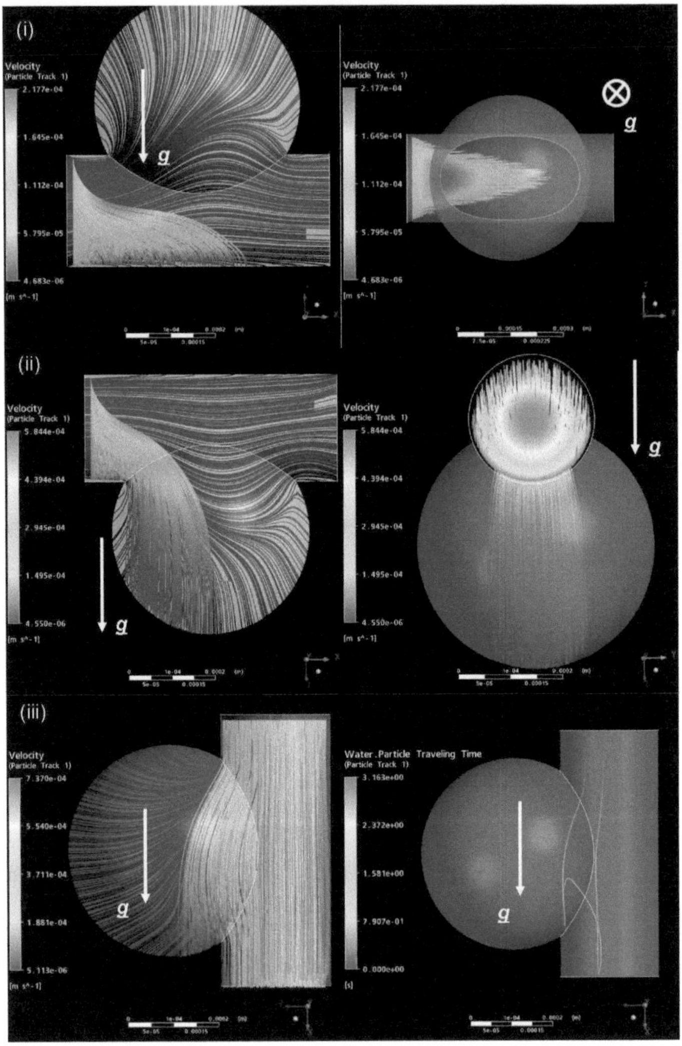

Figure 7.21: 3 μm particle trajectories, with velocity magnitude (scale in m/s) along trajectories (particle residence time is illustrated in the bottom right in seconds). Cases (i)–(iii) correspond to cases (i)–(iii) illustrated in Fig. 7.17 (b).

occurs solely at the bottom of the duct.

In contrast, cases (ii) and (iii) exhibit particle deposition inside the alveolus (after long residence times). This is again due to the specific gravity orientation which enables particles to be ultimately "trapped" within the alveolar cavity, due to the slow convective flows and small effects of gravitational settling. For example, individual trajectories in case (ii) of generation 8 (see Fig. 7.19) illustrate analogous paths seen earlier in case (ii) of generation 5 (see Fig. 6.6), where particles describe oscillating and undulating trajectories due to the coupled transport mechanisms. It is interesting to note that similar complex trajectories of fine 1 μm aerosols are now observed in case (iii) of generation 8 (see Fig. 7.19), for particles which have entered the alveolar cavity.

Aerosol Kinematics: 3 μm Particles

Results obtained for 3 μm trajectories in the simple alveolated model at generation 8 (Fig. 7.21) compare qualitatively well with findings obtained earlier in generation 5 of the acinus (see discussion in section 6.4.1 and Fig. 6.7). In particular, for cases (i) and (ii), particle trajectories recover those exhibited earlier in generation 5. Namely, aerosols describe characteristic sedimentation profiles, where trajectories are nearly vertical. In case (i), this leads to a deposition pattern similar to the one observed in laminar pipe flow (see Appendix D), where deposition occurs at the bottom of the pipe wall and particles are not influenced by the presence of the alveolus. In case (ii), we observe vertical trajectories inside the alveolus, analogous to the ones observed for the same gravity orientation in the simple alveolated duct model of generation 5. Here again, the alveolar flow is too weak to influence the sedimentation fall of relatively heavy 3 μm particles. Consequently, the curves for deposition efficiencies of 3 μm particles in cases (i) and (ii), shown in Fig. 7.17, illustrate qualitatively similar profiles as those seen earlier in generation 5 (see Fig. 6.5 (b)). However, since ductal flow in generation 8 is relatively weaker than the one occurring in generation 5, particles do not travel quickly enough to exit the flow domain before deposition. Hence, for cases (i) and (ii), efficiencies yield $n(t)/N = 1$ within the end of the first inhalation phase.

For case (iii), aerosol trajectories of 3 μm particles show a generally similar trend to those observed in generation 5. However, since the flow topology within the alveolar cavity of generation 8 is fundamentally different than the one observed in generation 5 (see Fig. 5.8 of chapter 5), the resulting kinematics do in fact differ slightly, despite the identical orientation of gravity with respect to the geometry. In particular, a significant amount of particles enter the alveolar cavity from the duct and sedimentate nearly vertically to deposit on the distal side of the alveolus wall (Fig. 7.21, bottom row). While the bulk of particles is convected out of the computational domain during sedimentation though the duct, deposition efficiency reaches $n(t)/N \approx 0.2$ within $t \approx 1.2T$ (compare with $n(t)/N < 0.05$ in Fig. 6.5 (b)) due to particles deposited inside the alveolus. The profile of the deposition curve obtained for 3 μm aerosols in generation 8 is nevertheless similar to the one observed in generation 5.

Part III

Insights on the Control of Alveolar Flows

Chapter 8

Low-Reynolds Boundary-Driven Cavity Flows in Thin Liquid Shells

Classic examples of low-Reynolds recirculating cavity flows are typically generated from lid-driven boundary motion at a solid-fluid interface, or alternatively result from shear flow over cavity openings. In the present study, we are interested in an original family of boundary-driven cavity flows occurring, in contrast to classic setups, at fluid-fluid interfaces. Particle image velocimetry (PIV) is used to study the structure of internal convective flows observed inside thin liquid shells. Under the specific soap bubble orientation investigated, our results reveal that the liquid shell exhibits motion described by local sporadic "bursts" due to surface tension gradients. These bursts induce transient flows within the cavity on the order of $Re \approx O(1)$. The combination of PIV and proper orthogonal decomposition (POD) is used to extract the dominant flow structures present within bubble cavities. In a subsequent step, we show that thermally-induced Marangoni flows in the liquid shell can lead to forced, (quasi) steady-state recirculating flows inside the cavity, in contrast to the "bursts" observed earlier. In particular, we will show in chapter 10 that the measured planar flow patterns may be captured analytically by considering the solution of the creeping motion equations in the region interior to the sphere. The present findings illustrate an original example of low-Reynolds boundary-driven cavity flows governed by creeping motion.

8.1 Introduction

In classic fluid dynamics examples of cavity flows, flow separation and internal recirculation may be generated by movements of external solid boundaries or fluid shear layers. Such flows may include eddies, secondary flows, complex three-dimensional (3D) patterns, and chaotic particle motions [238]. In the limit of low Reynolds numbers, cavity flows occur under conditions of creeping motion such that their structure is governed by the equations of Stokes flow [181]. Slow internal recirculation may then be induced by the translation of one or more of the containing walls [133,181,237], driven by a shear flow over the cavity [101,239], or generated by the action of surface tension gradients [200]. Experimentally, these reverse and separating flows have drawn considerable interest: from the pioneering photographic visualizations of Taneda [260] to more recent studies using liquid crystal techniques [203] or PIV [174]. While in two-dimensional (2D) rectangular cavities, recirculating Stokes flows may exhibit corner vortices

[236], the extension to 3D shapes involves a number of features that are absent from corresponding 2D motions [266], such as the occurrence of saddle points and the formation of open stream lines, present in recirculating flows in spherical cavities, that spiral into singular points [195].

In analogy to the examples of low-Reynolds flows in cavities with solid boundaries, it is hypothesized that similar internal flow structures may possibly arise within thin liquid shells, such as simple air-filled soap bubbles. Indeed, film dynamics of such liquid shells are influenced, amongst other, by the interaction between (i) liquid thinning under the influence of gravity and (ii) the presence of local surface tension gradients which create flowing fluid layers (i.e. Marangoni flows [231]) in opposite direction to film draining [34,215] (Fig. 8.1). At the interface between the liquid shell and the resident gas, the no-slip boundary condition holds such that internal flows would be induced during the motion of the shell. This would effectively yield an analogous configuration to the one found in lid-driven cavity flows or to Marangoni flow patterns in moving droplets and bubbles under the action of temperature gradients. Such examples of cavity flows illustrating a liquid-gas boundary, rather than a solid-fluid one, are of particular relevance in biological processes. For example, pulmonary alveoli constitute the millions of sub-millimeter gas exchange units necessary for oxygen and carbon-dioxide exchange between the lung and blood capillaries (typical diameter of a human alveolus is $\sim 250\ \mu m$ [90]). These cavities, analogous in some ways to soap bubbles, are lined with a thin aqueous liquid layer containing surfactant ($\approx 0.1 \mu m$ thick [8]), and generate boundary-driven flows during breathing [87].

The present work therefore constitutes a first step in characterizing experimentally boundary-driven cavity flows at a liquid-gas interface, for a given orientation of the liquid shell. Our experimental approach is primarily based on PIV measurements carried out on particle-seeded soap bubbles, where detailed 2D velocity vector maps of the internal airflows are obtained in two different measurement planes. Furthermore, the proper orthogonal decomposition (POD) technique is implemented to identify the dominant structures in the flow carrying the largest portion of energy, by performing a decomposition on the measured fluctuating velocity fields, obtained from PIV data. In a final step, we experimentally illustrate how thermally-induced Marangoni flows can be manipulated to generate forced recirculating motion within the soap bubble cavities. Such low-Reynolds forced cavity flows illustrate experimentally solutions of the creeping motion equations in the region interior to the sphere (see chapter 10).

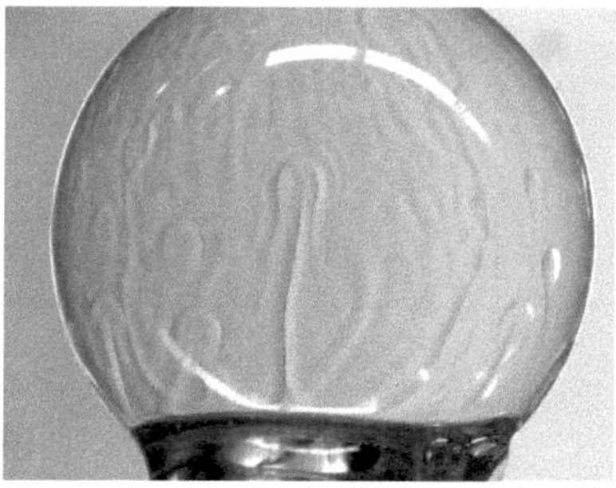

Figure 8.1: Instantaneous photographic visualization of vertical buoyant vortices on the liquid shell of a soap bubble.

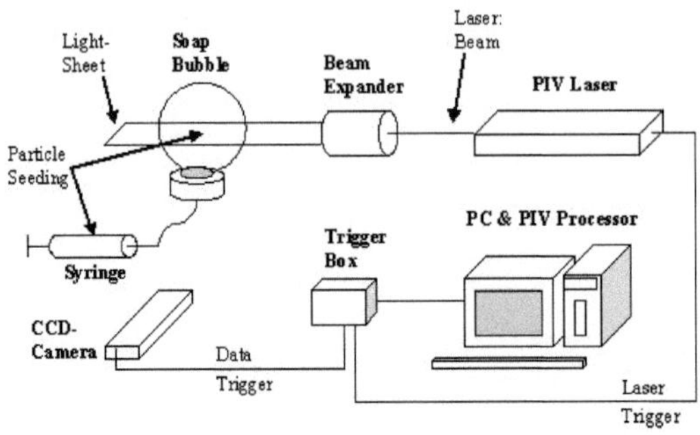

Figure 8.2: Sketch of the experimental setup.

8.2 Experiments and data processing

8.2.1 Experimental setup

A sketch of the experimental setup is depicted in Fig. 8.2. Soap bubbles were generated at an orifice of radius $r_o = 1.5$ mm, by the expansion of a soap film into a thin liquid shell, through the use of a graduated syringe. The radius, R, of the soap bubble may be estimated based on the volume, V, pushed through the syringe using a spherical cap model (see Fig. 8.3). The syringe was filled with smoke particles, or alternatively with oil droplets, such that the cavity flow was effectively seeded. The syringe plunger was slowly displaced with volumes in the range $V = 0.2 - 0.7$ ml, corresponding to bubbles with a radius $R = 3.5 - 5.5$ mm (see Fig. 8.3). The internal pressure within the bubble is slightly greater than the external atmospheric pressure. The pressure difference across the shell may be estimated as $\Delta P = 4\sigma/R$, where σ is the surface tension of the soap film [206]. To increase the stability and life expectancy of the generated soap bubbles (bubbles could be maintained for up to several hours), a mixture composed of 1/3 distilled water, 1/3 commercial liquid detergent, and 1/3 glycerine was used [112]. Typical soap bubbles have a film thickness on the order of 1 μm [112,215]. To avoid draining effects such as soap film accumulating in a pool at the bottom of the shell, bubbles were specifically oriented vertically upwards above a retaining ring with attached drainage reservoir, rather than hanging downwards.

The measuring equipment consisted of a progressive scan CCD camera with 120 Hz image acquisition rate and a resolution of 640×480 pixels (Pulnix TM-6710), equipped with a Nikon macro lens ($f/\# \ 2.8$, $f = 105$ mm). The laser sheet was generated by a 150 mW diode laser (Laseris Inc., Canada) making use of a Powell lens beam expander. Due to the lighting and flow conditions, a pulsed illumination was not required; rather, consecutive images were recorded with an exposure time of $1/120$ s each. To investigate, however, whether a continuous laser illumination scheme induced motion in the liquid shell or in the cavity due to thermal effects, a pulsed illumination approach was also performed using a timing unit (LabSmith LC880 Programmable Experimental Controller). Over the measurement times considered, no significant changes in the bubble motion were observed. In particular, under thermal forcing the characteristic flow patterns observed first with a continuous laser illumination were preserved

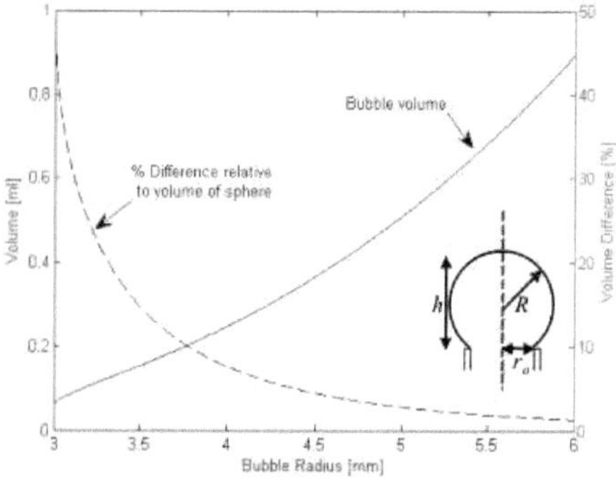

Figure 8.3: Volume, V, of bubble as function of radius R (–); Difference in volume relative to that of a sphere (– –). Inset: spherical cap model. For a soap bubble of height, h, blown at an opening of radius, r_o, the volume, V, of the liquid shell may be described using a spherical cap model such that [96] $V = \pi\left(h^3/6 + hr_o^2/2\right)$, where $h = R + \sqrt{R^2 - r_o^2}$. As can be seen from the figure, for any given bubble radius, R, in the range of volumes considered, the difference in volume relative to that of a sphere, where $V = 4/3\pi R^3$, remains below 10%.

(see section 8.3.3, Fig. 8.14). The soap bubble is geometrically described by a spherical cap and is therefore axisymmetric along the out-of-plane z-axis only. PIV measurements were then conducted for two different planes cutting through the center of the bubble, as illustrated in Fig. 8.4(a): (i) a horizontal x-y plane (top view) and (ii) a vertical x-z plane (side view). The coordinate system was specified, where the origin was placed at the center of the spherical cavity (see Fig. 8.4(b)). Measurements in the horizontal and vertical plane were performed asynchronously.

Planar vector displacement maps in each measurement plane were obtained with a standard PIV algorithm (see Appendix F for a brief overview of the method) based on cross-correlation pattern matching with subpixel interpolation [209]. An interrogation window size of 32×32 pixels was chosen with a maximum window search size in x- and y-direction of 5×5 pixels and a window shift of 16×16 pixels, respectively. Given a CCD size of 640×480 pixels, and an image size of about 108×84 mm (which varied slightly depending on the bubble sizes investigated), the spatial resolution was approximately 0.017 mm and the total number of velocity vectors obtained was approximately ≤ 1000, depending on the measurement plane considered. The exact scaling of the images was made possible by recording before each measurement, the image of a fixed reference scale. The temporal resolution was limited by the image acquisition rate (120 Hz) and series of image pairs were acquired for POD analysis over a length of up to several minutes.

8.2.2 POD Analysis

The principal orthogonal decomposition (POD), also referred to as the Karhunen-Loeve expansion, was first introduced by Lumley [143] into the field of fluid dynamics and is a pattern analysis method based on energy considerations. In particular, the snapshot form suggested by Sirovich [244] is useful in helping to recognize and characterize coherent structures and to analyze comparatively small ensembles of large

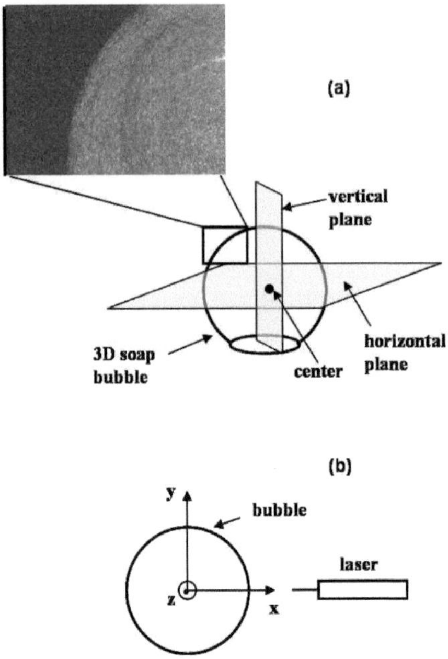

Figure 8.4: (a) PIV measurement planes. Inset: visualization of particle seeding inside cavity. (b) Top view of the measurement field inside the membrane, including coordinate system. The origin is located at the center of the bubble.

data vectors. For its application, spatio-temporal data are needed (i.e. a series of simultaneous 2D flow fields), which is provided by PIV. The following POD procedure follows closely that employed in previous PIV studies [11,185].

Any 2D field at time t_n is referred to as a snapshot, where the total number of snapshots is M. The data exist at discrete points on a rectangular grid in the spatial plane, with N_x points in the x-direction and N_y points in the y-direction (or similarly N_z points in the z-direction when considering measurements in a vertical x-z plane). The average snapshot was calculated and subtracted from each member of the ensemble such that only the fluctuating part of all velocities in the domain for the n-th snapshot remained. The average snapshot of the velocity field, $\underline{\overline{u}}(\underline{x})$, is calculated using:

$$\underline{\overline{u}}(\underline{x}) = \frac{1}{M}\sum_{n=1}^{M} \underline{u}(\underline{x}, t_n) \,, \tag{8.1}$$

where $\underline{u}$ is the velocity field at t_n and $\underline{x}$ represents the discrete 2D spatial coordinates, (x, y), or respectively (x, z), in any snapshot. The resulting adjusted snapshots of the data representing the deviations from the mean are given by:

$$\underline{u}'(\underline{x}, t_n) = \underline{u}(\underline{x}, t_n) - \underline{\overline{u}}(\underline{x}) \,. \qquad n = 1, 2..., M.. \tag{8.2}$$

Following the established procedure, a representation of the fluctuating PIV vector maps, $\underline{u}'(\underline{x}, t_n)$, is found based on an eigenvector/-value decomposition (i.e. single value decomposition) of the covariance matrix, $[\underline{u}'(\underline{x}, t_n)]^T \underline{u}'(\underline{x}, t_n)$,:

$$R(t_i, t_n) = \sum_{j=1}^{N} \underline{u}'(x_j, t_i) \cdot \underline{u}'(x_j, t_n), \tag{8.3}$$

such that:

$$\underline{u}'(\underline{x}, t_n) = \sum_{k=1}^{m} \lambda^{(k)} \theta^{(k)}(t) \sigma^{(k)}(\underline{x}) \,. \tag{8.4}$$

In this notation, temporal(θ) and spatial(σ) eigenvectors are introduced, as well as the eigenvalues λ. The eigenvalues permit the identification of energetically significant modes, and the following equation holds for the total kinetic energy present in the data,

$$E = \sum_{n=1}^{M} \left\| \underline{u}'(\underline{x}, t_n) \right\|^2 = \sum_{k=1}^{m} \lambda^{(k)^2} \,, \tag{8.5}$$

where the value of m specifies the number of basis modes included in the reconstruction. The POD decomposition is mathematically rigid, and the eigenmodes $\sigma(\underline{x})$ often show a strong "physical" appearance. Nevertheless, a direct interpretation of the eigenmodes in terms of relevant flow patterns is not always warranted. A more complete analysis would perhaps use some form of pattern recognition (e.g. adaptive clustering) to detect recurring combinations of the POD projection coefficients $\theta(t)$ and use these in a conditional averaging step. Applying this procedure to the present data did not, however, yield any significant change / improvement in the extracted flow patterns and the POD modes were kept as the basis of further interpretations.

8.3 Results and discussion

8.3.1 Instantaneous flow fields

Instantaneous velocity vector maps reveal the existence of internal flows within the bubble cavity as shown in Figs. 8.5 and 8.6, in the vertical and horizontal planes, respectively. In particular, the liquid shell exhibits sporadic "bursts", which under the no-slip boundary condition at the liquid-gas interface induce locally the internal motion of the air residing in the proximity of the shell. Transient "bursts" observed along the shell generate tangential displacements which, in turn, induce internal air flows circulating around the perimeter of the bubble. As a net result, the entire flow within the cavity must be displaced to fulfill the requirements of mass conservation since the soap bubble approximates closely a closed spherical control volume (i.e. over the measurement times considered, the bubble volume remains unchanged, see also section 8.3.3), giving rise to slow recirculation motion bounded by the liquid shell. Local velocity gradients, $d\underline{u}/dr$, in the radial direction ($r = 0$ at center of bubble), are clearly visible, where the velocity magnitude is largest at the shell surface ($r = R$) and $d\underline{u}/dr > 0$ in the direction spanning from the bubble center to the location of the burst. With PIV, we are able to study the origin and velocity of these "bursts" present on the shell by investigating the induced internal velocity field and recognizing that internal airflow motion results indeed from Marangoni driven fluid layers in the thin film (i.e. bursts) due to surface tension gradients as acknowledged in the literature [34,215] (see discussion at the end of section 8.3.1). Nevertheless, a direct correlation between motion in the gas and in the liquid is not available.

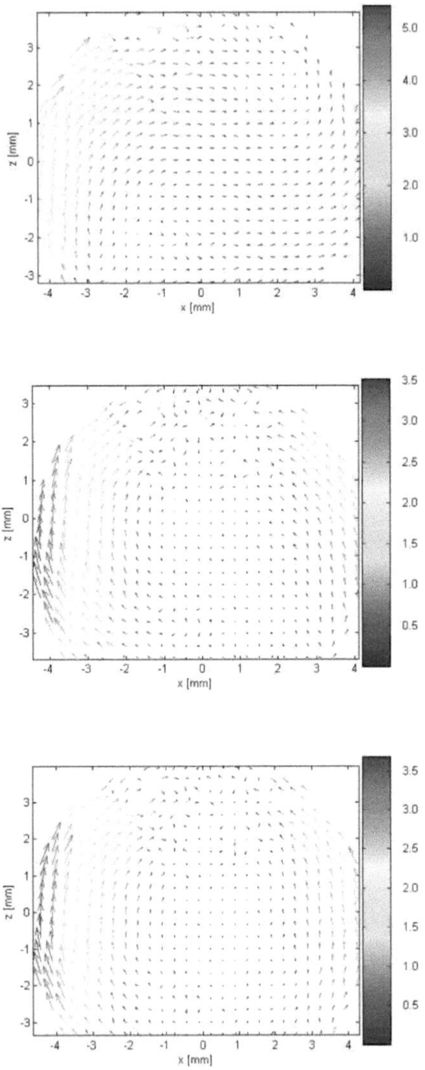

Figure 8.5: From top to bottom : sequence of instantaneous vector maps (vertical plane). Scale is in [mm/s].

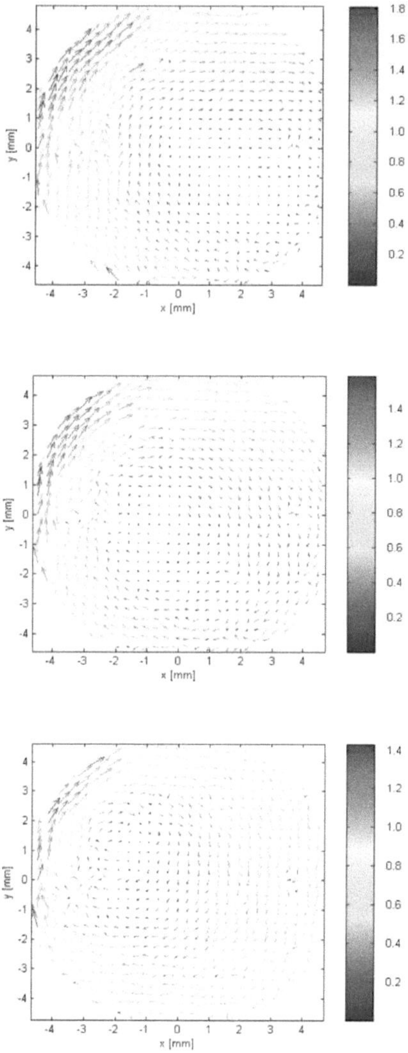

Figure 8.6: From top to bottom : sequence of instantaneous vector maps (horizontal plane). Scale is in [mm/s].

Under the specific bubble configuration and dimensions investigated here ($R < 6$ mm), local velocities near the shell may yield, during the transient of a burst, a magnitude of up to several mm/s (Figs. 8.5 and 8.6), depending on the measurement plane considered. At any time t_n, the mean spatial velocity magnitude in the measurement field considered may be given by:

$$\overline{|\underline{u}(\underline{x}, t_n)|} = \frac{1}{N_x N_y} \sum_{i=1}^{N_x} \sum_{j=1}^{N_y} (u_i^2(t_n) + v_j^2(t_n))^{1/2} , \tag{8.6}$$

(or respectively using w for measurement in the x–z plane), as illustrated experimentally in Fig. 8.7 (a). The resulting time-averaged value of the mean velocity magnitude may then be expressed as:

$$\overline{|\underline{u}|} = \frac{1}{t_M - t_1} \sum_{n=1}^{M} \overline{|\underline{u}(\underline{x}, t_n)|} , \tag{8.7}$$

where $t_1 = 0$. As seen in Fig. 8.7 (a), the internal cavity of these thin liquid shells is effectively characterized by the existence of net non-zero convective flows which persist over time. For the measurements illustrated here, the time-averaged mean planar velocity magnitude is on the order of $\overline{|\underline{u}|} \approx O(1.5 \times 10^{-3})$ m/s both in the horizontal and vertical plane. Qualitatively, flow recirculation is a transient process exhibiting temporal fluctuations in flow magnitude, due to the sporadic but repetitious motion of the liquid shell. One may note that locally, magnitudes of planar flow fields are observed to be slightly larger in the vertical plane compared to those seen in the horizontal plane, which may be due to the predominance of the shell motion in the vertical direction under the specific configuration investigated here (see discussion at end of section 8.3.1). Concurrently, the vertical motion inside the cavity appears to be typically restricted to a local region near the shell (Fig. 8.5), whereas flow motion in the horizontal plane is maybe weaker in magnitude but simultaneously extends perhaps more globally over a larger region inside the bubble (Fig. 8.6).

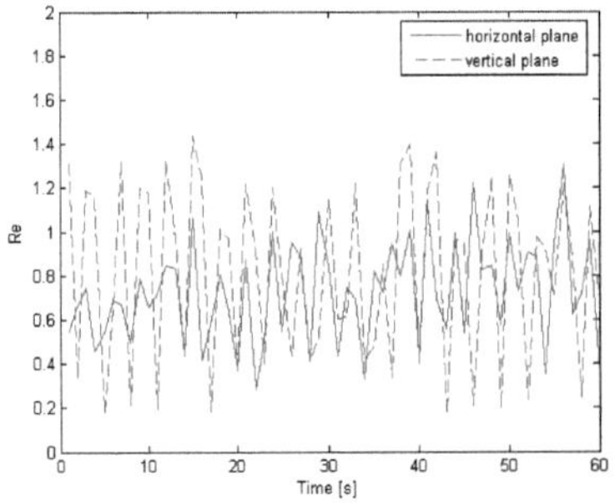

(a)

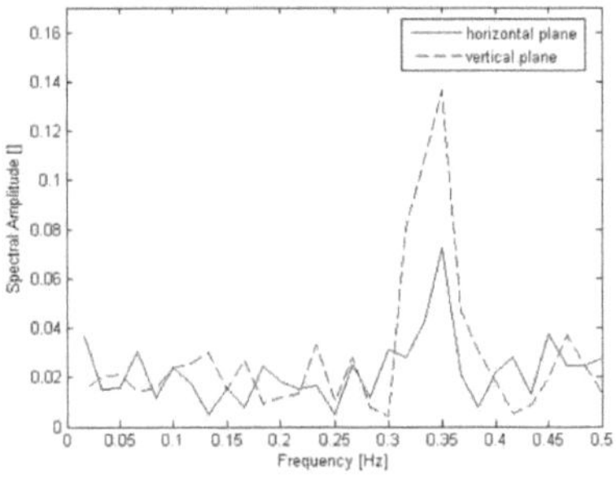

(b)

Figure 8.7: (a) Temporal evolution of the the Reynolds number, $Re = \overline{|\underline{u}(\underline{x}, t_n)|}D/\nu$), in horizontal and vertical planes for a 0.3 ml bubble (measurements are asynchronous). (b) Corresponding spectral amplitude of the mean spatial velocity magnitude signal obtained with a Fast Fourier Transform (FFT), respectively in the horizontal and vertical planes.

Defining here the Reynolds number as $Re = D\overline{|u|}/\nu$ following Pan & Acrivos for a cavity flow [181], where, $D = 2R$ and ν is the kinematic viscosity of air, one sees that for the time-averaged mean velocity field measured ($\overline{|u|} \approx 1.5$ mm/s), values of the Reynolds number are generally on the order of $Re \approx O(1)$ (for a 0.3 ml bubble $D \approx 8.5$ mm, see Fig. 8.3). This result suggests that cavity flows within soap bubbles are indeed slow and governed by Stokes flow, where inertial effects are negligible. Hence, internal flows will be driven provided local motion of the liquid shell persists over time, as experimentally observed (see Fig. 8.7 (a)). In particular this is also illustrated in the ensemble averaged velocity maps which yield a non-zero velocity field (Fig. 8.8) both in the horizontal and vertical planes. Moreover, Fig. 8.7 (b) illustrates in both measurement planes a dominant frequency near 0.35 Hz ($\approx$ 3 s). The existence of such discernable frequency may plausibly be interpreted as a "turnover time," τ, representing the approximate duration of a "burst" moving along a quarter of the shell's diameter, i.e. $\tau = \pi D/4\overline{|u|} \approx O$ (4 s).

We open a short parenthesis to discuss briefly recirculating flow motion observed inside the soap bubble cavity in relation to the specific experimental configuration and orientation of the bubble. In the present study, soap bubbles are positioned vertically sitting on a base (i.e. ring) such that bubbles are truncated spheres (i.e. spherical caps), as discussed in detail in section 8.2.1 (see schematic of setup Fig. 8.2). The vertical flowing fluid layers we observe here and refer to as "bursts" have been described previously in detail by Couder *et al.* [34]. In particular, the buoyant motion seen presently resembles qualitatively that which may be observed for example in 2D vertical soap films, due to surface tension gradients resulting from spatially inhomogeneous distribution of surfactant in the film (compare Fig. 8.1 with vortices in Figs. 10 and 11 from [34]). While liquid film motion observed here (Figs. 8.5–8.8) may perhaps be a specificity resulting from the particular choice of the soap bubble orientation, Kumar Sarma & Chattopadhyay [215] have reported, nevertheless, similar liquid film motion both in vertically as well as horizontally blown soap

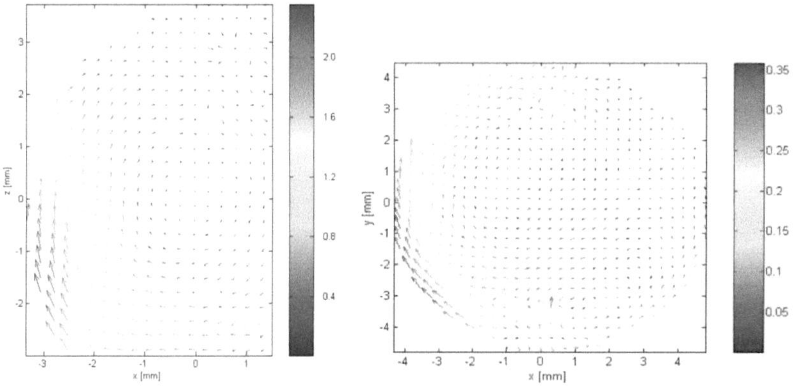

(a) (b)

Figure 8.8: Ensemble averaged vector maps of the flow field obtained from 100 instantaneous PIV vector maps in the (a) vertical and (b) horizontal plane. Scale is in [mm/s].

bubbles, where Marangoni convection driven fluid flow due to surface tension gradients created by the stretching of the film to form a bubble was measured using spectrophotometry [26,27]. In the present study, rather than monitoring the film motion evolution through its thickness, we illustrate the feasibility of studying instead the resulting flows generated inside the soap bubble cavity, as a result of the no-slip boundary condition at the liquid-gas interface.

8.3.2 Dominant structures

We have made use of the POD technique to extract the dominant structures of the internal flows measured. The relative energy, ${\lambda^{(k)}}^2$, of POD modes 1 through 20 is compared to the total energy, E (Eq. (8.5)), of the data set in Fig. 8.9 for asynchronous measurements in the horizontal and vertical planes of a 0.3 ml bubble. The first 20 modes capture, for both measurement planes, approximately 95% of the total energy. In particular, the first two modes capture over 85% of the total energy while modes greater than number 3 remain under 1%. The curves decay rapidly at the beginning and become less steep for the higher mode numbers. The lower energy levels indicate smaller flow structures or noise, whereas the first, most energetic modes, represent the dominant, large structures of the flow. In particular, the first mode alone captures slightly over 60% of the total energy, as shown in Fig. 8.9.

A selection of POD modes is shown, respectively for the vertical and horizontal planes, in Figs. 8.10 and 8.11, where $\sqrt{\lambda^{(k)}}\sigma^{(k)}$ from Eq. (8.4) is plotted ($k = 1$ through 4). Hence, for each mode k plotted, $\sqrt{\lambda^{(k)}}\sigma^{(k)}$ has dimensions of a velocity magnitude and illustrates the relative importance of each mode, according to the magnitude of the eigenvalue $\lambda^{(k)}$. The first two modes relate to the relatively large-scale flow structures and in particular, large vectors are visible near the region of the shell which is in motion. Moreover, recirculation regions are present within the core of the bubble. Namely, a relatively large vortex structure is present in the vertical plane (Fig. 8.10, mode 1) due to the local motion of the shell vertically upward, which induces a recirculation region in its proximity. A relatively less energetic recirculation region is present in the horizontal plane, in the proximity of the shell motion, and therefore

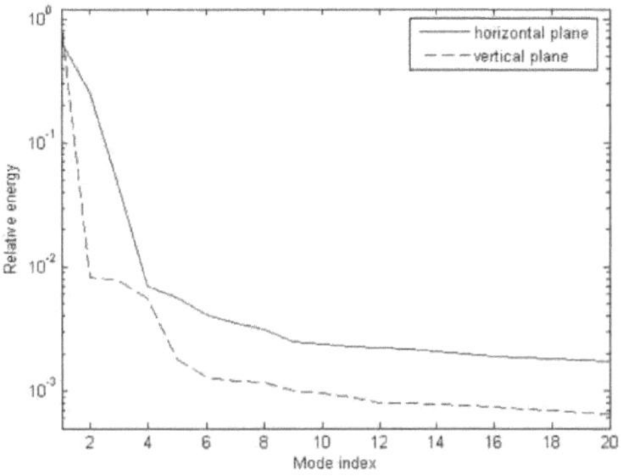

Figure 8.9: Relative energy, ${\lambda^{(k)}}^2/E$, of first 20 POD modes for horizontal and vertical planes of a 0.3 ml bubble.

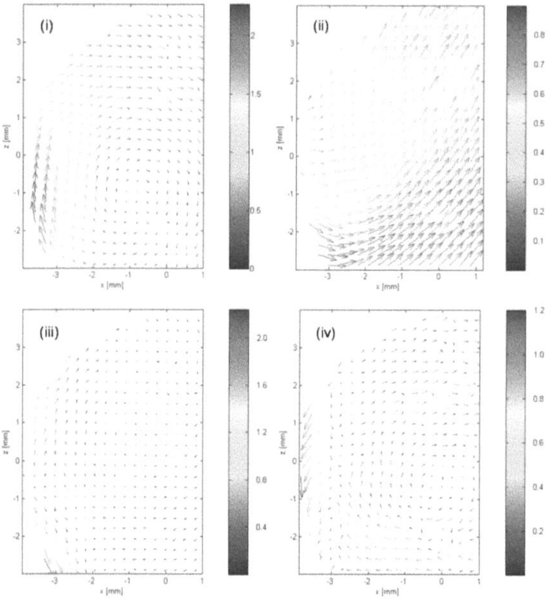

Figure 8.10: POD modes (i) through (iv) for a 0.3 ml bubble (vertical plane). Small regions of flow obstruction are due to laser reflection on bubble surface. We have plotted $\sqrt{\lambda^{(k)}}\sigma^{(k)}$ from Eq. (8.4), with $k = 1$ to 4. Scale is in [mm/s].

slightly off-centered relative to the origin of the bubble (Fig. 8.11, mode 2). In Fig. 8.11 (modes 2 and 3), it becomes more clear in fact that the entire flow along the shell interface is circulating in the horizontal plane.

8.3.3 Thermally-induced Marangoni flows and forced cavity recirculation

As observed experimentally here and reported previously for soap bubbles [215], the Marangoni effect may induce local upward flow of liquid along the bubble film, depending on the orientation of the shell. This flow is driven by surface tension gradients that arise due to local gradients in surfactant concentration on the shell [215], as discussed earlier (see section 8.3.1). Under the no slip condition at the liquid-gas interface, this phenomenon induces a boundary-driven flow inside the cavity. Similarly, it is well known that surface tension driven (i.e. Marangoni) flows may be utilized for thin liquid film spreading in technological and biological processes [23,117], by applying thermal gradients. Because most liquids maintain a negative and constant value of $\partial\sigma/\partial T$ where T is the temperature, the application of a constant thermal gradient produces a fixed viscous shear stress at the liquid surface given by $\tau = \nabla\sigma = (\partial\sigma/\partial T)\nabla T$ (where ∇ is the vector differential operator), which in turn may yield the driving of a film provided the

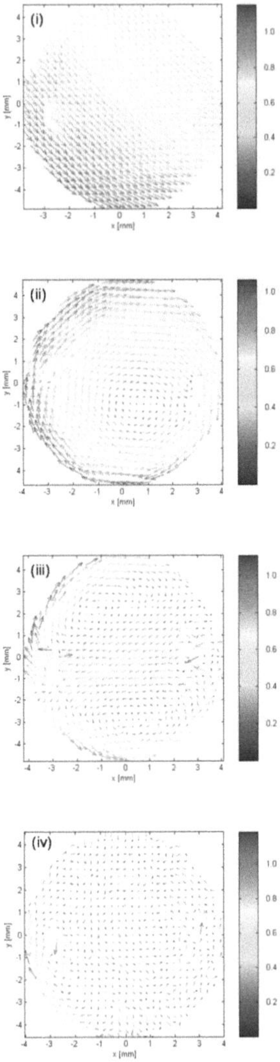

Figure 8.11: POD modes (i) through (iv) for a 0.3 ml bubble (horizontal plane). Small regions of flow obstruction are due to laser reflection on bubble surface. We have plotted $\sqrt{\lambda^{(k)}}\sigma^{(k)}$ from Eq. (8.4), with $k = 1$ to 4. Scale is in [mm/s].

upward flux due to thermal stresses is larger than the downward flux due to gravitational drainage, for the specific bubble orientation investigated here.

While soap bubbles may exhibit the existence of sporadic, yet persisting, internal cavity flows, as has been shown for the present configuration, thermally-induced Marangoni flows in a soap bubble film may potentially lead to constant forced cavity recirculation. This may be achieved for example by applying locally a heat source in the vicinity of the liquid shell, such that a temperature gradient, ∇T, is effectively generated on the surface of the liquid shell. To support this hypothesis, we experimentally provide a heating source near the liquid shell at approximately $(x = -R, y = 0, z = 0)$ (coordinates are also specified in Figs. 8.12 and 8.13), using a 3.3 Ω resistor connected to a power supply delivering a voltage in the range 0.8-1.2 V. The resistor yields a local temperature gradient, with respect to the ambient surrounding, which is set between approximately 6^oC and 13^oC (caution is taken not to apply a too large temperatures near the thin film, which may lead to bubble rupture).

To guarantee that internal flow motion is generated by thermally-induced surface tension gradients, rather than by buoyancy effects, a qualitative visualization of the liquid shell motion was first performed by seeding the thin film with titanium dioxide particles (TiO_2). This simple visualization scheme (not shown

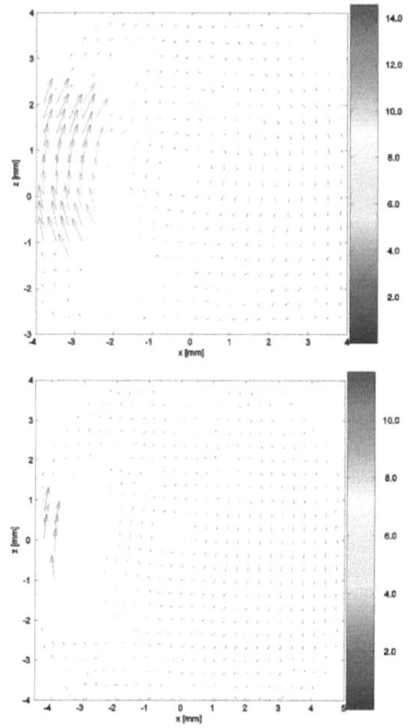

Figure 8.12: Two examples of bubbles under thermal forcing. Heating source is located approximately at $(x = -4$ mm, $z = -1$ mm). Vector maps are obtained in the vertical plane from ensemble averaged PIV of 100 instantaneous vector maps. Scale is in [mm/s].

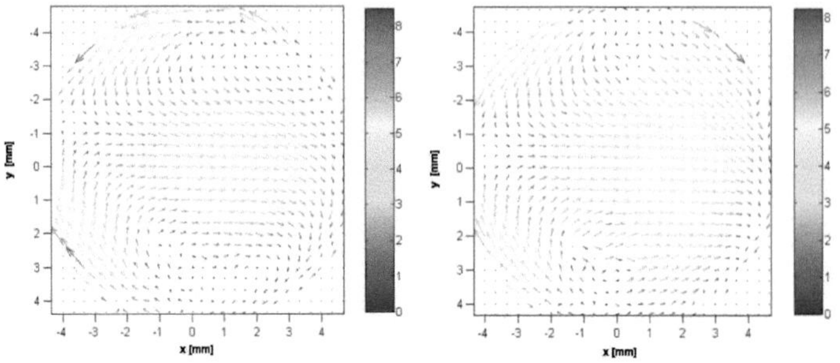

Figure 8.13: Two examples of bubbles under thermal forcing. Heating source is located approximately at ($x = -4$ mm, $y = 0$ mm). Vector maps are obtained in the horizontal plane from ensemble averaged PIV of 100 instantaneous vector maps. Scale is in [mm/s].

here) was useful to illustrate two important features: (i) thermal forcing in the present configuration yields the driving of the liquid film (rather than directly inducing the motion of the internal flow); and (ii) over the short measurement times considered, the thin liquid film represents approximately a shell of constant mass, as no accumulation of the fluid is observed near the base.

Examples of ensemble averaged velocity fields illustrating the internal flows under thermal forcing are shown in Figs. 8.12 and 8.13, respectively in the vertical and horizontal plane. Thermally-induced Marangoni flows in the liquid film lead to forced boundary-driven recirculation inside the cavity. In particular, an approximately constant temperature heat source leads to a relatively constant shear stress along the shell, such that flow fields are rather invariant over time. The cavity exhibits a strong recirculation

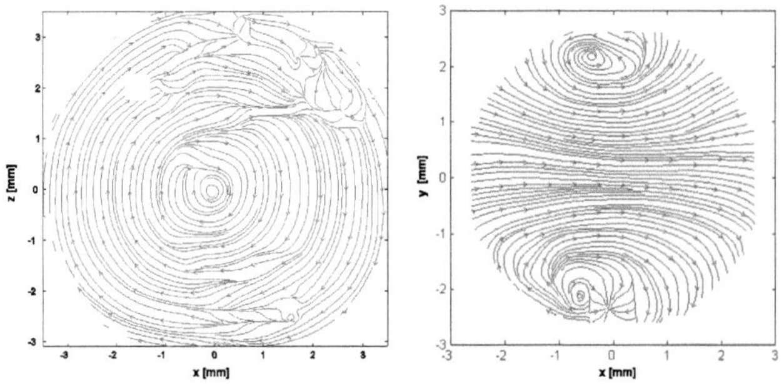

Figure 8.14: Reconstructed internal stream line patterns under thermal forcing in the vertical (left) and horizontal plane (right) plane. Results (right) are obtained using a pulsed laser illumination (see section 8.2.1) and illustrate no significant differences in the flow patterns obtained in comparison with a continuous illumination approach (see Fig. 8.13).

region in the vertical plane which rotates about the center of the bubble (Fig. 8.14 (a)) while the horizontal plane is characterized by two closely symmetrical eddies (Fig. 8.14 (b)). Heating a spot on the side of the liquid shell reduces locally the surface tension of the soap film and drives it, thus, towards regions of higher surface tension. However, since the liquid film represents approximately a shell of constant mass, as discussed above, the fluid flowing away from the heat source must induce, following continuity, a reverse flow in the opposite direction. This, in turn, leads to the characteristic recirculation regions observed, which follow directly from the no-slip condition at the liquid-gas interface.

In Fig. 8.15 (a), the temporal evolution of the mean spatial velocity magnitude, $\overline{|\underline{u}(\underline{x}, t_n)|}$, is illustrated for the thermal forcing configuration, in both measurement planes (plotted here as $Re = \overline{|\underline{u}(\underline{x}, t_n)|} D/\nu$, where $D \approx 9$ mm for an 0.4 ml bubble). The resulting mean flow magnitude appears to be slightly larger in the vertical plane, compared with that measured in the horizontal plane. In particular, for both measurement planes, the time-dependent Reynolds number is on the order of $Re \sim O(3)$ (see Fig. 8.15 (a)), which is indeed larger than values obtained earlier under no thermal forcing conditions (see Fig. 8.7 (a)). Moreover, a spectral analysis of the temporal mean velocity magnitude seems to suggest that a distinct frequency peak in the signal is no longer discernable (see Fig. 8.15 (b)), illustrating strong contrast with the behavior observed earlier due to sporadic "bursts" of motion (Fig. 8.7 (b)). Indeed, the spectral amplitude plots obtained under thermal forcing are relatively noisy with very low amplitudes (< 0.1). Hence, qualitatively speaking, it appears that a constant shear stress applied on the liquid shell generates rather clearly a (quasi) steady-state recirculating flow inside the cavity, where no apparent oscillatory behavior persists.

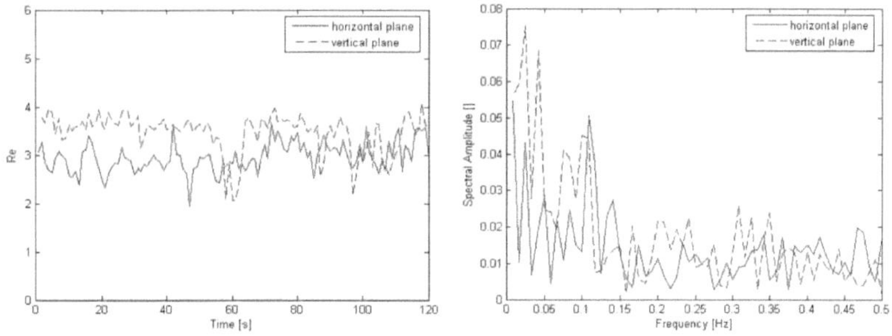

(a) (b)

Figure 8.15: (a) Temporal evolution of the Reynolds number, $Re = \overline{|\underline{u}(\underline{x}, t_n)|} D/\nu$) in horizontal and vertical planes under thermal forcing (measurements are asynchronous) for an 0.4 ml bubble. (b) Corresponding spectral amplitude obtained with a Fast Fourier Transform (FFT) in the horizontal and vertical plane.

8.4 Qualitative Model for Marangoni Forcing in a Liquid Shell

In section 3.3.3, we argued using a simple 1D steady-state model that the velocity field (Eqs. (3.55) and (3.56)) in the continuous gas phase inside acinar airways is not influenced by the thin liquid lining layer under normal physiological considerations, in particular without the presence of surface tension gradients $\nabla\sigma$. Based on the experimental results for Marangoni forcing in a soap bubble presented above in section 8.3.3, we open a short parenthesis to revisit the analysis carried in section 3.3.3 and derive an insightful qualitative model for thermocapillary motion of a liquid film in a soap bubble (i.e. free film). We compare this result with one obtained for thermocapillary motion in the liquid layer lining in a model alveolus (i.e. liquid film at a solid wall).

Thermocapillary Motion: Vertical Free Soap Film

We attempt to build a simplified model for thermocapillary motion in a free soap film, such as in a soap bubble (Fig. 8.16). Our model is based on a draining model for a vertical soap film [164], where locally we may consider the soap bubble to be a vertical free film. The film thickness is given by $2h$ and a symmetry line lies at $y = 0$ (see Fig. 8.16 for choice of coordinate system). During film motion, the thickness remains continuous over the whole length, L, of the film, and since $2h \ll L$, curvature effects in the film are assumed to be negligible. For simplicity, we assume that the liquid film is incompressible (with viscosity μ_l), and the flow obeys the lubrication approximation in the film (as discussed earlier in section 3.3.3). Furthermore, we assume that thermocapillary motion is symmetrical about $y = 0$.

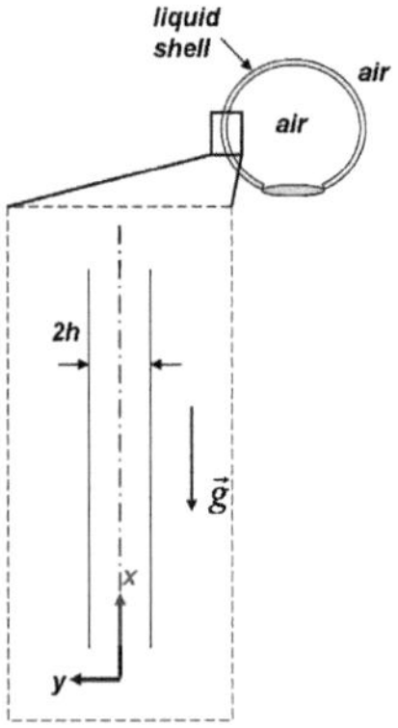

Figure 8.16: Schematic of thin liquid film in a soap bubble.

The Navier-Stokes equations describing unidirectional flow reduce to:

$$\frac{\partial p}{\partial x} = \mu_l \frac{\partial^2 u_x}{\partial y^2} - \rho_l g, \quad (8.8)$$

$$\frac{\partial p}{\partial y} = 0. \quad (8.9)$$

The above equations are solved subject to the following boundary conditions,

$$\left.\frac{\partial u_x}{\partial y}\right|_{y=0} = 0, \quad (8.10)$$

$$u_x|_{y=\pm h} = V_s, \quad (8.11)$$

where V_s is the velocity of the interface in the x-direction. Using the appropriate boundary conditions and assuming that the thickness, $2h$, remains constant such that $u_y = -\partial h/\partial t = 0$, the steady-state velocity profile, $u_x(y)$, yields upon integration

$$u_x(y) = \frac{1}{2\mu_l}\left(\frac{\partial p}{\partial x} + \rho_l g\right)(y^2 - h^2) + V_s. \quad (8.12)$$

For the conditions evaluated here, it is reasonable to assume that $\partial p/\partial x \ll \rho g$, such that the velocity in the vertical film is given by:

$$u_x(y) = \frac{\rho_l g}{2\mu_l}(y^2 - h^2) + \left(\frac{\partial \sigma}{\partial T}\right)\left(\frac{dT}{dx}\right)\frac{h}{\mu_l}, \quad (8.13)$$

where the second term on the right-hand side corresponds to the velocity, V_s, at the free surface. Note here that surface tension gradients are assumed to be dependent solely on temperature gradients (see Eq. (3.58)). Hence, the steady-state velocity profile in the free vertical film results qualitatively from the balance between gravitaty forces and thermocapillary motion induced at the free surface.

Thermocapillary Motion: Alveolus Model

Based on the above derivation, we consider the influence of gravity and thermocapillary motion of a liquid film in a model alveolus. We assume here that the thin liquid layer is spread uniformly and continuously over the alveolar wall (Fig. 8.17). The Navier-Stokes equations describing unidirectional flow in the thin liquid layer lining remain identical to Eqs. (8.8) and (8.9). However, the boundary conditions are now slightly altered [142]. The no-slip condition applies at the alveolar wall ($y = 0$):

$$u_x|_{y=0} = 0. \quad (8.14)$$

At the free surface, the boundary condition is given as:

$$\mu_l \left.\frac{\partial u_x}{\partial y}\right|_{y=h} = \tau = \left(\frac{\partial \sigma}{\partial T}\right)\left(\frac{dT}{dx}\right). \quad (8.15)$$

Note that the liquid layer thickness is now given as h (see coordinate system in Fig. 8.17). Since $h << L$ (h is assumed to remain constant), we may assume again that both surface curvature and the pressure gradient, $\partial p/\partial x$, are negligible. Upon integration, the velocity profile, $u_x(y)$, is then given by:

$$u_x(y) = \frac{\rho_l g}{\mu_l}\left(\frac{y^2}{2} - hy\right) + \left(\frac{\partial \sigma}{\partial T}\right)\left(\frac{dT}{dx}\right)\frac{y}{\mu_l}. \quad (8.16)$$

Comparing Eqs. (8.13) and (8.16), velocity profiles are indeed similar. In particular we will now briefly look at the applicability of these equations.

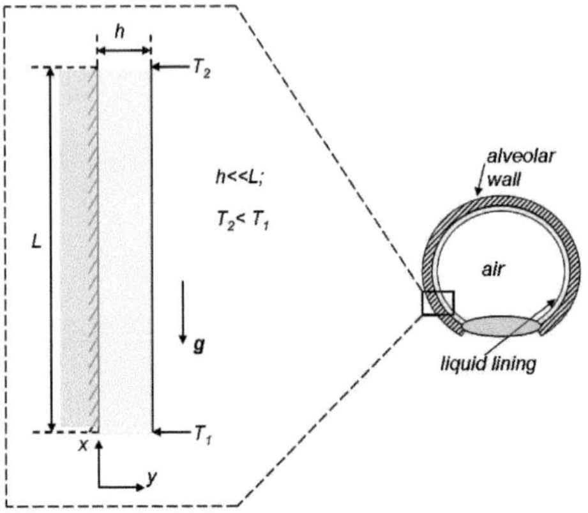

Figure 8.17: Schematic of vertical thin liquid lining in alveolus model.

Applicability and Dimensionless Parameters

The applicability of our solutions Eqs. (8.13) and (8.16) depends on the following two conditions [134]:

$$h^3 \ll \frac{4\nu_l^2 \rho L}{\left|\frac{\partial \sigma}{\partial x}\right| \left|\frac{dT}{dx}\right|}, \tag{8.17}$$

$$Re = \frac{u_x|_{y=0}\, h}{\nu} << 1. \tag{8.18}$$

We can now identify the dimensionless parameters which characterize both thin liquid film configurations. The Reynolds number, Re, which relates inertial to viscous forces is based on the maximum velocity at the free surface of the liquid lining:

$$Re = \frac{u_x|_{max}\, h}{\nu_l}. \tag{8.19}$$

The Capillary number, Ca, represents the relative effect of viscous forces and surface tension acting across the interface between the liquid and the gas, and is defined as:

$$Ca = \frac{\mu_l\, u_x|_{max}}{\sigma}. \tag{8.20}$$

The Bond number, Bo, which characterizes the thin liquid lining under a static configuration expresses the ratio of gravitational forces to surface tension forces and may be expressed as:

$$Bo = \frac{\rho_l g h^2}{\sigma}. \tag{8.21}$$

Finally, the Weber number, We, can be thought of as a measure of the relative importance of the thin liquid's inertia compared to its surface tension and may be written as:

$$We = \frac{\rho_l\, u_x^2|_{max}\, h}{\sigma}. \tag{8.22}$$

The list of parameters and associated values used in the present estimations are presented in Table 8.1. As a first approximation, we assume that the temperature gradient, dT/dx, is linearly dependent on the length scale x, with:

$$\sigma = \sigma(T_2) + \left(\frac{\partial \sigma}{\partial T}\right) \frac{T_2 - T_1}{L} x, \tag{8.23}$$

such that:

$$\frac{dT}{dx} \approx \frac{T_2 - T_1}{l}, \tag{8.24}$$

where l is the length scale involved in determining the magnitude of dT/dx. A perhaps feasible way of inducing physically a temperature gradient is between the external skin and the alveoli inside the thoracic cavity. Therefore, we may assume for simplicity that $l = O(10^{-2})$ m, which corresponds approximately to the thickness of the tissue residing between the exterior of the body and the alveoli. One may note that it is most likely unphysical to assume, on the other hand, that $l = L$, which would correspond to a temperature gradient of multiple degrees ^oC applied over the alveolar diameter, d_a, without considering conduction effects in the liquid lining.

Estimates for the dimensionless parameters for film motion in the alveolus model (Eq. (8.16)) are presented in Table 8.2. Results illustrate that the alveolar liquid lining is entirely dominated by viscous and surface tension forces, while gravitational influence may be completely disregarded, as expected. Therefore, velocity profiles respectively for the vertical free film and the liquid film in the alveolus model reduce effectively to:

$$u_x(y)|_{free\ film} = \left(\frac{\partial \sigma}{\partial T}\right)\left(\frac{dT}{dx}\right)\frac{h}{\mu_l}, \tag{8.25}$$

$$u_x(y)|_{alveolus} = \left(\frac{\partial \sigma}{\partial T}\right)\left(\frac{dT}{dx}\right)\frac{y}{\mu_l}, \tag{8.26}$$

which match at the free surface ($y = h$). We have computed velocity profiles for two (thin and thick) alveolar wall thicknesses, h (Table 8.1), as illustrated in Fig. 8.18. For the thin film ($h = 0.1$ μm), we find that maximal velocities (at the fluid-gas interface) are on the order of $u_{max} \approx 0.01$ mm/s for $|\Delta T| < 10^oC$ (temperature gradients need to remain physiologically feasible). For the thick film ($h = 0.9$ μm), we find $u_{max} 0.1$ mm/s.

Similarly, results for the thin and thicker film in the vertical free film configuration are presented in

Table 8.1: Parameters for analytical thermocapillary motion in thin film model.

lining length	$L \approx d_a$	200 μm
lining thickness [8]	h	thin: 0.10 μm thick: 0.9 μm
lining density	ρ_l	998 kg/m^3
lining viscosity	μ_l	$0.8 \cdot 10^{-3}$ N-s/m^2
lining viscosity	ν_l	$0.8 \cdot 10^{-6}$ m^2/s
reference surface tension	σ	$2 \cdot 10^{-2}$ N/m
	$\partial\sigma/\partial T$	$-0.15 \cdot 10^{-3}$ J-K/m^2
gravitational acceleration	g	9.81 m/s^2
reference temperature	T_2	37^oC

Table 8.2: Dimensionless numbers for thermocapillary motion of the liquid layer lining in the alveolus model.

	Thin Wall	Thick Wall
Re	$O(10^{-6})$	$O(10^{-5})$
Ca	$O(10^{-7})$	$O(10^{-6})$
Bo	$O(10^{-9})$	$O(10^{-7})$
We	$O(10^{-13})$	$O(10^{-10})$

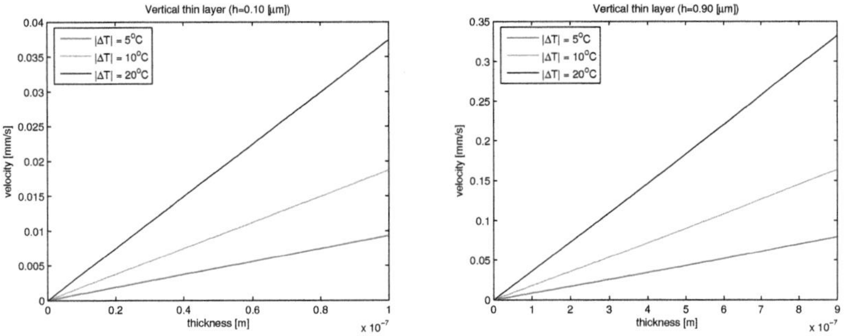

(a) $h = 0.1\ \mu m$ (b) $h = 0.9\ \mu m$

Figure 8.18: Velocity profile for motion of a thin (left) and thick (right) liquid lining under thermocapillary motion in the alveolus model.

Fig. 8.19. The results yield convective time scales on the order of:

$$t = \frac{L}{v_{max}} \approx 2 - 10\ s, \tag{8.27}$$

which are approximately on the same order of magnitude as quiet tidal breathing, where a breathing period is $T \approx 3$ s for an average adult human being (see details in section 4.6 and Fig. 4.3). Hence, the theoretical application of thermocapillary motion in the liquid lining layer towards gas flow generation inside an alveolus would probably require important temperature gradients if we wish to reduce significantly the time scales necessary to compete against gravitational sedimentation or diffusion processes in the process of particle deposition. However, the generation of such temperature gradients in the lung septa over small length scales does not seem to be easily feasible for medical purposes. Nevertheless, recirculating flows, as shown here, induced inside thin liquid shells under thermocapillary motion may possibly find future applications in the field of microfluidics [23,117].

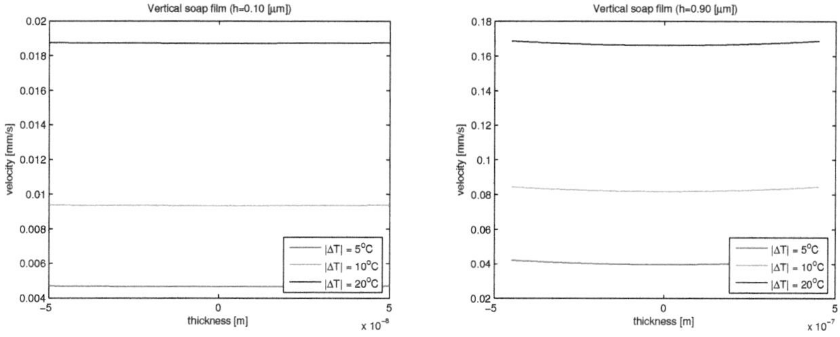

(a) $h = 0.1\ \mu$m (b) $h = 0.9\ \mu$m

Figure 8.19: Velocity profile for motion of a vertical free thin (left) and thick (right) film of a soap bubble.

8.5 Conclusions

We have shown using PIV measurements for the present soap bubble configuration that slow recirculating cavity flows may indeed exist inside a bubble under no thermal forcing, due to sporadic yet persisting "bursts" in the liquid film, resulting from surface tension gradients. Additional information on the flow structures present inside the liquid shell was extracted using a POD analysis. The flow patterns appear to be governed by the motion of the liquid shell such that recirculation regions are effectively induced in different planes of the bubble. Their location and strength are dependent upon the velocity magnitude and exact location of the local displacements of the liquid shell. The internal flows observed here at a liquid-gas interface exhibit similarities with classic setups of low-Reynolds number boundary-driven cavity flows at solid-fluid interfaces.

Under thermal forcing, Marangoni induced flow motion in the liquid shell may yield (quasi) steady-state flow recirculation inside the soap bubble cavity. As will be shown in chapter 10, the resulting low-Reynolds flows may indeed be captured by considering analytical solutions of the creeping motion equations in the region interior to the sphere. While a straightforward implementation of such techniques for the enhancement of acinar gas flows for increased alveolar deposition appears difficult, the present findings may give further insight on flows induced at the interface between two fluids, where surface tension effects, such as Marangoni flows, play an important role.

Chapter 9

Visualization of Acoustic Streaming Inside Thin Elastic Spherical Cavities

Acoustic streaming occurring in a fluid outside an oscillating solid body or gas bubble has been extensively investigated. In contrast, experimental investigations of streaming flows generated inside oscillating spherical cavities are scarce. In the present study, flow visualizations are presented for acoustic streaming inside transparent hemispherical elastic cavities oscillating in an acoustic field. Streaming flows are visualized using particle image velocimetry (PIV) and results are presented for a range of values of a dimensionless frequency parameter, $M = 120 - 306$. Over the frequency range investigated, $f = 3 - 20$ kHz, diverse streaming flow fields are encountered. Generated flows are inherently three-dimensional, while the magnitude of the flow circulating inside the cavity remains small (< 1 mm/s) and non-linearly dependent on the acoustic power of the incoming sound wave. The present boundary-driven cavity flows may enhance particle fluid transport mechanisms, leading ultimately to potential fluid mixing applications.

9.1 Introduction

It is well-known that the propagation of sound waves in a fluid may lead to a bulk non-periodic motion of the fluid. This nonlinear phenomenon is called acoustic streaming and is directly related to the quadratic convective terms of the flow field.

Acoustic streaming flows have been reviewed extensively [137,169,204] and numerous well-developed theoretical studies exist. In particular, the theory for streaming flows around oscillating bodies has been developed for gas bubbles undergoing harmonic translating and volume oscillation modes in a liquid. The important difference between oscillating solid bodies and gas bubbles occurs in the boundary conditions. Solid walls have a no-slip boundary condition on their surfaces, whereas for bubbles, there is no radial velocity and zero shear-stress at the gas-liquid interface. Davidson and Riley [45] considered small-scale acoustic streaming (i.e. microstreaming) in a liquid outside an isolated gas bubble induced by the translational harmonic oscillation of the bubble. More recently, Wu & Du [294] extended this work by studying the streaming behavior of a (micro) gas bubble simultaneously undergoing translating oscillations and volume oscillations seen as radial pulsations of the bubble wall. In particular, they demonstrated that the streaming velocity inside a bubble is much greater than that outside the bubble, with microstreaming most pronounced for a bubble undergoing volume resonance (monopole motion). In parallel, theoretical descriptions for the acoustic streaming occurring near a fluid-solid interface, rather than a fluid-gas one, have been developed [21,168], giving rise to flow patterns outside solid spheres similar to those observed in the vicinity of gas bubbles [127,130].

Although acoustic streaming has been studied for over half a century now, there are limited flow visualization data and experimental studies on how the mode of oscillation affects the type of flow patterns generated. Experimentally, streaming flows are difficult to evaluate because of their small velocities and displacements. Kolb & Nyborg [122] were the first to observe vortex motions in the vicinity of small vibrating sources in liquids. Since then, qualitative [84] and recent quantitative studies [123,263] have completed the literature. However, these studies have mainly concentrated on resolving the streaming flows occurring outside the oscillating cavity, rather than inside. This has been in part motivated by bio-engineering applications, such as soluminescence, ultrasound contrast agents [84], DNA degradation [197] and sonoporation as a result of the shearing action of microstreaming flows [295]. In particular, it has been experimentally shown that streaming in a fluid outside a gas bubble, generated by a bubble-scattered sound field, may be used for microfluidic applications, such as in the transport of particles [146] or in the mixing of fluids at the microscale [139]. Finally, acoustic streaming has been found to have practical utility in various diagnostic and therapeutic medical ultrasound applications. Examples include amongst others (i) distinguishing between stagnant blood and tissue as well as clotted and unclotted blood [241]; (ii) diagnosis of fluid-filled breast cysts and lesions [165]; and (iii) lithotripsy (i.e. noninvasive disintegration of kidney stones and gallstones with focused shock waves [212]), where nonlinear acoustical effects are associated not only with propagation of the shock wave but also with the generation of cavitation activity near the stones.

While there exist theoretical investigations for streaming flows generated inside an oscillating gas bubble

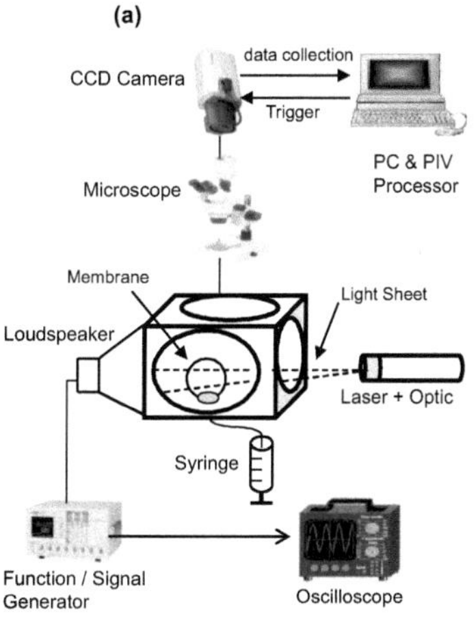

Figure 9.1: Schematic of the experimental apparatus.

[294] or a levitated drop [302], there is however to our knowledge, few if any experimental visualizations of internal streaming flows generated at a solid-fluid interface. One reason may be the difficulty of choosing an appropriate experimental setup illustrating internal streaming flows generated at a solid-fluid boundary while simultaneously allowing sufficient optical access for modern measurement techniques. Therefore, in an effort to complete existing flow-visualization studies on the topic, we have investigated acoustic streaming flows generated by a sound wave inside transparent, air-filled, thin elastic spherical cavities. Our experimental approach is based on particle image velocimetry (PIV) measurements carried out inside elastic membranes inflated into spherical cavities and seeded with particles. Our results suggest that multiple modes of membrane oscillations exist, leading to a variety of complex acoustic streaming flow patterns. It is our belief that these boundary-driven cavity flows may enhance the transporting mechanisms of a fluid inside the elastic chamber, leading to potential applications in micromixing, similar to designs involving peristatically induced flow motion in closed micro-cavities with vibrating walls [160, 297]. In particular, the elastic cavities investigated here constitute a confined airspace in some sense analogous to pulmonary alveoli, suggesting that acoustic streaming could potentially be used as a means for convective flow enhancement possibly leading to increased particle deposition in the lung.

9.1.1 Review of Acoustic Streaming

In low-Reynolds number flow applications (i.e. microfluidics, alveolar flows, etc.), small feature sizes typically prevent flow velocities from being high enough. High-frequency acoustic waves can serve as a means to circumvent such difficulties. While periodic wave motion might seem at first to be of little use for fluid manipulation, the inertial nonlinearity can, however, rectify oscillatory fluid motion to give a tie-averaged flow called steady or acoustic streaming. One may define three broad classes of steady streaming: quartz wind, boundary-induced streaming (of particular relevance here), and cavitation microstreaming [248].

The simplest manifestations of acoustic streaming corresponds to the quartz wind (named for the wind observed to blow away from oscillating quartz crystals). Dissipation causes acoustic waves to decay over an attenuation length $\alpha^{-1}(\omega)$, resulting in an oscillatory velocity field $u_\omega \sim U_o e^{-\alpha z} e^{i\omega t} \underline{z}$ (U_o is the amplitude) with zero time average. However, the oscillation amplitude of a fluid particle decreases in one half cycle as it moves away from the source. Conversely, its amplitude increases as it moves towards the source. Oscillating fluid particles this constantly impart momentum to the fluid, driving a secondary streaming flow away from the acoustic source [137]. This rectified forcing comes from the nonlinear inertial term in the Navier-Stokes equations (see Eq. (3.1)) which may be neglected for low-Re flows. In particular, time averaging Eq. (3.1) yields a steady body force:

$$\underline{f}_{QW} = \rho < \underline{u}_\omega \cdot \nabla \underline{u}_\omega > \sim \rho \alpha U_0^2 e^{-2\alpha z} \underline{z}, \tag{9.1}$$

which drives the wind felt in front of stereo loudspeakers.

While quartz wind occurs in the bulk of the fluid, steady streaming flows occur around solid boundaries as well, with an amplitude that is independent of viscosity. An oscillatory flow with an amplitude U_0 over a solid surface must vanish on the surface due to the no-slip condition. In unsteady viscous flows, vorticity generated at the wall spreads diffusively with diffusivity ν, so that wall effects are effectively confined to a distance over which vorticity can diffuse in one cycle before it is annihilated. An oscillatory boundary layer (also known as a Stokes layer) of size:

$$\delta \sim \left(\frac{\nu}{\omega}\right)^{1/2} \tag{9.2}$$

contains all of the vorticity in the flow.

If the amplitude of oscillatory flow U_0 above the Stokes layer varies with length scale L along the boundary, the nonlinear inertial term $\rho\underline{u} \cdot \nabla\underline{u}$ rectifies the oscillatory flow to give a steady inertial forcing, similar to the quartz wind. The steady inertial force, $f_i \sim \rho U_0^2/L$, is balanced by steady viscous forces, $f_v \sim \mu u_s/\delta^2 \sim \rho\omega u_s$, that are, surprisingly, independent of viscosity. This results in a velocity scale for steady boundary-driven streaming,

$$u_s \sim \frac{U_0^2}{\omega L}. \tag{9.3}$$

The acoustic boundary-driven slip velocity outside the Stokes layer is given by [259]:

$$u_s \sim= -\frac{3U_0}{4\omega}\frac{dU_0}{dx_{||}}, \tag{9.4}$$

and flows in the direction of decreasing free-stream velocity.

In boundary-induced acoustic streaming, body forces localized near a surface give rise to an effective slip velocity and streaming flows reserve direction within the Stokes layer, causing recirculating rolls. The flow outside the Stokes layer obeys the Navier-Stokes equations with a slip velocity given in Eq. (9.4). The external flow due to this slip velocity may be associated with a streaming Reynolds number $Re_s = u_sL/\nu = U_0^2/\omega\nu$, giving two regimes of acoustic streaming, for large and small Re_s [207,259].

9.2 Experimental Methods and Procedures

9.2.1 Apparatus

The experimental apparatus (Fig. 9.1) consists of a test cell enclosing an inflated elastic membrane, a loudspeaker and an imaging system. The test cell is made of a cubic-shaped ($\sim 5 \times 5 \times 5$ cm) aluminum frame with detachable cover plates, each of which may be mounted on five of the faces of the cube (four side faces and the top face). Each plate guarantees hermetical sealing of the test volume. Side plates may either be painted black to minimize scattering of laser light, or designed with a circular glass

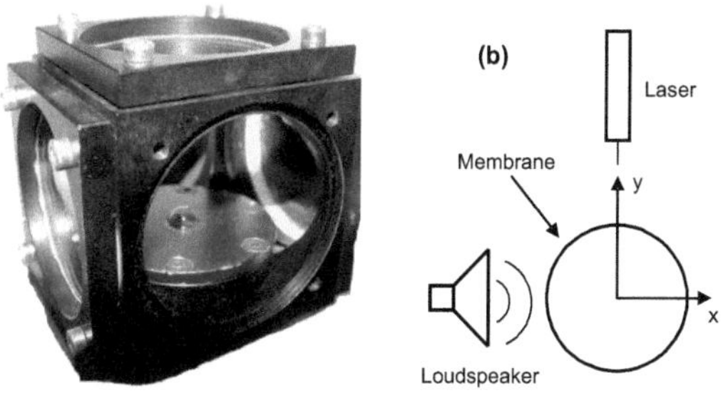

Figure 9.2: Close-up of the test cell with an inflated hemispherical membrane in the center. (b) Top view of the measurement field inside the membrane, including coordinate system.

window for optical access into the chamber (Fig. 9.2). The remaining bottom face of the cube is fitted with a thin transparent silicone elastomer film (50 μm thickness, $\rho = 1260$ kg/m^3, Goodfellow Cambridge Limited, UK) sandwiched between a bottom cylindrical slab and an exchangeable upper plate designed with different circular orifice opening sizes with a rounded edge. In this way, the silicone membrane is tightly clamped between both plates, and a silicone paste is first applied at the contact between the elastic membrane and the bottom slab to guarantee negligible air leakage upon inflation. The bottom slab is drilled with a central hole connected to a graduated syringe. In turn, thin elastic bubbles may be inflated by injecting air which distends the silicone membrane through the orifice opening into a spherical cap-shaped volume. Typical elastic cavities are generated at a 6 mm circular orifice opening, by inflating $\sim 1.5-2$ ml of air, resulting in a spherical cap with a characteristic diameter of $D \sim 6.5-7$ mm. A schematic of the measurement plane is illustrated in Fig. 9.2 (b).

Acoustic excitation is generated with a piezoelectric loudspeaker mounted onto one of the test cell faces and connected to a signal generator which delivers a sinusoidal electrical waveform. The waveform frequency may be varied from 0 to 20 kHz in increments of approximately 0.01 kHz and the voltage amplitude (peak-to-peak, V_{pp}) between 3 and 20 V_{pp} in increments of 0.1 V. These input parameters are verified by an oscilloscope (Agilent 54622A MegaZoom) connected to the signal generator. Sound pressure levels emitted by the loudspeaker vary nonlinearly with its excitation frequency. To determine the actual acoustic power delivered inside the chamber, the power (dB) was measured as a function of the input frequency, f, and voltage amplitude, V_{pp}. These were recorded using a sound level meter (Voltcraft SL-100) with a resolution of 0.1 dB and accuracy of $\pm$ 2 dB. The microphone head was placed directly above the orifice opening, at a distance of ~ 25 mm away from the loudspeaker, where elastic cavities are inflated. Results are plotted in Fig. 9.3 over the principal range of frequencies investigated.

The imaging system consists of a progressive scan CCD camera (Pulnix TM-1010) with 15 Hz image acquisition rate and a resolution of 1008 x 1008 pixels triggered via computer control. The CCD camera is fitted onto a microscope such that typical inflated cavities are imaged with a field of view of about 7

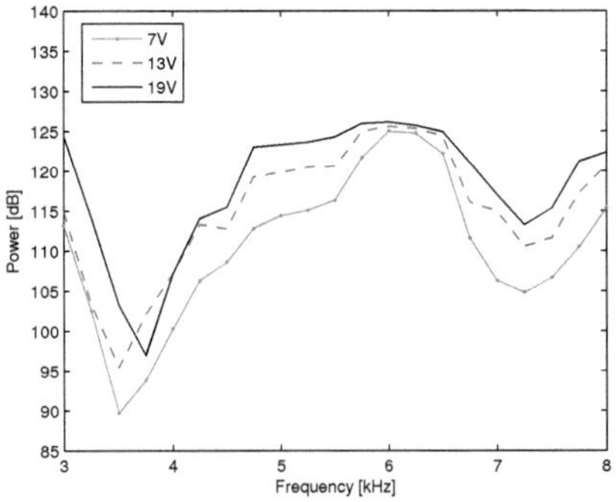

Figure 9.3: Acoustic power delivered by the loudspeaker vs. excitation frequency for voltage amplitudes of 7, 13 and 19 V_{pp}. Each curve results from the averaging of three independent measurements and displays the main range of frequencies investigated.

x 7 mm, resulting in a spatial resolution of $\sim 6.9\mu m$. The laser sheet is generated by a 150 mW diode laser (Laseris Inc., Canada) making use of a light sheet optic. Due to the lighting and flow conditions (driven flow is typically $\ll$ 1 mm/s for the given output power range), a pulsed illumination is not required. Rather, consecutive images are recorded with an exposure time of 1/15 s each.

For the present setup, image recordings are obtained in a horizontal plane cutting through the inflated membrane at approximately its maximal diameter. Due to the finite thickness of the elastic membrane, its curvature upon inflation into a spherical cavity, as well the fact that the material is not perfectly transparent, light sheets cutting horizontally through the cavity at other heights result in strong scattering effects compromising successful flow visualization. Similarly, a light sheet cutting vertically through the inflated hemisphere results in strong scattering, limiting our optimal measurements to a horizontal plane.

9.2.2 Analysis

Different solid particle seedings were evaluated, including smoke, talc (hydrated magnesium silicate) and titanium dioxide particles. However, the deposition of solid particles on the transparent membrane quickly resulted in significant optical obstruction to the measurement plane. Different liquid solutions were tested as well and the best results for flow visualization were obtained with olive oil liquid droplets generated using an airbrush nozzle.

The syringe barrel is filled with air seeded with liquid droplets such that the cavity flow is completely seeded upon inflation. Two-dimensional vector displacements are obtained with a custom PIV algorithm (see Appendix F for a brief overview of the method) based on cross-correlation pattern matching with sub-pixel interpolation [209]. To reduce the noise level present in the raw data, while preserving detail in the image, an edge preserving median filter with a window size of 3 x 3 pixels is first applied to each recorded frame prior to the correlation algorithm. Cross-correlations were obtained with an interrogation window size of 128 x 128 pixels, with a maximum window search size in x- and y-direction of 30 x 30 pixels and a window shift of 16 x 16 pixels. Typical measurements consist in the acquisition of 100 consecutive frames, representing a physical time of ~6.67 s. The PIV velocity vectors obtained from independent

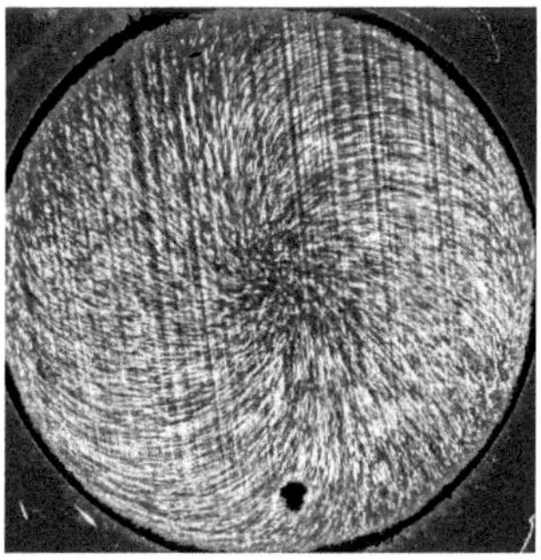

Figure 9.4: Pathline visualization (i.e. streaks) of steady streaming flow at $M = 120$.

image pairs are then time-averaged following an average correlation method [154] (see Appendix F) and resulting maps typically consist of ~ 2100 velocity vectors. Finally, pathline visualizations (i.e. streaks) are obtained following a short routine based on a repetitive comparison and integration method (see Appendix F).

9.3 Results and Discussion

9.3.1 Pathline Visualizations

For the range of excitation frequencies, f, investigated, we found several well-defined internal steady streaming flows. Examples of pathline visualizations (i.e. streaks) of some of the flows found are illustrated in Figs. 9.4 - 9.6. Such flow fields may be categorized using a dimensionless frequency parameter, M, defined as [302]:

$$M = d\sqrt{\frac{\omega}{\nu}}, \tag{9.5}$$

where d is the characteristic diameter of the hemispherical cavity, $\omega = 2\pi f$ the angular frequency of oscillation, and ν the kinematic viscosity of air. The parameter M may be interpreted as the ratio of a body length scale, d, to a viscous length scale $(\nu/\omega)^{1/2}$ (see Eq. (9.2). For the cavity sizes and frequencies investigated, the resulting frequency parameter ranges between $M \approx 120 - 306$, and the generated flows are steady and reproducible.

The first qualitative observation which may be made is that each streaming flow shows strong evidence of three-dimensionality. This is particularly noticeable at $M = 120$ (Fig. 9.4) where a nearly axisymmetric spiraling flow with a source or sink (direction a priori unknown) is present at the center of the plane. The source/sink suggests that fluid is leaving the measurement plane and flowing in the out-of-plane z-axis of the cavity, while the flow remains bounded at the membrane interface such that mass conservation

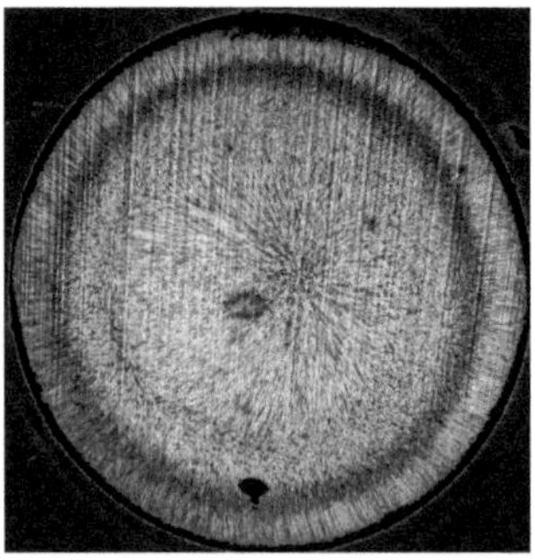

Figure 9.5: Pathline visualization (i.e. streaks) of steady streaming flow at $M = 178$.

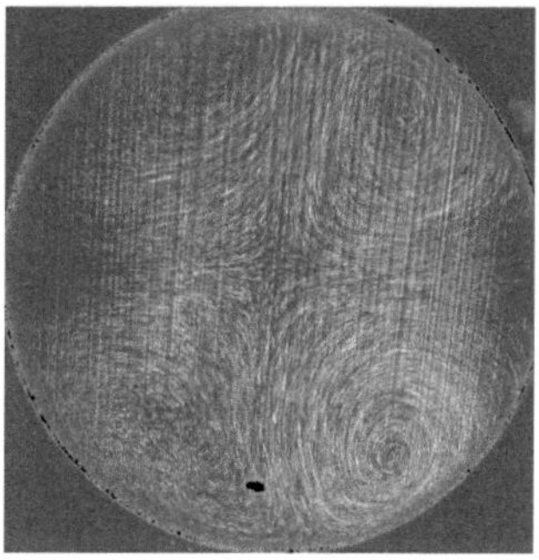

Figure 9.6: Pathline visualization (i.e. streaks) of steady streaming flow at $M = 287$.

applies inside the cavity. This is also true at $M = 178$ (Fig. 9.5), where the flow is again axisymmetric in the measurement plane and consists of two distinct regions: (i) a thin outer region near the membrane wall, separated (i.e. dark ring with no flow) from (ii) a central region with a radially oriented in- or outward flow (direction to be determined). Here flow is leaving/entering the measurement plane both at the center of the cavity ($x \approx 0, y \approx 0$) as well as in the region described by the dark ring, suggesting again the inherent three-dimensionality of the flow field. PIV analysis (following section) will help elucidate some of these flow features, and in particular the direction of the flow.

Figure 9.6 reveals the existence of internal circulation in the shape of four vortices. Experimentally, one

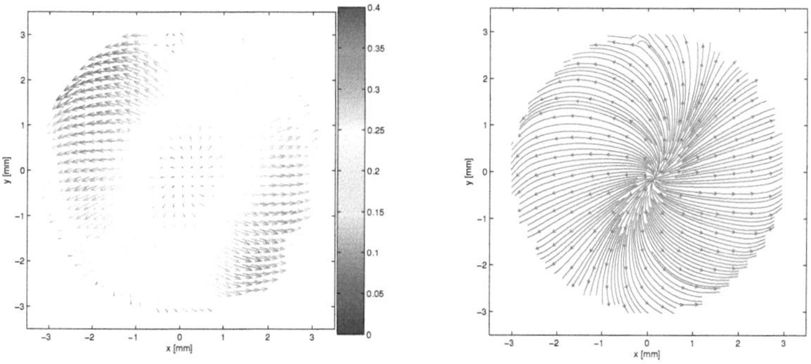

Figure 9.7: (Left) PIV vector plot and (right) reconstructed streamlines for an elastic membrane at $M = 134$ ($V_{pp} = 19.7$ V). Scale is in [mm/s] (top).

observes here a slight asymmetry in the generated vortices. Generally, we have observed a degree of asymmetry in many of the internal streaming flows (see following PIV vector maps), obtained at different values of M. We suspect this may result from the fact that the inflated elastic membranes are not perfectly axisymmetric in nature caused by local differences in the tension present when inflated at the orifice opening. Furthermore, in contrast to theoretical studies describing streaming in and/or outside spherical bodies (i.e. oscillating solid spheres or gas bubbles) [127,294,302], these latter geometries are perfect spheres illustrating axisymmetry in all spatial directions, while the present cavities are, rather, spherical caps or hemispheres, illustrating at best axisymmetry along the out-of-plane z-axis only. Therefore, we expect resulting flow patterns to be influenced by such geometrical differences.

9.3.2 Velocity Fields

Figures 9.7 - 9.11 illustrate PIV vector maps and resulting stream lines of the flow field for a range of dimensionless frequency values M. Quantitative results are obtained after time averaging over 50 image pairs. As a side remark, one may note a slight distortion in some of the resulting flow fields (and consequently in the reconstructed stream lines) obtained in the region of the measurement plane nearest the laser light source ($x \approx 0, y \approx D/2$). This problem arises from slight scattering effects on the membrane surface, which as mentioned previously is both curved and simultaneously not perfectly transparent.

Generally, we observed a rich diversity in the steady streaming flows generated inside the elastic cavity as seen in the pathline visualizations. From the PIV map and the resulting stream lines, it now becomes clear that the flow at $M = 134$ (Fig. 9.7) is moving radially from the center of the measurement plane towards the membrane wall, with a swirling motion. The general topology of the flow observable in the measurement plane bears strong qualitative resemblance with a potential flow resulting from the superposition of a counter-clockwise vortex flow with a source flow. At $M = 200$ (Fig. 9.10), the flow

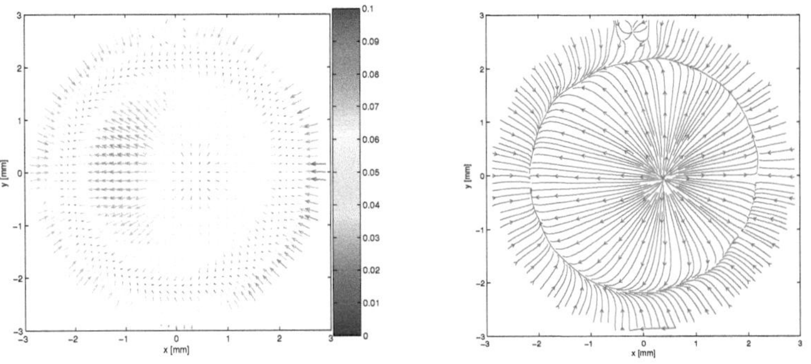

Figure 9.8: (Left) PIV vector plot and (right) reconstructed stream lines for an elastic membrane at $M = 180$ ($V_{pp} = 19.1$ V). Scale is in [mm/s] (top).

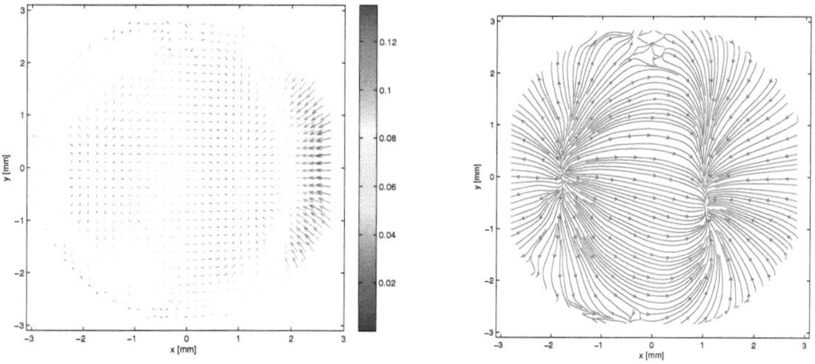

Figure 9.9: (Left) PIV vector plot and (right) reconstructed stream lines for an elastic membrane at $M = 193$ ($V_{pp} = 16$ V). Scale is in [mm/s] (top).

looks strikingly similar to that at $M = 134$, but here the direction of motion has changed. Indeed, fluid travels now radially inwards, again with a slight swirling motion, while the location of the two-dimensional sink is slightly off-centered here.

Finally, at $M = 306$ (Fig. 9.11), we observed internal recirculation made of four characteristic vortices. In particular, the stream surfaces form a nested family of tori and a circle of elliptic fixed (stagnation) points

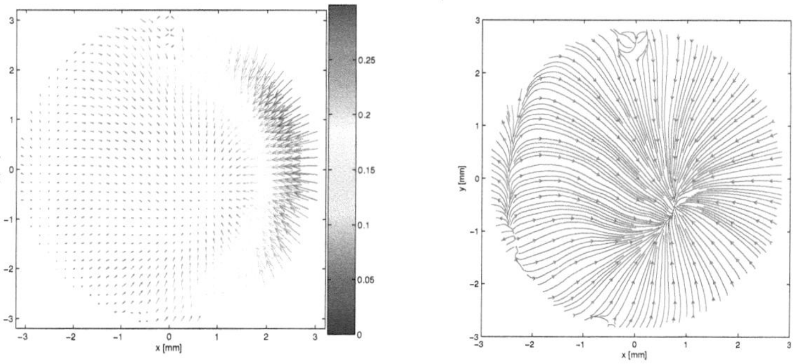

Figure 9.10: (Left) PIV vector plot and (right) reconstructed stream lines for an elastic membrane at $M = 200$ ($V_{pp} = 19.4$ V). Scale is in [mm/s] (top).

lies at the center of each of the fours vortices. In the language of dynamical systems theory [258], one expects a saddle fixed point at the origin, $r = 0$ (this is a stagnation point of the flow). The poles are then also saddle fixed points. In addition, there is a ring of saddle fixed points along the equator. A very important role is played by trajectories that connect saddle points; such trajectories are known as heteroclinic orbits. For example, in the stream line pattern at $M = 306$ in Fig. 9.11, heteroclinic orbits connect the origin to the pole, the pole to the equator, and the equator back to the origin. Taken together these heteroclinic orbits form a heteroclinic cycle. Perturbations of such cycles are known to provide a classic mechanism for the generation of chaos.

For the range of voltages investigated, $V_{pp} = 3 - 20$ V, resulting flows in the measurement plane were found to be < 1 mm/s. Reynolds numbers are then characterized by $Re = DU/\nu < 1$, where U is taken as the mean flow velocity in the measurement plane obtained from the time-averaged PIV vector maps. For several streaming flow fields, we investigated the relationship between the mean flow, U, and the acoustic power delivered by the loudspeaker. Results are shown in Fig. 9.12. We found that the acoustic power followed a nearly logarithmic profile as a function of the applied voltage Fig 9.12 (a). This is particularly true for frequencies where the acoustic power was found to be the lowest (i.e. 3.3 kHz). Fitting the data with a curve of the form $P \propto \ln V_{pp}$, where P is the acoustic power (dB), yields $R^2 > 0.99$. For increasing power levels, however, the curves level off. Curves for P vs. V_{pp} follow the loudspeaker characteristic illustrated earlier in Fig. 9.3.

Correspondingly, results for the mean flow, U, suggest that the flow magnitude follows approximately an exponential growth, $U \propto e^P$, as a function of the delivered acoustic power. This is illustrated in Fig. 9.12 (b) where each set of points is fitted with an exponential curve. One may note that since $P \propto \ln V_{pp}$ (Fig. 9.12 (a)) and $U \propto e^P$, it follows that $U \propto e^{\ln V_{pp}} \propto V_{pp}$ as illustrated in Fig. 9.12 (c). Hence, while the magnitude of the flow in the measurement plane remains relatively small (< 1 mm/s), it is foreseeable that the magnitude of the generated streaming flows may be substantially augmented using a different setup with a signal generator coupled with a loudspeaker delivering higher acoustic power.

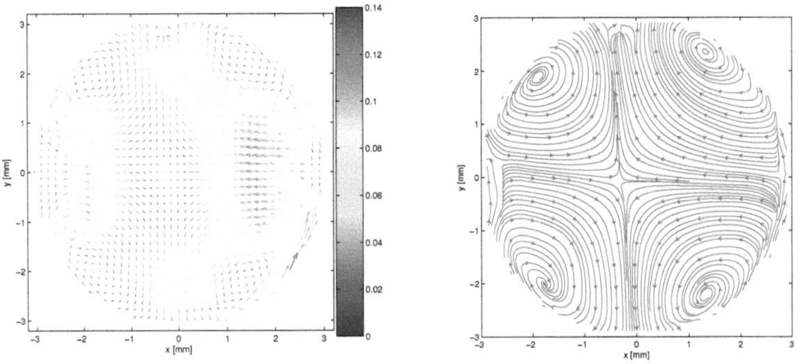

Figure 9.11: (Left) PIV vector plot and (right) reconstructed stream lines for an elastic membrane at $M = 306$ ($V_{pp} = 7$ V). Scale is in [mm/s] (top).

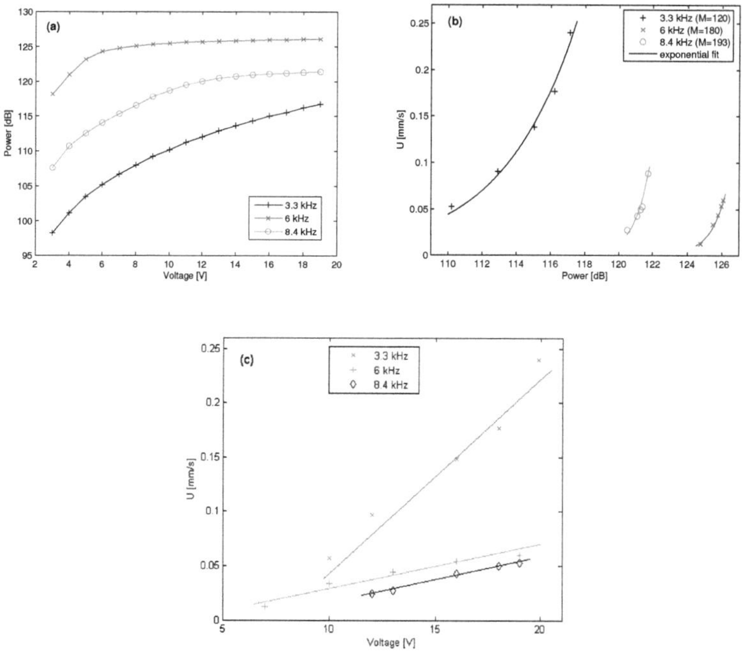

Figure 9.12: (a) Loudspeaker characteristic for frequencies where streaming flows were found for a 1.5 ml (~ 6.5 mm diameter) cavity. Each curve results from the averaging of three independent measurements. (b) Mean streaming flow vs. loudspeaker power. Data is illustrated with exponential fits of the form $U = C_1 e^P + C_2$. (c) Mean streaming flow vs. voltage with linear fits ($R^2 > 0.97$).

It is interesting to note, however, that the velocity magnitude is found to be largest for streaming flows occurring at the lowest excitation frequency (i.e. 3.3 kHz, Fig. 9.12 (b) and (c)). As the excitation frequency is increased, the magnitude of the streaming flows decreases (Fig. 9.12 (b) and (c)). This trend follows qualitatively well with theoretical modelling of acoustic streaming, where the streaming velocity $\propto \omega^{-1}$ [130,168], such that the amplitude of resonance oscillations decreases with increasing frequency.

In the present study, the mean velocity magnitude, U, was found to be highest at $M = 134$ (Fig. 9.7), corresponding to the swirling flow with a source at the center. A qualitative inspection of the flow generated in the vertical z-axis (not shown here), perpendicular to the measurement plane, further reveals that flow motion describes two nearly symmetrical vortices which meet along the hemisphere's centerline, corresponding to the source in Fig. 9.7. The combination of observations at $M = 134$, relating both to the velocity magnitude and the topology of the flow, seem to suggest that the membrane is undergoing here a volume resonance as described by Wu & Du [294]. Indeed, for streaming generated by a gas bubble in an ultrasound field [294], microstreaming velocities are most pronounced at volume resonance ($n = 0$ mode) and the internal flow is depicted as being made of two counter-rotating vortices analogous to a Hill spherical vortex.

9.4 Conclusions

Experimental visualizations were performed using PIV and particle pathlines of the streaming flows generated inside a thin elastic cavity placed in an acoustic sound field. We observed well-defined time-independent flow fields, generated at different values of the dimensionless frequency parameter M. Under the conditions tested, streaming flows exhibited small velocities (< 1 mm/s) such that $Re \ll 1$. The resulting flows suggest that fluid motion inside the cavity is inherently three-dimensional, due to the existence of sources/sinks in the observed two-dimensional vector maps. In particular, the existence of internal streaming flows illustrating well-defined recirculating vortices may be useful in the mixing of fluids on small scales and may potentially exhibit characteristics of chaotic motion, useful in the design of microfluidic devices. In particular, streaming flows observed inside elastic cavities may be interpreted as a precursor to acoustic streaming inside alveolar airspaces. These could potentially lead to enhanced convective flows possibly useful in the transport and deposition of inhaled particles.

We include a short parenthesis on comparing velocity magnitudes obtained under Marangoni forcing (chapter 8) and those observed under acoustic excitation. In both scenarios, cavities are on the order of $D \sim O(10^{-2}$ m). While magnitudes of streaming flows are below <1 mm/s, average Marangoni-driven flows reached several mm/s under thermal forcing conditions. This difference may be explained by the relatively high temperature difference (several degrees ^oC) imposed on the surface of the liquid shell. Indeed, increasing the acoustic power delivered yields quicker flows, and conversely, decreasing the heating temperature at the surface of the soap bubble reduces the effective surface tension gradient driving the liquid shell. Note that while our simple 1D steady-state model for Marangoni forcing (see section 8.4) suggests that the steady velocity of the liquid layer is directly proportional to ΔT, on the other hand, the streaming velocity is proportional to square of the oscillation amplitude U_0.

Chapter 10

Creeping Motion Solutions Inside Spherical Cavities

Low-Reynolds number flows are typically described by the equations of creeping motion (i.e. Stokes flow, see section 3.3.1), where viscous forces are dominant. In the previous chapters, we illustrated using particle image velocimetry (PIV) two examples of small-scale boundary driven cavity flows, where forcing relies on viscous mechanisms at the boundary but the resulting flow patterns are, however, inviscid: (i) Marangoni-driven flows inside a thin liquid shell (see chapter 8), and (ii) acoustic streaming inside an elastic spherical cavity (see chapter 9). Here, the inviscid equations of fluid motion are not used as an approximation, but rather come as a result from the general solution of the creeping motion equations solved in the region interior to a sphere.

10.1 Solution to Creeping Motion in Spherical Coordinates

Lamb [126] outlines a general solution of the creeping motion equations in spherical coordinates. As described earlier in section 3.3.1, the pressure field, p, is harmonic, satisfying the Laplace equation $\nabla^2 p = 0$ (see Eq. (3.25)). This suggests expanding the pressure field in a series of solid spherical harmonics:

$$p = \sum_{n=-\infty}^{\infty} p_n. \tag{10.1}$$

This expansion forms the basis of Lamb's general solution, such that in spherical coordinates (r, θ, ϕ) the velocity field may be given as [94]:

$$\underline{u} = \sum_{n=1}^{\infty} \left[\nabla \times (\underline{r}\chi_n) + \nabla\Phi_n + \frac{(n+3)\,|r|^2\,\nabla p_n - n\underline{r}p_n}{2\mu(n+1)(2n+3)} \right], \tag{10.2}$$

with the assumption of finite velocities at the origin ($r = 0$), and where the scalar functions p_n, χ_n and Φ_n are solid spherical harmonics of order n defined as:

$$\begin{aligned}\chi_n &= \frac{1}{n(n+1)}\left(\frac{r}{a}\right)^n Z_n^m(a,\theta,\phi),\\ \Phi_n &= \frac{a}{2n}\left(\frac{r}{a}\right)^n\left[(n+1)X_n^m(a,\theta,\phi) - Y_n^m(a,\theta,\phi)\right],\\ p_n &= \frac{\mu(2n+3)}{na}\left(\frac{r}{a}\right)^n\left[Y_n^m(a,\theta,\phi) - (n-1)X_n^m(a,\theta,\phi)\right].\end{aligned} \tag{10.3}$$

The functions χ_n and Φ_n arise from the solution of the associated homogeneous equations:

$$\nabla^2\underline{u} = 0, \tag{10.4}$$

$$\nabla\cdot\underline{u} = 0. \tag{10.5}$$

The formulation in Eq. (10.3) makes use of the surface harmonics $Z_n^m(r,\theta,\phi)$, $Y_n^m(r,\theta,\phi)$, and $X_n^m(r,\theta,\phi)$ of degree m and order n. Each harmonic function takes the form :

$$\begin{aligned}Z_n^m(r,\theta,\phi) &= r^n P_n^m(\cos\theta)\, e^{im\phi}\\ Y_n^m(r,\theta,\phi) &= r^n P_n^m(\cos\theta)\, e^{im\phi}\\ X_n^m(r,\theta,\phi) &= r^n P_n^m(\cos\theta)\, e^{im\phi},\end{aligned} \tag{10.6}$$

where $P_n^m()$ are the associated Legendre functions. The solution of a boundary value problem is effected when these three harmonic functions, namely p_n, χ_n and Φ_n, are determined, for each n, from the prescribed boundary conditions. In particular, the unknown scalar functions are determined by matching the appropriate velocity and vorticity boundary conditions at the surface of the sphere ($r = a$). These conditions are described as follows:

$$\begin{aligned}u_n = \frac{1}{|r|}\left(\underline{r}\cdot\underline{u}_s\right)\Big|_{r=a} &= \sum_{n=1}^{\infty} X_n^m(a,\theta,\phi),\\ -|r|\left(\nabla\cdot\underline{u}_s\right)\big|_{r=a} &= \sum_{n=1}^{\infty} Y_n^m(a,\theta,\phi),\\ |r|\,\underline{\omega}_n = \underline{r}\cdot\left(\nabla\times\underline{u}_s\right)\big|_{r=a} &= \sum_{n=1}^{\infty} Z_n^m(a,\theta,\phi),\end{aligned} \tag{10.7}$$

where the velocity vector $\underline{u}_s(\theta,\phi)$ describes the surface velocity field at $r = a$ and ω_n is the vorticity component normal to the surface. For the problem at hand, one may use the fact that there is no normal velocity component, $u_n = 0$, at the surface of the sphere, such that:

$$X_n^m(a,\theta,\phi) \equiv 0\,. \tag{10.8}$$

As a consequence, the full 3D velocity field, $\underline{u}(r,\theta,\phi)$, in the region interior to the sphere can be described in terms of its surface normal vorticity, ω_n, and any contribution of source/sink distributions on the surface of the sphere resulting from $\nabla\cdot\underline{u}_s \neq 0$. Note that $\underline{u}(r,\theta,\phi)$ is independent of viscosity μ, following Eqs. (10.2) and (10.3).

10.2 Marangoni–Driven Flows in a Thin Liquid Shell

The planar flow fields measured inside the soap bubble cavity under thermal forcing (Figs. 8.12 and 8.13 in section 8.3.3) correspond to 2D sections obtained from the 3D velocity field, $\underline{u}$, respectively at $z \approx 0$

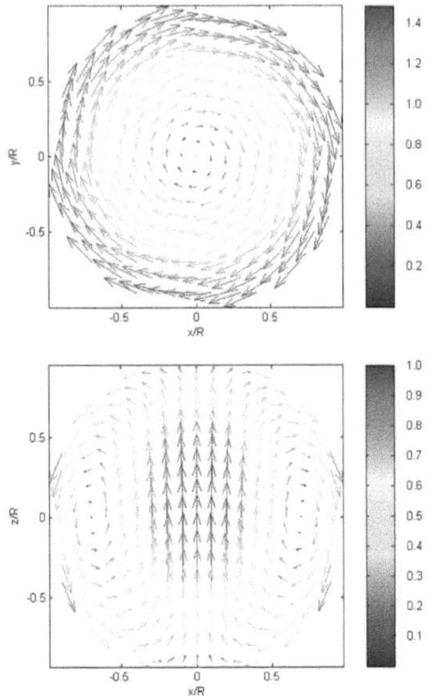

Figure 10.1: Planar flows obtained from solutions of the creeping motion equations, through the superposition of Eqs. (10.9) and (10.10). Top: In the x-y plane ($z = 0$), only the the "solid body rotation" contributes to the 2D flow field. Bottom: In the x-z plane ($y = 0$), the 2D flow field results solely from Hill's spherical vortex. Velocity scale is arbitrary, with $K = -1.5$ and $U_0 = -1$.

(horizontal plane) and $y \approx 0$ (vertical plane), in cartesian coordinates. Qualitatively, flow patterns in the horizontal plane (Fig. 8.14, left) resemble that of a simple vortex flow, while in the horizontal plane (Fig. 8.14, right), the flow field illustrates some similarities with Hill's spherical vortex [102]. To reconstruct analytically the 2D flows measured in each plane from a 3D creeping flow solution (Eq. (10.2)) in the region interior to the cavity, we may first consider a single surface harmonic $Z_1^0(R, \theta, \phi)$. This boundary condition is equivalent to applying in Eq. (10.7) a vorticity field, $\omega_n = \Omega \cos \theta \underline{e}_r$, on the surface of the sphere, where Ω is a constant and a radius of unity is arbitrarily chosen ($R = 1$). Solving Eq. (10.2) in cartesian coordinates, where $\Phi_n = p_n = 0$ (Eq. 10.3), yields an inviscid velocity field, $\underline{u}$, of the form:

$$\begin{bmatrix} u \\ v \\ w \end{bmatrix} = Kr\sin\theta \begin{bmatrix} -\sin\phi \\ \cos\phi \\ 0 \end{bmatrix} = K \begin{bmatrix} -y \\ x \\ 0 \end{bmatrix}, \tag{10.9}$$

where K is a constant. Physically, this 3D flow is analogous to a clockwise ($K < 0$) or counter-clockwise ($K > 0$) "solid body rotation" of the sphere in the x-y plane, where the velocity distribution is independent of z. Note, however, that the general analysis described above does not follow in particular the arbitrary coordinate system chosen for our experiments (see Fig. 8.4 (b) in section 8.2.1).

For measurements obtained in the horizontal plane (Figs. 8.13 and 8.14), flow patterns may be under-

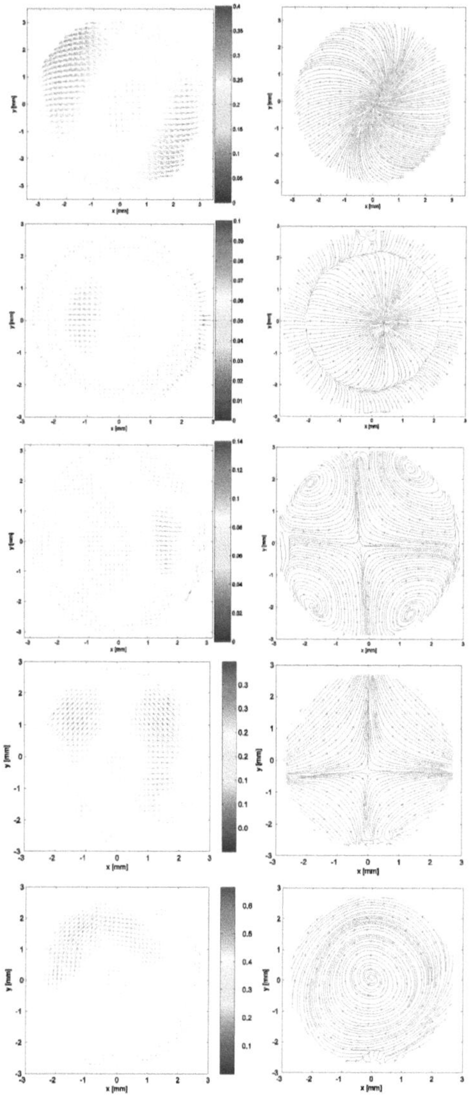

Figure 10.2: Acoustic streaming flows inside the elastic cavity. Left column: Time averaged PIV (scale in mm/s). Right column: Reconstructed stream lines. From top to bottom: $M = 134, 180, 306, 405$, and 454.

stood by considering the boundary condition imposed by $\nabla \cdot \underline{u}_s = 2U_0 \cos\theta$ from Eq. (10.7), where U_0 is a constant. This functional shape matches with the solid spherical harmonic $Y_1^0(R, \theta, \phi)$. The resulting inviscid velocity field is then calculated from Eqs. (10.2) and (10.3), such that:

$$\begin{bmatrix} u \\ v \\ w \end{bmatrix} = U_0 \begin{bmatrix} -xz \\ -yz \\ 2(x^2 + y^2) + z^2 - 1 \end{bmatrix}, \quad (10.10)$$

in cartesian coordinates. Physically, this flow corresponds to Hill's spherical vortex, where internal flow may result for example from the slow translation of a liquid sphere in an external fluid.

Under the specific thermal forcing configuration investigated here, internal flow patterns inside the soap bubble may possibly be understood as being analogous to the 3D superposition of a "solid body rotation" in one plane with Hill's spherical vortex in an orthogonal plane. The superposition of both flows is by definition a solution of the creeping motion Eqs. (3.23) and (3.24) of section 3.3.1. In particular, the resulting 3D flow field inside the cavity corresponds to the sum of Eqs. (10.9) and (10.10). In the x–y plane ($z = 0$), velocity components u and v from Hill's spherical vortex vanish (see Eq. (10.10)) such that a net velocity contribution results solely from the "solid body rotation". Correspondingly, in the orthogonal x–z plane ($y = 0$), the opposite occurs and only velocity components u and w from Hill's spherical vortex

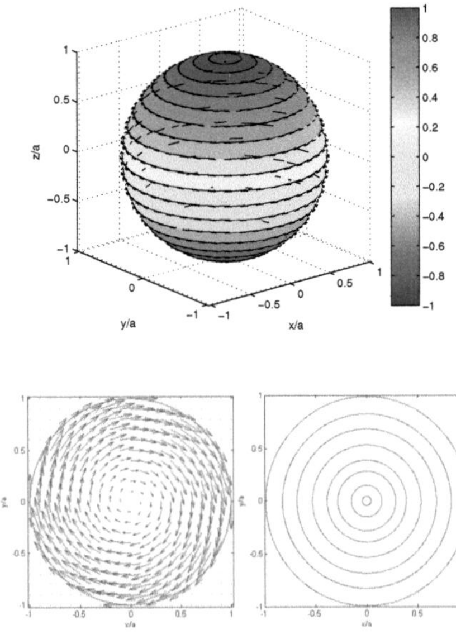

Figure 10.3: Top: Velocity field on the sphere from Eq. (10.9) (colorbar: vorticity ω_n). Bottom: Corresponding velocity field (left) and stream lines (right) at $z = 0$ ($K = -1$).

yield a contribution, while $u = w = 0$ from Eq. (10.9). The resulting analytical planar flows are illustrated in Fig. 10.1 and match qualitatively well PIV flows measured under thermal forcing in the vertical (Fig. 8.12) and horizontal plane (Fig. 8.13). In particular, the ratio K/U_0 governs the relative strength of the "solid body rotation" compared to the recirculating vortex flow.

10.3 Acoustic Streaming Inside an Elastic Spherical Cavity

Recalling PIV results obtained for acoustic streaming flows inside an elastic spherical cavity (see section 9.3), we illustrate again a selection of such streaming flows in Fig. 10.2. The simplest flow perhaps observed in the measurement plane was encountered at $M = 454$ (Fig. 10.2, bottom row), resembling the structure of a simple vortex flow (i.e. 2D potential flow theory). Analytically, the 2D flow measured in the plane is described again by the "solid body rotation" given above in Eq. (10.9). The velocity distribution is independent of z and holds directly in the equatorial x-y plane ($z = 0$). The analytical flow field (Fig. 10.3) bears striking resemblance with the experimental measurement.

At $M = 120$, the resulting streaming flow in the equatorial plane resembles qualitatively a spiraling counter-clockwise vortex flow with a source located approximately at the origin (Fig. 10.2, top row).

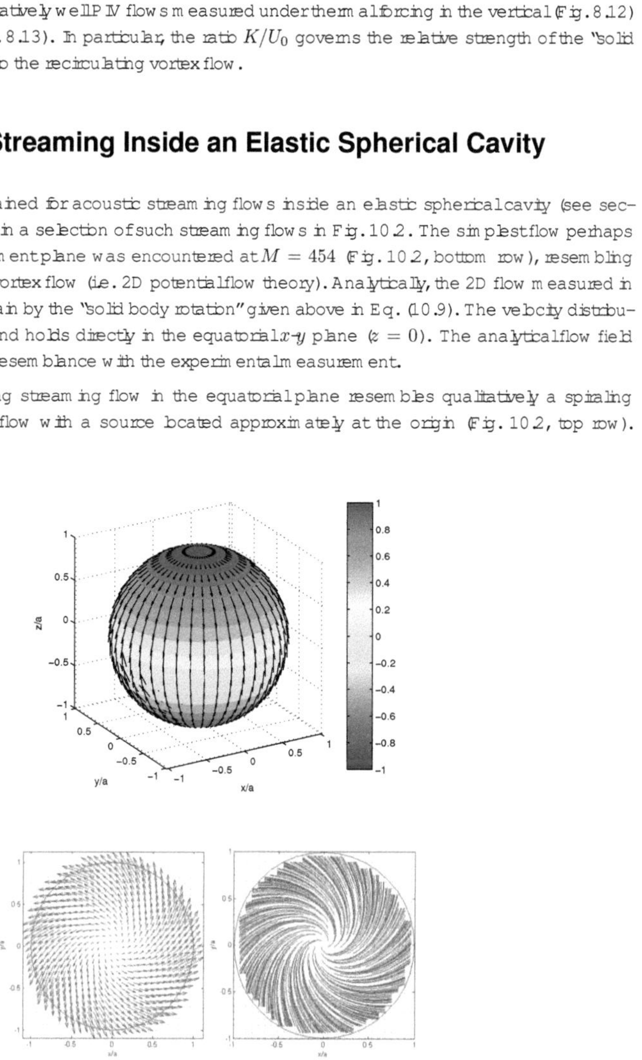

Figure 10.4: Top: Velocity field on the sphere from Eq. (10.11) (colorbar: vorticity ω_n). Bottom: Corresponding velocity field (left) and stream lines (right) at $z = 0.01$ ($K/U_0 = 0.01$).

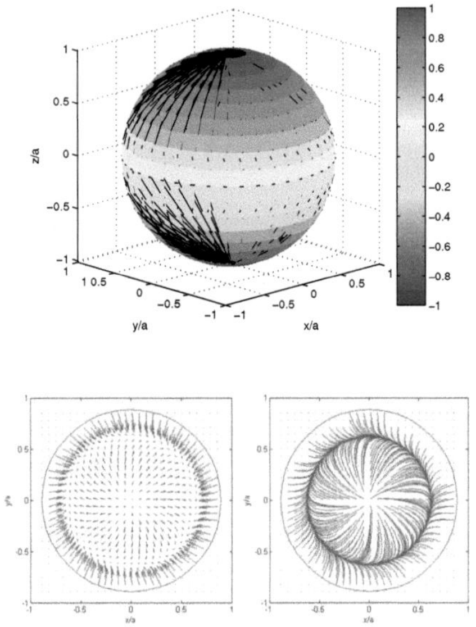

Figure 10.5: Top: Velocity field on the sphere from Eq. (10.12) (colorbar: vorticity ω_n). Bottom : Corresponding velocity field (left) and stream lines (right) at $z = 0.4$ ($K/U_0 = -0.05$).

Analytically, the flow inside the cavity may be constructed by superimposing a "solid body rotation", $Z_1^0(a,\theta,\phi)$, as described in Eq. (10.9), with a surface harmonic $Y_1^0(a,\theta,\phi)$. This latter boundary condition is equivalent to imposing a surface velocity, $\underline{u}_s = U_o \sin\theta \underline{e}_\theta$, from Eq. (10.7), where U_0 is a constant. The resulting inviscid 3D velocity field is found from Eqs. (10.2) and (10.3) and takes the form :

$$\begin{bmatrix} u \\ v \\ w \end{bmatrix} = U_0 \begin{bmatrix} xz \\ yz \\ 1-2(x^2+y^2)-z^2 \end{bmatrix} + K \begin{bmatrix} -y \\ x \\ 0 \end{bmatrix}, \qquad (10.11)$$

in cartesian coordinates. Note that in the equatorial plane ($z = 0$), $u = v = 0$ and only an out-of-plane w velocity component remains. However, since the elastic cavity is a spherical cap, as mentioned earlier, and thus not entirely axisymmetric, we evaluate $\underline{u}$ at a small finite value $z = \epsilon$, slightly off the symmetrical plane. The resulting analytical velocity field, $\underline{u}$ (Eq. (10.11)), captures qualitatively well the planar experimental measurement at $M = 120$, with $K/U_0 = 0.01$ (Fig. 10.4).

At $M = 178$, the planar flow is approximately axisymmetric (Fig. 10.2, second row) and consists qualitatively of two distinct regions: (i) a thin annular shaped region near the membrane wall, separated from (ii) a central circular region with a radially oriented flow. Fluid flows in the plane towards the discernable ring, originating both from the center of the cavity where it moves radially outwards, and from the outer wall where it flows inwards. Analytically, the 3D flow inside the cavity may be constructed by considering

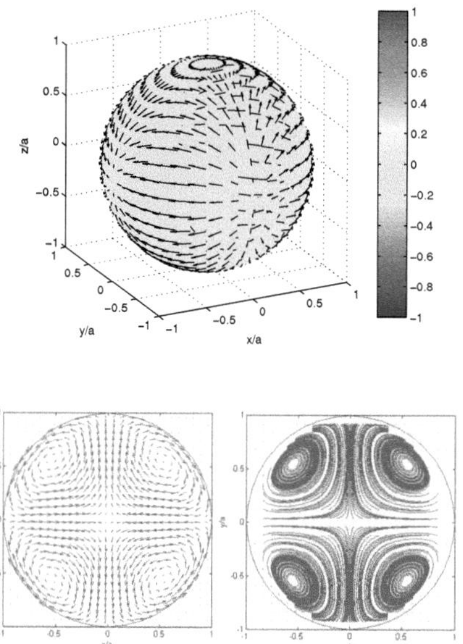

Figure 10.6: Top: Velocity field on the sphere from Eq. (10.13) (colorbar: vorticity ω_n). Bottom: Corresponding velocity field (left) and stream lines (right) at $z = 0$ ($U_0 = 1$).

the surface harmonic $Y_2^0(a,\theta,\phi)$, which is equivalent to imposing a surface velocity, $\underline{u}_s = U_o \cos\theta \sin\theta \underline{e}_\theta$, in Eq. (10.7). To capture the slight rotational motion observed in the experimental planar flow field, we superimpose again $Z_1^0(a,\theta,\phi)$ (Eq. (10.9)). The resulting inviscid 3D velocity field is solved in cartesian coordinates from Eqs. (10.2) and (10.3):

$$\begin{bmatrix} u \\ v \\ w \end{bmatrix} = U_0 \begin{bmatrix} -\frac{x}{4}(x^2+y^2+3z^2-1) \\ -\frac{y}{4}(x^2+y^2+3z^2-1) \\ \frac{z}{2}(2x^2+2y^2+z^2-1) \end{bmatrix} + K \begin{bmatrix} -y \\ x \\ 0 \end{bmatrix}. \tag{10.12}$$

Here, we evaluate again $\underline{u}$ at $z = \epsilon$. The resulting analytical velocity field, $\underline{u}$ (Eq. (10.12)), resembles closely the planar flow at $M = 178$, with $K/U_0 = -0.05$ (Fig. 10.5).

At $M = 306$, the stream surfaces form a nested family of tori and a circle of elliptic fixed (stagnation) points lies at the center of each of the four vortices (Fig. 10.2, third row). For this characteristic streaming flow, the stream line patterns resemble closely internal circulation flows described for a levitated drop in an acoustic field [302] or similarly for an immersed drop in Stokes flow [258]. The measured planar flow

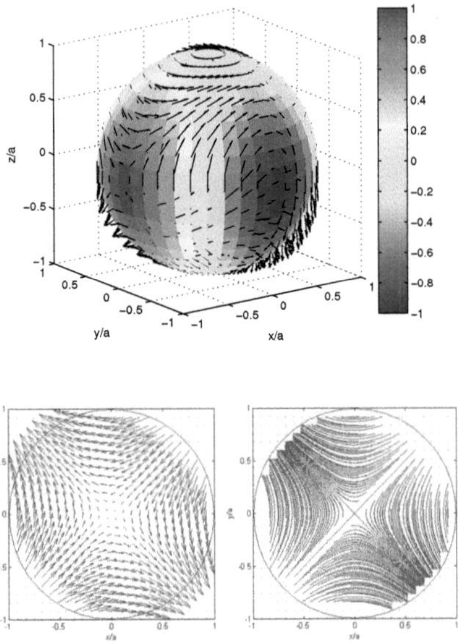

Figure 10.7: Top: Velocity field on the sphere from Eq. (10.14) (colorbar: vorticity ω_n). Bottom : Corresponding velocity field (left) and stream lines (right) at $z = 0.01$ ($K = 1$).

may be reconstructed by considering the boundary condition $\nabla \cdot \underline{u}_s = Y_2^2(a, \theta, \phi) = \sin^2\theta(2\cos^2\phi - 1)$ in Eq. (10.7). This leads to the inviscid 3D velocity field:

$$\begin{bmatrix} u \\ v \\ w \end{bmatrix} = U_0 \begin{bmatrix} \frac{x}{2}(3x^2 + 7y^2 + 5z^2 - 3) \\ -\frac{y}{2}(7x^2 + 3y^2 + 5z^2 - 3) \\ -z(x-y)(x+y) \end{bmatrix}. \quad (10.13)$$

Evaluated at the equatorial plane ($z = 0$), the resulting analytical planar flow, $\underline{u}(x, y)$, captures closely the experimental flow pattern (Fig. 10.6).

Finally at $M = 405$, the four vortices have now disappeared, giving place to open stream lines in each quadrant of the plane (Fig. 10.2, fourth row). The stagnation (saddle) point at $r = 0$ is preserved and the poles remain saddle fixed points. This planar flow may be captured by imposing the boundary condition $\omega_n = Z_2^2(a, \theta, \phi) = \sin^2\theta(2\cos^2\phi - 1)\underline{e}_r$ in Eq. (10.7). Solving Eqs. (10.2) and (10.3) leads to the inviscid

3D velocity field:

$$\begin{bmatrix} u \\ v \\ w \end{bmatrix} = K \begin{bmatrix} -zy \\ -zx \\ 2xy \end{bmatrix}. \tag{10.14}$$

Note again that $u = v = 0$ in the equatorial plane ($z = 0$), where only w subsides. Hence, $\underline{u}$ is evaluated at $z = \epsilon$, slightly off the equatorial plane. The resulting analytical flow field (Fig. 10.7) resembles closely the experimental measurement, although here the orientation of the flow in the plane is slightly altered with respect to Fig. 10.2 (fourth row). This difference may perhaps result from the arbitrary location of the acoustic source (i.e. loudspeaker/transducer) relative to the cavity.

10.4 Conclusions

We have illustrated, using PIV, two original examples of low-Reynolds boundary-driven cavity flows: (i) Marangoni-driven recirculating flows in a thin liquid shell and (ii) acoustic streaming inside elastic spherical cavities. While the generation of such flows relies on viscous mechanisms at a fluid-fluid or solid-fluid boundary, in the bulk of the fluid, however, flow patterns are steady and inviscid. Analytically, the measured planar flows may be captured from the general solution of the creeping motion equations inside a sphere. Inviscid 3D flow patterns are constructed from the superposition of surface harmonics, defining the flow boundary conditions on the surface of the sphere. The inviscid equations of fluid motion are not used as an approximation here, but rather come as a result.

Referring again to alveolar flows and the control of such, the analytical results presented above suggest that since inviscid flows are generated in the bulk of cavities under acoustic streaming, their magnitude is not a priori limited by $Re \ll 1$. This observation may be useful when considering acoustic streaming as a forcing mechanism for the control and enhancement of alveolar flows.

Chapter 11

Conclusions and Outlook

Although, traditionally, convective respiratory flows in the pulmonary acinus have drawn comparatively little attention, as it was thought for very long that flows in the acinus were rather trivial due to their slow motion (i.e. low-Reynolds number flows), we have confirmed in the present work that characteristics of acinar fluid dynamics are, in fact, much more complex than previously anticipated. These observations come in large part as a direct result from the coupling between the specific geometrical structure of the acinus and the time-dependent rhythmical wall motion exhibited during respiration. Using computational fluid dynamics (CFD) techniques to model transient respiratory breathing in acinar models under moving wall motion, we were able to capture some of the intricate features of alveolar flows, such as the existence of flow separation and recirculation, using in a first step a rather abstract yet insightful simple model of an alveolated duct. In particular, we have shown that the resulting low-Reynolds convective flows in the acinar airways may play a decisive role in the fate of inhaled particles. Based on the original description of lung structure by Fung [71], we developed a novel space-filling model of a pulmonary acinar tree. This geometry was particularly useful to investigate the detailed trajectories as well as the deposition patterns and efficiencies of inhaled non-diffusing micron-sized aerosols. Amongst others, our findings suggest that if aerosols are fine enough while non-diffusive, their kinematics are strongly influenced by the specific time-dependent acinar flow structure in conjunction with gravitational sedimentation effects. These mechanisms may lead to complex irreversible trajectories which span throughout the entire acinar geometry and exhibit long residence times during which particles remain suspended in the bulk of the airspace. Hence, the present results suggest that not only could it take multiple breathing cycles before deposition finalizes, but moreover, deposition patterns are highly non-uniform, in particular when particles are heavier and thus governed by sedimentation processes, leaving important regions of the acinar geometry void of aerosols. These complex aerosol kinematics cannot be easily captured by simple models of isolated alveolar cavities or alveolated ducts. Moreover, the present findings imply that localized targeting of aerosols to specific sites in the acinus remains generally a difficult task.

While both the simple alveolated duct and space-filling model described above remain in essence reductionist versions of real acinar anatomy despite some of their complex features, we have shown that geometrical models of the acinus may nevertheless be successful at capturing essential characteristics of fluid dynamics in the pulmonary acinus and describing the resulting aerosol kinematics which follow. This modelling approach coupled with the use of computational fluid dynamics remains a relatively straightforward strategy to tackle the limited accessibility and complexity of the pulmonary acinus to assess acinar flow properties. Furthermore, we have shown that with the use of novel imaging techniques (i.e. X-ray

Tomographic Microscopy) which can resolve spatial resolutions of the acinar structure ($\sim O(1\ \mu m)$), it is now, in principle, feasible to conduct respiratory flow simulations in reconstructed three-dimensional alveolar models. This points towards future, more realistic acinar flow simulations and aerosol deposition studies, once technical limitations both in the imaging and reconstruction schemes are overcome.

Given the often low or insufficient amount of aerosol lung deposition achieved using state-of-the-art inhalation devices, in particular in young children [226], as well as the relative lack of precise control in targeting aerosols to localized sites [9,129], the potential development of novel strategies towards improved and enhanced particle deposition inside the lung is more than ever a relevant challenge. In particular, new strategies may involve in the future a departure from traditional methodologies largely based on the selection of aerosol particle size coupled with the limited flow controllability through patients' breathing patterns. Hence, we have attempted to investigate the use of non-invasive forcing mechanisms, namely (i) Marangoni driven thermocapillary motion and (ii) acoustic streaming, to generate and control forced convective flows within benchmark alveolar models. These experiments were conducted as a first milestone in view of future potential medical applications which we hope could lead one day towards enhanced particle mixing and lung deposition through forced alveolar flow excitation.

While we have shown that it is in principle possible to generate low-Reynolds number forced cavity flows as a result of thermocapillary motion induced in a thin liquid shell (i.e. soap bubble), this approach seems for the time being rather difficult to translate into a realizable clinical application using, e.g. selective microwave heating. In particular, relatively large temperature gradients (several degrees ^oC) in the alveolar liquid layer lining would be sought to generate sufficient airflow convection inside alveoli. Nevertheless, our findings may perhaps trigger more direct applications in microfluidic mixing devices. On the other hand, our benchmark model for acoustic streaming generated inside a thin elastic cavity seems a more likely candidate for direct medical implementation aimed at the enhancement of aerosol lung deposition. We have indeed illustrated that it is feasible to generate and control non-intrusively forced convective flows inside a soft extendable cavity, at a solid-fluid interface. The potential use of this technology to support inhalation therapy as well as possibly other pulmonary applications stems from the fact that acoustic streaming is already established in medical applications including for example the diagnosis of fluid-filled breast cysts and lesions [165] as well as lithotripsy (i.e. noninvasive disintegration of kidney stones and gallstones with focused shock waves [212]). Therefore, we strongly believe that research in the direction of acoustic streaming aimed at enhancing aerosol deposition in the lung should be pursued. Such technology could potentially support the use of inhalation devices to augment total lung deposition or, alternatively, to target deposition in localized or regional lung sites.

Appendix A

Laplace-Young Equation

Derivation of the Laplace-Young Equation

The present analysis follows the derivation of Isenberg [112] Consider a small curvilinear rectangular element of the surface separating two fluids, $ABCD$, of area S (Fig. A.1). The sides of the rectangle have lengths x and y. The radii of curvature of the sides of the rectangle are r_1 and r_2. The radii of curvature at A and B in the plane through the x-axis meet at O_1, and the radii of curvature at B and C in the plane through the y-axis meet at O_2. Now let the surface element $ABCD$ undergo a virtual displacement, δu, normal to the surface under the action of the excess pressure, p. The new position of $ABCD$ is $A'B'C'D'$. The radii of curvature will increase to $r_1 + \delta u$ and $r_2 + \delta u$, and the sides of the surface element will increase to $x + \delta x$ and $y + \delta y$, respectively. If this virtual displacement is performed under isothermal conditions, the work done by the excess pressure, δW, will be equal to the increase in the surface energy δF, due to the change in surface area of the element, δS. That is,

$$\delta W = pS\delta u. \tag{A.1}$$

The increase in energy on the surface

$$\delta F = \sigma \delta S, \tag{A.2}$$

where σ is the interfacial tension, or surface tension, between the two fluids. Expressing the above equation in terms of x and y yields:

$$\delta F = \sigma\left[(x + \delta x)(y + \delta y) - xy\right]. \tag{A.3}$$

The segment $O_1A'B'$ and O_1AB are similar, hence:

$$\frac{x + \delta x}{r_1 + \delta u} = \frac{x}{r_1}, \tag{A.4}$$

such that

$$x + \delta x = x\left(1 + \frac{\delta u}{r_1}\right). \tag{A.5}$$

Similarly for segments $O_1B'C'$ and O_1BC,

$$y + \delta y = y\left(1 + \frac{\delta u}{r_2}\right). \tag{A.6}$$

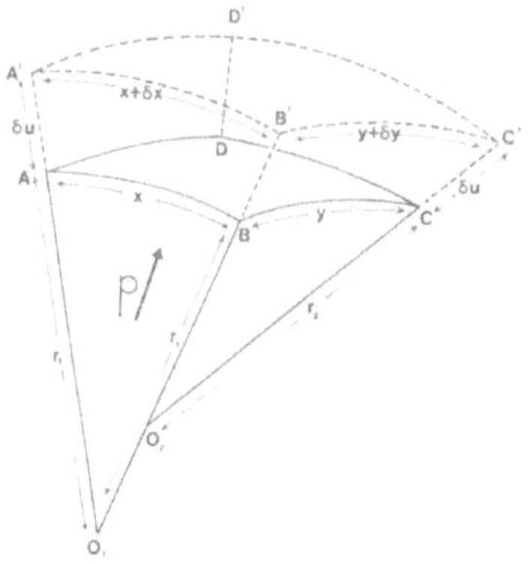

Figure A.1: A curvilinear rectangular element of a surface separating two fluids. From Isenberg [112]. With kind permission from Dover Publications.

Substituting the above two equations into (A.3) yields

$$\delta F = \sigma \left[xy \left(1 + \frac{\delta u}{r_1}\right)\left(1 + \frac{\delta u}{r_2}\right) - xy \right] \quad (A.7)$$

$$= \sigma xy \delta u \left(\frac{1}{r_1} + \frac{1}{r_2}\right) + O(\delta u^2) \quad (A.8)$$

$$= \sigma S \delta u \left(\frac{1}{r_1} + \frac{1}{r_2}\right) + O(\delta u^2), \quad (A.9)$$

as $S = xy$. For small displacements, δu, terms of $O(\delta u^2)$ may be neglected. Equating δW and δF, respectively from (A.1) and (A.7) yields:

$$pS\delta u = \sigma S \delta u \left(\frac{1}{r_1} + \frac{1}{r_2}\right). \quad (A.10)$$

Therefore

$$p = \sigma \left(\frac{1}{r_1} + \frac{1}{r_2}\right). \quad (A.11)$$

This result is valid for any orthogonal curvilinear system of coordinates in which x and y are measured in the interfacial surface. If we choose the coordinate system which forms the principal, maximum and minimum, radii of curvature R_1 and R_2 at any point in the surface, then (A.11) becomes

$$p = \sigma \left(\frac{1}{R_1} + \frac{1}{R_2}\right). \quad (A.12)$$

This is the well known Laplace-Young equation [128]. If a radius of curvature R_1 or R_2 is in the opposite direction that shown in Fig. A.1, it will have a negative sign. That is, a radius of curvature is positive if it is convex in the direction of the pressure, and negative is it is concave in this direction.

A soap film has two parallel surfaces. Thus, applying the Laplace-Young equation to each surface, the excess pressure, p_f, across the film is:

$$p_f = \sigma_f \left(\frac{1}{R_1} + \frac{1}{R_2} \right), \quad (A.13)$$

where $\sigma_f = 2\sigma$. The weight of the soap film element is negligible compared within the surface tension forces acting on the element. In thermodynamic equilibrium its thickness will be typically in the range of 50–300 Angstroms. Consequently, the weight of the film may be neglected. This is also true of the interfacial layer between two immiscible fluids.

The Laplace-Young equation determines the shape of the interfacial surface providing the excess pressure, p, is known at all points on the surface.

Equilibrium of Soap Bubbles

A soap bubble consists of a thin spherical shell which is composed of water and soap ions. Inside the shell is air or gas at a greater pressure than the external atmospheric pressure. For a spherical bubble, the principle radii of curvature, R_1 and R_2 are equal to its radius, that is $R_1 = R_2 = r$. The excess pressure across each surface of the bubble is obtained from (A.13) (a bubble has two surfaces):

$$p = \frac{4\sigma}{r}, \quad (A.14)$$

as $\sigma_f = 2\sigma$.

It is instructive to examine the equilibrium of two bubble, A and B (Fig. A.2), both of radius r connected by a pipe. We assume that the concentration of the surfactant soap ions (i.e. surface ions) is sufficiently great to ensure that σ_f remains constant for variations in r. The pressure in the two bubbles will be initially equal. Small fluctuations in the air pressure will cause a small quantity of air to be transferred from A to B. The radius of B will increase and so the excess pressure in B will decrease (see (A.14)). The converse will be true for bubble A. The radius of A will decrease with a consequent increase in the excess pressure. Thus, the pressure difference between A and B will continue to increase. The bubble B will grow whilst bubble A shrinks. The system of bubbles is unstable, and the radius of curvature of the smaller bubble will continue to decrease until it becomes equal to the diameter of the pipe to which it is connected. Beyond this state, the radius of curvature of the bubble will increase as it now forms the minor spherical cap of a sphere bounded by the orifice of the pipe. The excess pressure will thus begin to decrease in bubble A. Eventually a radius of curvature A will be reached that is equal to that of B, and the stable equilibrium will be attained. The broken curves in Fig. A.2 indicate this final state.

In order for two bubbles, A and B, to be in stable equilibrium, a small transfer of air from A to B must be associated with a pressure increase in B, so that air flows back to restore the equilibrium and vice versa. This condition is satisfied by the final equilibrium state of the two bubbles examined above, under the constraints imposed by the radii of curvature of the exit outlets of the pipe. Thus, for stable equilibrium, we require that the excess pressure, p, and radius r of each bubble satisfy:

$$\frac{dp}{dr} > 0. \quad (A.15)$$

It has been assumed that σ_f remains constant in investigating the behavior of the bubbles. For soap films with low surfactant concentrations, σ_f will not remain constant. As the radius of the bubble decreases

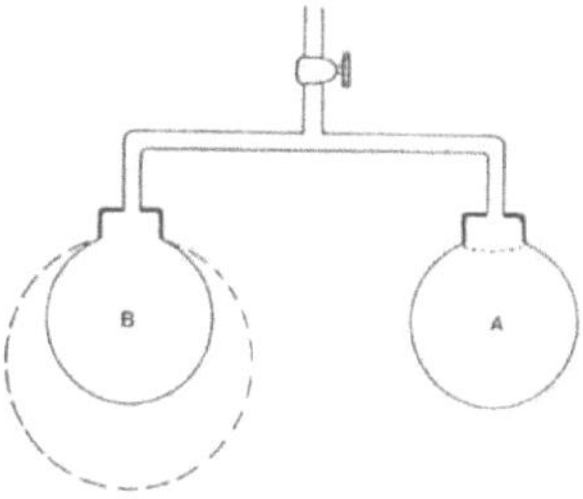

Figure A.2: Two bubble in equilibrium. The full curves represent the initial unstable position, the broken curves represent the final stable equilibrium position. From Isenberg [112]. With kind permission from Dover Publications.

more soap ions will be adsorbed into the surface, which will decrease σ_f. By increasing the radius of the bubble, the film will become more water-like, as the surface density of surfactant ions will decrease. Hence σ_f will increase as water has a higher surface tension than soap solution. Under these conditions, a bubble will stay in stable equilibrium if the condition in Eq. (A.15) is satisfied. That is, from (A.14), if:

$$\frac{d}{dr}\left(\frac{2\sigma_f}{r}\right) > 0. \tag{A.16}$$

Differentiating the above, where σ_f may depend on r yields:

$$\frac{2}{r^2}\left(-\sigma_f + r\frac{d\sigma_f}{dr}\right) > 0, \tag{A.17}$$

$$\frac{d\sigma_f}{d\log r} > \sigma_f. \tag{A.18}$$

The area of the bubble is $A = 4\pi r^2$. So (A.18) can be rewritten as:

$$2\frac{d\sigma_f}{d\log A} > \sigma_f. \tag{A.19}$$

The quantity

$$\gamma = \frac{d\sigma_f}{d\log A} \tag{A.20}$$

was first introduced by William Gibbs and is called the ***surface elasticity*** of the film. The condition for two or more bubbles to co-exist in stable equilibrium with the same excess pressure is, from (A.19) and (A.20),

$$2\gamma > \sigma_f. \tag{A.21}$$

Similarly, the surface elasticity of the surface of a soap solution can be defined by replacing σ_f in (A.19) by σ.

Appendix B

Stokes Law for Small Spherical Particles

In the following pages, we review Stokes law [257] for small spherical particles, based on the non-dimensionalized Navier-Stokes equations in the creeping flow regime, where Reynolds numbers are low, i.e. $Re \ll 1$.

Governing Equations for the Creeping Flow Regime

Assuming incompressible flow in the pulmonary airways [47,66], the Navier-Stokes equations may be written in tensor and indicial notation, respectively, as follows:

$$\frac{\partial \underline{u}}{\partial t} + (\underline{u} \cdot \nabla)\underline{u} = -\frac{1}{\rho}\nabla p + \nu \nabla^2 \underline{u} + \underline{f}, \tag{B.1}$$

$$\frac{\partial u_i}{\partial t} + u_j \cdot \frac{\partial u_i}{\partial x_j} = -\frac{1}{\rho}\frac{\partial p}{\partial x_i} + \nu \frac{\partial^2 u_i}{\partial x_j \partial x_j} + f_i, \tag{B.2}$$

where $\underline{u}$ is the velocity field, t the time, ρ the density of the fluid, and $\nu = \mu/\rho$ is the kinematic viscosity of the fluid (μ is the dynamic viscosity). Here, $\underline{f}$ represents externals force acting on the fluid (e.g. gravity). We neglect such forces in the following analysis, and derive the dimensionless form of the Navier-Stokes equations by introducing the following dimensionless variables [125]:

$$x_i' = \frac{x_i}{L}; \quad t' = \frac{U}{L}t; \quad u_i' = \frac{u_i}{U}; \quad p' = p\frac{L}{\mu U},$$

where U is a characteristic velocity and L a characteristic length scale. Substituting the above dimensionless variables into the index form of the Navier-Stokes equations yields:

$$Re\left(\frac{\partial u_i'}{\partial t'} + u_j' \cdot \frac{\partial u_i'}{\partial x_j'}\right) = -\frac{\partial p'}{\partial x_i'} + \frac{\partial^2 u_i'}{\partial x_j' \partial x_j'}, \tag{B.3}$$

where the Reynolds number is defined as $Re = UL/\nu$. In tensor form, the non-dimensionalized equation reads as:

$$Re\left(\frac{\partial \underline{u}'}{\partial t'} + (\underline{u}' \cdot \nabla')\underline{u}'\right) = -\nabla' p' + \nabla'^2 \underline{u}', \tag{B.4}$$

where $\nabla' = L\nabla$. Considering a creeping flow regime, governed by low Reynolds numbers, i.e. $Re \ll 1$, for small spherical particles, the left-hand side terms of the above equation may then be neglected such that $\nabla' p' = \nabla'^2 \underline{u}'$. Therefore, we can express the governing equations for the creeping flow regime by neglecting inertial and transient terms altogether reducing effectively to:

$$\nabla p = \mu \nabla^2 \underline{u}. \tag{B.5}$$

Due to the low Reynolds numbers involved, the flow is effectively incompressible such that mass conservation is preserved. The equations of incompressible creeping (Stokes) flow motion are then expressed as:

$$\nabla p - \mu \nabla^2 \underline{u} = 0, \tag{B.6}$$

$$\nabla \cdot \underline{u} = 0. \tag{B.7}$$

Applying the divergence operator, $\nabla\cdot$, to Eq. (B.6), while making use of Eq. (B.7), yields:

$$\triangle p = \nabla^2 p = 0. \tag{B.8}$$

The strategy consists in solving the above second order Laplace equation, Eq. (B.8), for the pressure field, p, from which the velocity field, $\underline{u}$, may then be solved using mass continuity, Eq. (B.7).

Velocity and Pressure Fields of Creeping Flow Around a Sphere

We consider a sphere of diameter D placed in a uniform flow field, $\underline{U}$, under creeping flow assumptions. The problem is axisymmetric and thus independent of angle ϕ (Fig. B.1).

For this problem, the no-slip boundary condition applies at the surface of the sphere:

$$\underline{u}(r = R, \theta) = 0 \tag{B.9}$$

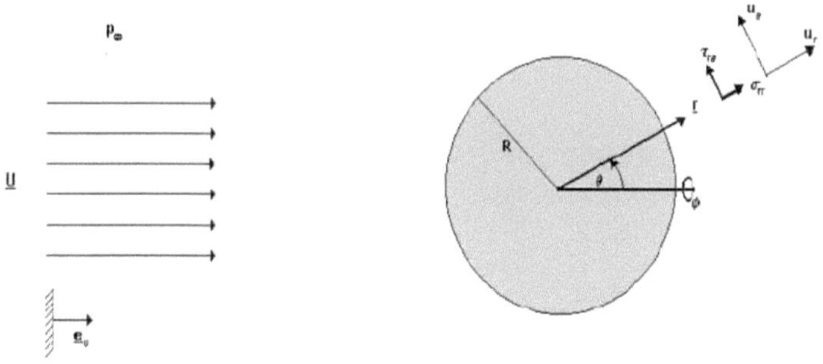

Figure B.1: Schematic of a small sphere placed in a uniform flow.

Far from the sphere, the boundary conditions are given as:

$$\lim_{r\to\infty}(\underline{u}(r,\theta)) = \begin{pmatrix} U\cdot\cos\theta \\ -U\cdot\sin\theta \end{pmatrix} \quad (B.10)$$

$$\lim_{r\to\infty}(\overline{p}(r,\theta)) = \lim_{r\to\infty}(p(r,\theta)-p_\infty) = 0. \quad (B.11)$$

The last two boundary conditions are imposed by symmetry with respect to the angle θ:

$$\underline{u}(r,\theta) = \underline{u}(r,-\theta), \quad (B.12)$$

$$\underline{p}(r,\theta) = \underline{p}(r,-\theta). \quad (B.13)$$

The first step consists in solving the Laplace equation, Eq. (B.8), for the pressure field, $\overline{p}(r,\theta) = p(r,\theta) - p_\infty$, since the Laplace equation is linear and p_∞ = constant represents a solution of $\Delta p = 0$. In spherical polar coordinates, the Laplace equation reads as (neglecting terms in ϕ):

$$\frac{1}{r^2}\frac{\partial}{\partial r}\left(r^2\frac{\partial\overline{p}(r,\theta)}{\partial r}\right) + \frac{1}{r^2\sin\theta}\frac{\partial}{\partial\theta}\left(\sin\theta\frac{\partial\overline{p}(r,\theta)}{\partial\theta}\right) = 0. \quad (B.14)$$

To solve the above partial differential equation, dependent on two variables, namely r and θ, a useful approach consists in assuming the following separation of variables:

$$\overline{p}(r,\theta) = f(r)\cdot g(\theta).$$

In particular, it may be shown that $f(r)$ is of the form $f(r) = Ar + B/r^2$ where A and B are constants. Assuming that the function $g(\theta)$ may be approximated with a Fourier series $g(\theta) = \sum_{i=1}^{\infty}(k_i\sin i\theta + l_i\cos i\theta)$ with both k_i and l_i constants, $g(\theta)$ reduces effectively to $l_i\cos\theta$.

Considering the boundary condition in the far-field, Eq. (B.10), it follows that $\lim_{r\to\infty}(f(r)) = 0$ and therefore the constant $A = 0$. This results leads to the following pressure field:

$$\Leftrightarrow \overline{p}(r,\theta) = K\frac{\cos\theta}{r^2}. \quad (B.15)$$

To calculate the velocity field $\underline{u}(r,\theta) = u_r\underline{e}_r + u_\theta\underline{e}_\theta$, we proceed as follows. We first transform the equations of momentum, Eq. (B.6), and continuity, Eq. (B.7), into spherical polar coordinates. The continuity equation will be used to cancel out the term $u_\theta(r,\theta)$ to obtain a single partial differential equation for $u_r(r,\theta)$. Following [125], the governing expressions for mass conservation is:

$$\frac{1}{r^2}\frac{\partial}{\partial r}\left(r^2u_r\right) + \frac{1}{r\sin\theta}\frac{\partial}{\partial\theta}(u_\theta\sin\theta) = 0, \quad (B.16)$$

while the radial and circumferential components of the momentum equation are described as:

$$\frac{\partial\overline{p}}{\partial r} = \mu\left(\frac{1}{r^2}\frac{\partial}{\partial r}\left(r^2\frac{\partial u_r}{\partial r}\right) + \frac{1}{r^2\sin\theta}\frac{\partial}{\partial\theta}\left(\sin\theta\frac{\partial u_r}{\partial\theta}\right) - \frac{2u_r}{r^2} - \frac{2}{r^2\sin\theta}\frac{\partial}{\partial\theta}(u_\theta\sin\theta)\right), \quad (B.17)$$

$$\frac{1}{r}\frac{\partial\overline{p}}{\partial\theta} = \mu\left(\frac{1}{r^2}\frac{\partial}{\partial r}\left(r^2\frac{\partial u_\theta}{\partial r}\right) + \frac{1}{r^2\sin\theta}\frac{\partial}{\partial\theta}\left(\sin\theta\frac{\partial u_\theta}{\partial\theta}\right) + \frac{2}{r^2}\frac{\partial u_\theta}{\partial\theta} - \frac{u_\theta}{r^2\sin^2\theta}\right). \quad (B.18)$$

Again, we attempt a separation of variables to solve for $u_r(r,\theta)$:

$$u_r(r,\theta) = R(r)\Theta(\theta).$$

Substituting this "Ansatz" into the u_r-component of the momentum equation, it may be shown that the functions $R(r)$ and $\Theta(\theta)$ are of the form $R(r) = \alpha + \beta/r^3 + K/\mu k$ and $\Theta(\theta) = k\cos\theta$. Considering the no-slip boundary condition at $r = R$ from Eq. (B.9) and Eq. (B.10) yields:

$$u_\theta(r,\theta) = \left(U + \frac{K}{\mu r} - R^2\left(\frac{K}{\mu} + RU\right)\frac{1}{r^3}\right)\cos\theta, \quad \text{(B.19)}$$

where K remains unknown. To determine the θ velocity component, $u_\theta(r,\theta)$, the continuity equation, Eq. (B.16), is regrouped and partially integrated with respect to θ, where an integration constant, $h(r)$ is defined ($\partial h(r)/\partial\theta = 0$), such that:

$$u_\theta(r,\theta)\sin\theta = \int\left(-\frac{\sin\theta}{r}\frac{\partial}{\partial r}(r^2 u_r(r,\theta))\right)d\theta + h(r),$$

such that:

$$u_\theta(r,\theta) = -\sin\theta\left(U + \frac{K}{2\mu r} + \frac{UR^3}{2r^3} + \frac{KR^2}{2\mu r^3}\right). \quad \text{(B.20)}$$

The unknown constant K may now be determined by applying the appropriate boundary conditions at the surface of the sphere, such that:

$$\begin{aligned} u_\theta(r = R,\theta) &= 0, \\ \Leftrightarrow K = -\frac{3\mu UR}{2}. \end{aligned} \quad \text{(B.21)}$$

Therefore the resulting pressure and velocity fields are:

$$p(r,\theta) = p_\infty - \frac{3}{2}\mu UR\frac{\cos\theta}{r^2}, \quad \text{(B.22)}$$

$$u_r(r,\theta) = U\cos\theta\left(1 - \frac{3R}{2r} + \frac{R^3}{2r^3}\right), \quad \text{(B.23)}$$

$$u_\theta(r,\theta) = -U\sin\theta\left(1 - \frac{3R}{4r} + \frac{R^3}{4r^3}\right). \quad \text{(B.24)}$$

We illustrate an example of the pressure and velocity field obtained for a spherical particle with a diameter $D = 2$ μm, $U = 1$ mm/s and $Re = 1.3 \cdot 10^{-4}$ in Fig. B.2.

Stokes Law

Considering Fig. B.1, we can write the component of the drag force per unit area, $\underline{f}_D$, in the direction of the uniform flow, $\underline{U}$, as follows:

$$\underline{f}_D = (-p(R,\theta)\cos\theta + \sigma_{rr}(r,\theta)\cos\theta - \tau_{r\theta}(r,\theta)\sin\theta)\underline{e}_U, \quad \text{(B.25)}$$

where the pressure field, $p(r,\theta)$ is given in Eq. (B.23) and may be evaluated at $r = R$. The viscous stress components, $\sigma_{rr}(r = R,\theta)$ and $\tau_{r\theta}(r = R,\theta)$, evaluated at $r = R$ are expressed in spherical polar coordinates as follows [125]:

$$\sigma_{rr}(r = R,\theta) = 2\mu\left(\frac{\partial u_r(r,\theta)}{\partial r}\right)_{r=R} = 3\mu U\cos\theta\left(\frac{R}{r^2} - \frac{R^3}{r^4}\right)_{r=R} = 0, \quad \text{(B.26)}$$

$$\tau_{r\theta}(r,\theta) = \mu\left(r\frac{\partial}{\partial r}\left(\frac{u_\theta(r,\theta)}{r}\right) + \frac{1}{r}\frac{\partial u_r(r,\theta)}{\partial\theta}\right)_{r=R} = \frac{3\mu U}{2R}\sin\theta. \quad \text{(B.27)}$$

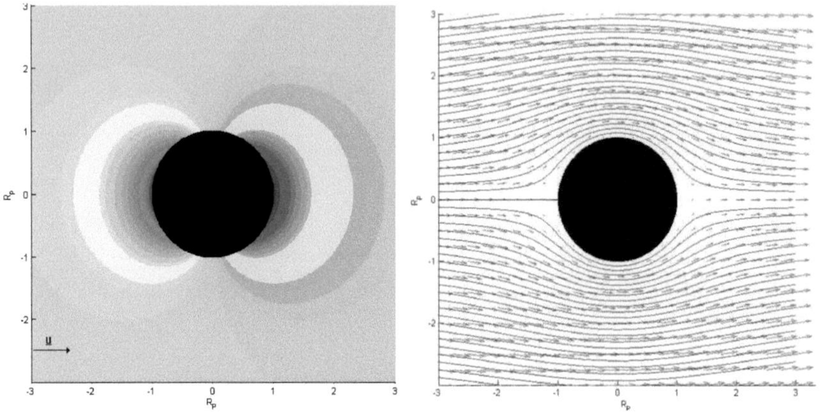

Figure B.2: Left: Pressure field around a sphere under creeping flow. Red color corresponds to higher pressure. Right: Corresponding velocity vector field and stream lines.

This leads to:

$$\underline{f}_D = \left(\frac{3\mu U}{2R} - p_\infty \cos\theta\right) \underline{e}_U. \tag{B.28}$$

To obtain the drag force, $\underline{F}_D$, exerted on the sphere, $\underline{f}_D$ is integrated over the surface of the sphere:

$$\begin{aligned} \underline{F}_D &= \iint_{S_{sphere}} \underline{f}_D dS_{sphere}, \\ \Leftrightarrow \underline{F}_D &= = \int_{\theta=0}^{\theta=2\pi} \int_{\phi=0}^{\phi=\pi} \left(\frac{3\mu U}{2R} - p_\infty \cos\theta\right) R^2 \sin\phi d\phi d\theta, \\ \Leftrightarrow \underline{F}_D &= 6\pi\mu U R \underline{e}_U, \end{aligned} \tag{B.29}$$

Applying the definition of the drag coefficient, C_D, results in the well known form of Stokes law:

$$\begin{aligned} C_D &= \frac{|\underline{F}_D|}{\frac{1}{2}\rho_f v_{rel}^2 A}, \\ \Leftrightarrow C_D &= \frac{3\pi\mu U D}{\frac{1}{2}\rho_f U^2 \frac{\pi}{4} D^2}, \\ \Leftrightarrow C_D &= \frac{24}{Re}. \end{aligned} \tag{B.30}$$

Note that Oseen [171] discovered the nonuniform character of Stokes solutions and proceeded to give a modified approximation that is uniformly valid. The failure of the Stokes equations occurs in the far field, where the convective term is just as large as the viscous term. Oseen reasoned that he could replace $(\underline{u} \cdot \nabla)\underline{u}$ by the linear approximation $U \partial u_i / \partial x$ where U corresponds to the free-stream velocity. Thus he proposed the momentum equation:

$$\rho U \frac{\partial u_i}{\partial x} = -\frac{\partial p}{\partial x_i} + \nu \frac{\partial^2 u_i}{\partial x_j \partial x_j}, \tag{B.31}$$

where x corresponds to the first index of x_i. This equation gives solutions which are uniformly valid for the whole field as $Re \to 0$. Near the spherical body the viscous terms are dominant and the linearized convective term above makes very little contribution to the flow. In fact, the Oseen approximation of $U\partial u_i/\partial x$ and the Stokes approximation of zero are errors of the same order in comparison with the true convective term $(\underline{u} \cdot \nabla)\underline{u}$. Therefore, both equations are acceptable in this region. Far away from the sphere, the velocity differs only slightly with U, so Oseen's linearized convection term is a valid approximation. The Oseen theory produces the drag law for a sphere:

$$\underline{F}_D = 6\pi\mu U R \left(1 + \frac{3}{8}Re\right) \underline{e}_U, \tag{B.32}$$

such that the drag coefficient yields effectively:

$$C_D = \frac{24}{Re}\left(1 + \frac{3}{8}Re\right) = \frac{24}{Re} + 9. \tag{B.33}$$

Appendix C

Error Estimation of Alveolus Model

In this section, the exact volume and surface of an alveolus placed on a duct (rather than on a plane) is calculated and compared to the volume and surface of an alveolus sitting on a plane (see Eqs. 5.10–5.13). The area/volume neglected is illustrated in Fig. C.1.

Volume Error Estimation

First, the volume of a sphere intersecting with a duct (Fig. C.1) is computed. To achieve the following, the area, $A(x)$, which forms the intersection of the sphere and the duct created by cutting cross-sectionally the body perpendicular to the x-axis is derived. Subsequently, the aforementioned volume is obtained through integration. A two-dimensional view of the problem is illustrated in Fig. C.2.

The area $A(x)$ obtained from the intersection of the circle k and the duct consists of two circle segments, one with radius R_d and height h_d, the other with radius $R(x) = \sqrt{{R_a}^2 - x^2}$ and height h_a. The area,

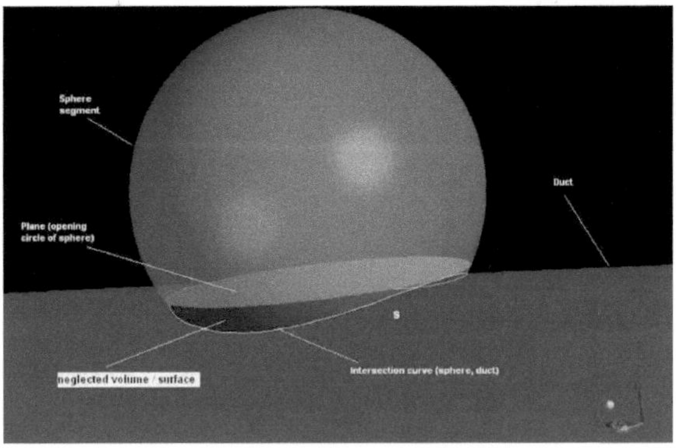

Figure C.1: Illustration of the neglected volume and surface area, indicated by the dark region between the plane and the intersection curve.

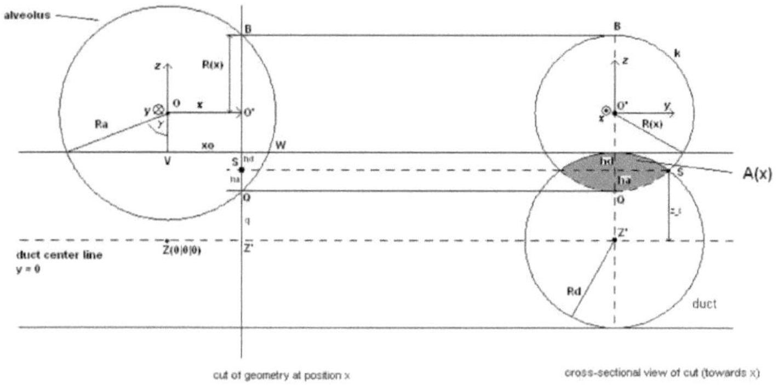

Figure C.2: Two dimensional illustration of sectioned body (see Fig. C.1). Left side: cut of geometry at position x; circle k with centre O' and radius $R(x) = \sqrt{R_a^2 - x^2}$; origin $Z(0|0|0)$. Right side: view towards x; circle with radius R_d and centre Z'. The figure shows the construction of a point S on the intersection curve s between the alveolus and duct. The intersection area, $A(x)$, consists of two circle segments, one of height h_a and radius $R(x)$, the other of height h_d and radius R_d. $q = \overline{Z'Q}$.

$A(x)$, can easily be calculated by adding the areas of these two circle segments. The calculation of a circle segment of radius r and height h is relatively straightforward and is illustrated in Fig. C.3 which also shows the construction of a point S of the intersection curve s. The z-coordinate, z_s, also has to be calculated in order to obtain h_d and h_a. With $A(x)$ known, it is then simple to calculate the volume of the intersection body of the sphere and the duct by integrating $A(x)$, with reference to x, from $x = 0$ to $x_0 = \overline{VW} = R_A \sin\alpha = \sqrt{3}/2 R_a$, where $\alpha = \pi/3$. The "real" volume of the alveolus, V_{alv}, can be calculated by taking the difference between the volume of the whole sphere and the approximation of the alveolar volume: $V_{alv} = 4/3\pi R_a^3 - V_a$. First, however, the area of a circle segment with radius r and height h is calculated.

The illustrated circle (Fig. C.3) can be described in the given coordinate system as:

$$(x - (h - r))^2 + y^2 = r^2 \iff y = \sqrt{r^2 - (x - h + r)^2}, \tag{C.1}$$

and the circle segment area defined as F is calculated as follows:

$$F = 2\int_0^h \sqrt{r^2 - (x - h + r)^2}dx = \pi/2r^2 + \sqrt{h(2r - h)}(h - r) - r^2 \arcsin\left(1 - \frac{h}{r}\right). \tag{C.2}$$

Before obtaining $A(x)$, h_a, h_d and z_s are first calculated. z_s may be found by equating the equations describing the circles for k and the "duct" (see Fig. C.2). The circle k is described as:

$$y^2 + (z - (R_d + R_a \cos\alpha))^2 = R^2(x) \tag{C.3}$$

and the duct is described by $y^2 + z^2 = R_d^2$. Substituting $y^2 = R_d^2 - z^2$ in the above equation for the circle k and solving for $z = z_s$ yields:

$$z_s = \frac{2R_d^2 + 2R_a R_d \cos\alpha + R_a^2 \cos^2\alpha - R^2(x)}{2(R_a \cos\alpha + R_d)}. \tag{C.4}$$

Therefore:

$$h_d = R_d - z_s \Longleftrightarrow h_d = \frac{R^2(x) - {R_a}^2 \cos^2\alpha}{2(R_a \cos\alpha + R_d)}. \tag{C.5}$$

To calculate h_a, we need $q = \overline{Z'Q} = \overline{OZ} - R(x) = R_d + R_a \cos\alpha - R(x)$, such that $h_a = R_d - h_d - q = z_s - q$, which leads then to:

$$h_a = \frac{2R(x)(R_a \cos\alpha + R_d) + R_a(R_a \cos\alpha + 2R_d)\cos\alpha - R^2(x)}{2(R_a \cos\alpha + R_d)}. \tag{C.6}$$

The surface area, $A(x)$, is then given by:

$$A(x) = \frac{\pi}{2}{R_a}^2 + (h_a - R_a)\sqrt{h_a(2R_a - h_a)} - {R_a}^2 \arcsin\left(1 - \frac{h_a}{r_a}\right) \tag{C.7}$$

$$+\frac{\pi}{2}{R_d}^2 + (h_d - R_d)\sqrt{h_d(2R_d - h_d)} - {R_d}^2 \arcsin\left(1 - \frac{h_d}{r_d}\right). \tag{C.8}$$

The volume is then found by integrating $2\int_{x=0}^{x=x_0=R_a \sin\alpha} A(x)dx$ and using the above results. This integral is evaluated numerically on a computer. The evaluated error between the "real" volume of an alveolus on a duct and our estimation of V_a from Eq. (5.11) is given in Table 5.3.

Surface Error Estimation

Now, we calculate the surface S_{alv} of the intersecting body. Formally, this surface may be expressed as:

$$S_{alv} = \iint R^2 \sin\theta \, d\phi \, d\theta. \tag{C.9}$$

The main difficulty lies in finding the appropriate elevation angle, θ, as a function of ϕ along the intersection curve s (see Fig. C.1). From Eq. (C.4), we already know the z-coordinate z_s where $R(x) = \sqrt{{R_a}^2 - x^2}$. Since S is a point on the sphere (or circle k), we can express y_s:

$$y^2 + (z - (R_d + R_a \cos\theta))^2 = R^2(x) \Longleftrightarrow y_s = \sqrt{{R_a}^2 - x^2 - (z_s - (R_d + R_a \cos\theta))^2}, \tag{C.10}$$

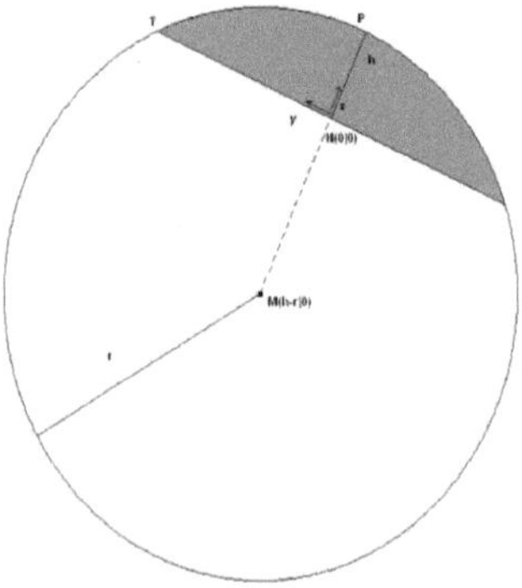

Figure C.3: Circle segment with radius r and height $h = \overline{HP}$; origin $H(0|0)$ and circle center is located at $M(h-r|0)$. $0 \le h \le 2r$.

where we can insert the expression for z_s into the equation for y_s. We know the coordinates of the point S with x as a parameter: $S(x|y_s|z_s)$. Now, we can express the angle ϕ with the projection of S in the x–y plane $S_0(x|y_s|0)$:

$$\cos\phi = \frac{\begin{bmatrix}1\\0\\0\end{bmatrix} \cdot \begin{bmatrix}x\\y_s\\0\end{bmatrix}}{\sqrt{x^2+{y_s}^2}} = \frac{x}{\sqrt{x^2+{y_s}^2}}. \tag{C.11}$$

Similarly, the elevation angle θ is given as:

$$\cos\theta = \frac{\begin{bmatrix}0\\0\\1\end{bmatrix} \cdot \begin{bmatrix}x\\y_s\\z_s\end{bmatrix}}{\sqrt{x^2+{y_s}^2+{z_s}^2}} = \frac{z_s}{\sqrt{x^2+{y_s}^2+{z_s}^2}}. \tag{C.12}$$

Substituting the equations for z_s and y_s, the parameter x can be eliminated from the two above equations such that θ may be expressed as a function of ϕ, namely $\theta(\phi) = f(\phi)$. Finally, the alveolar surface area, S_{alv}, is evaluated numerically on a computer:

$$S_{alv} = \int_0^{2\pi} \left(\int_0^{f(\phi)} {R_a}^2 \sin\theta d\theta \right) d\phi. \tag{C.13}$$

The error estimation between the "real" alveolus surface and the approximated alveolar surface is given in Table 5.3.

Appendix D

Gravitational Deposition in Horizontal Laminar Pipe Flow

To assess the accuracy of our computational schemes for gravitational deposition of non-diffusing particles in small airways (see chapter 6, section 6.3.2), we have investigated gravitational sedimentation of aerosols under laminar flow conditions in a straight horizontal pipe. For this test case, a horizontal duct was constructed with a length of 3.17 mm and a diameter of 0.317 mm making up a computational mesh containing approximately 1.4 million volume elements. The gravity direction was set perpendicular to the axial flow in the pipe. Flow conditions were investigated at $Re = 0.3$, representative of the 3rd acinar generation (see results in Fig. 5.4 in chapter 5). A time step of $\Delta t = 10^{-4}$ s was chosen such that the rms Courant number at any time step was $Co < 0.1$ [64]. A total of $N = 15'000$ particles were injected uniformly across the inlet at $t = 0$. To maintain the total computing time ($\approx T_s$) within reasonable to reach deposition of all injected particles within the computational domain, gravitational settling of spherical particles ($\rho_p = 997$ kg/m^3) with a diameter of 10 μm was investigated. For low-Reynolds number flows in ducts, the entrance length, L_e, for the flow to develop into a fully-developed parabolic profile is given in Eq. (5.43) and based on the duct diameter D_d. For the given flow conditions, the entrance length makes up $\approx 6.1\%$ of the duct length.

The vertical sedimentation motion is assumed to be independent from the axial flow and particle motion

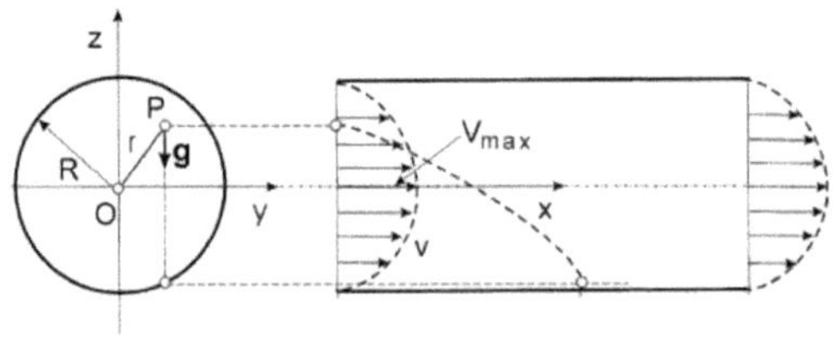

Figure D.1: Schematic of laminar pipe flow in a horizontal duct with particle sedimentation under gravity. Adapted from Kojic & Tsuda [121].

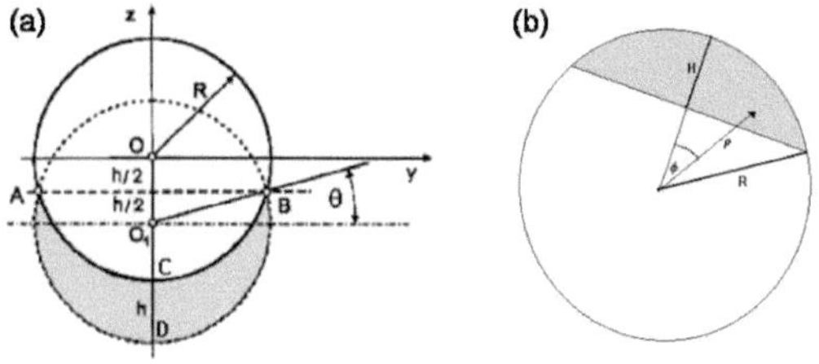

Figure D.2: (a) The number of particles, $n(t)$, which deposit during time t is represented by the gray shaded area, assuming that a total number of particles, N, is uniformly distributed over the cross-section of the pipe (shown as solid circle) [121]. The dotted circle is moving vertically downwards with a terminal sedimentation velocity u_t. (b) Grey circular segment of height H.

can be decomposed into an axial and vertical trajectory (Fig. D.1). Imagining that all particles distributed uniformly over the inlet are attached to a circular plate (shown as dotted circle in Fig. D.2), the total number of particles that deposit during the time interval, t, are represented by the grey shaded area in Fig. D.2 (a). The distance covered by the dotted circle within the time interval, t, is simply given by $h = u_t t$, where particles may be assumed to fall at terminal sedimentation velocity (see Eq. (6.11)). In order to calculate the grey shaded area shown in Fig. D.2 (a), it is useful to first calculate the area of an arbitrary circular segment (Fig. D.2 (b)). Using polar coordinates, it is easy to derive an expression for the grey shaded area, A, i.e. the area of the circular segment, based on the radius R of the circle and the segment height H (Fig. D.2 (b)). This leads to:

$$A(R,H) = 2 \int_{\phi=0}^{\phi=\arccos\left(\frac{R-H}{R}\right)} \int_{r=\frac{R-H}{\cos\phi}}^{r=R} r\,dr\,d\phi, \tag{D.1}$$

$$= \frac{1}{2}\pi R^2 - (R-H)\sqrt{H(2R-H)} - \arcsin\left(\frac{R-H}{R}\right)R^2. \tag{D.2}$$

Using the above result, one can derive an expression for the grey shaded area in Fig. D.2 (a). We subtract the area of the circular segment ABC in the solid circle, $A_{ABC}(R, R-h/2)$, from the segment ABD in the dotted circle, $A_{ABD}(R, R+h/2)$. This finally yields:

$$A(t) = A_{ABD}\left(R, R+\frac{h}{2}\right) - A_{ABC}\left(R, R-\frac{h}{2}\right), \tag{D.3}$$

$$= \frac{1}{2}h(t)\sqrt{4R^2-h^2(t)} + 2R^2\arcsin\left(\frac{h(t)}{2R}\right). \tag{D.4}$$

The total number of particles, $n(t)$, deposited during time t is then given by:

$$n(t) = N\frac{A(t)}{\pi R^2} = \frac{2N}{\pi}\left(\Theta(t) + \frac{1}{2}\sin(2\Theta(t))\right), \tag{D.5}$$

where $\sin\Theta(t) = h(t)/2R = h(t)/D_d = u_t t/D_d$. The above result has been similarly derived by Kojic & Tsuda [121]. Note that the vertical sedimentation motion of particles is entirely independent from the

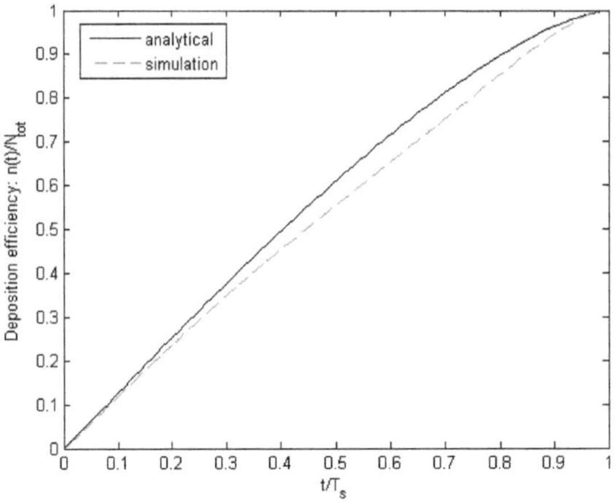

Figure D.3: Analytical and simulation results for the deposition efficiency, $n(t)/N$, during gravitational settling of 10 μm spherical particles in laminar horizontal pipe flow ($Re = 0.3$).

axial flow such that the rate of deposition does not depend on the nature of carrier fluid flow. In contrast, flow will influence the axial motion of particles (axial distribution of deposition depends both on constant vertical motion of particles and axial motion of the carrier fluid). At time $t = 0$, particles are at rest such that the time-dependent particle sedimentation velocity, u_s, is found by solving Eq. (6.3) along the direction of gravity:

$$u_s(t) = u_t \left(1 - e^{\frac{gt}{u_t}}\right) \tag{D.6}$$

In the present test case, we investigate a configuration where particles reach their terminal velocity, u_t, at

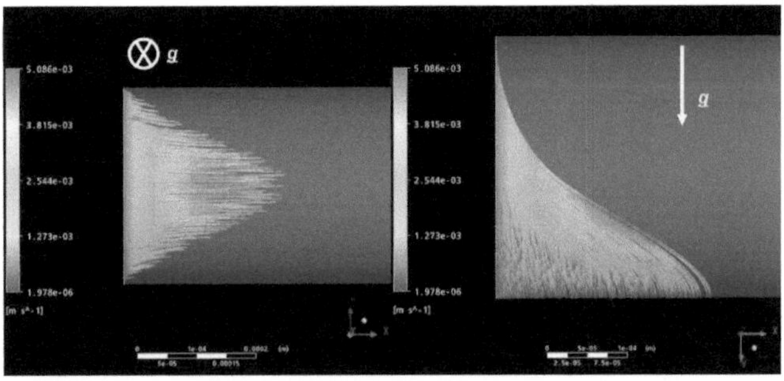

Figure D.4: Particle trajectories (10 μm diameter) with velocity magnitude along trajectories (scale in [m/s]), viewed from below (left) and from the side (right).

a finite time, $t \gg \Delta t$, and Eq. (D.6) reduces effectively to Eq. (6.11) for $gt/u_t \gg 1$. Figure D.3 compares the deposition efficiency, $n(t)/N$, of deposited particles, $n(t)$, with respect to the non-dimensionalized time, t/T_s, between analytical predictions and simulation results. Figure D.4 illustrates trajectories of the deposited particles inside the horizontal duct. The simulation follows rather well the analytical solution, with a maximum difference between solutions on the order of $\leq 9\%$. The cause of small deviation of the numerical results may arise due to several factors. First, there is an error the numerical method makes in calculating the velocity of the surrounding fluid compared to the prescribed Poiseuille flow profile used in the analytical exact solution for steady, fully-developed laminar pipe flow. Unstructured discretization of the domain using CFX-11 results in a disturbance of the flow, and small particles will predominantly follow the fluid, and therefore may not drop steadily, as recently reported by de Jongh *et al.* [50]. The analytical model also disregards the small entrance effects before achieving fully developed flow (see Eq. (5.43)). Furthermore, the analytical solution assumes that a particle reaches terminal sedimentation velocity, u_t, instantaneously, while particles in the simulation reach their terminal velocity after $\approx 40\Delta t$. In the present study, the analytical solution is based on a friction factor derived from Stokes law ($C_D = 24/Re$, see Appendix B), rather than the correlation proposed by Schiller & Neumann (Eq. (6.5) [219]), giving rise to a difference in terminal velocities, u_t, on the order of an additional $\sim 2\%$. Despite these small discrepancies, results for sedimentation in a horizontal laminar pipe flow appear to confirm the validity of our computational scheme.

Appendix E

Alveolar to Ductal Flow Rate Ratio

Each alveolus in the space-filling geometry consists of an identical truncated octahedron (14-hedron). The alveolar flow rate, $\dot{Q}_a$, is therefore independent of acinar generation and given by:

$$\dot{Q}_a = \frac{dV_a(t)}{dt} = V_{a,0}\frac{d\lambda^3(t)}{dt}, \tag{E.1}$$

which was previously given in Eq. (5.25) for a spherical cap alveolus, where $\lambda(t)$ was defined in Eq. (5.5). Substituting the length scale displacement function, $\lambda(t)$, the above equation yields:

$$\dot{Q}_a = 3(8\sqrt{2}s_0^3)\lambda^2\pi f\beta\sin(2\pi ft), \tag{E.2}$$

where $V_{a,0} = 8\sqrt{2}s_0^3$ is the alveolar volume for a tetrahedron alveolus. $s(t) = \Lambda(t)/6$ and s_0 is the edge length at FRC ($t = 0$). At the entrance of any acinar generation, z', the ductal flow rate, $\dot{Q}_T$, may be expressed as the rate of change with respect to time of the acinar volume located distally from the duct considered. This volume constitutes the network of airways and alveoli fed by the duct considered at location z'. For our specific space-filling geometry, $\dot{Q}_T$ is expressed as:

$$\dot{Q}_T(z') = \sum_{i=z'}^{8} n_i\frac{dV_a(t)}{dt}, \tag{E.3}$$

where n_i represents the total number of 14-hedra found at generation z'. One should note that the duct flow rate is computed at the entrance of an airway generation, along the longitudinal path length leading from the acinar tree entrance to alveolar sacs (gen. 8) [90]. Therefore, the ratio, $\dot{Q}_a/\dot{Q}_T$, does not describe flow phenomena past asymmetrical bifurcations leading abruptly to an airway end (e.g. gen. 4). Bearing this in mind, at any generation z, $\dot{Q}_a/\dot{Q}_T$ is then given by:

$$\frac{\dot{Q}_a}{\dot{Q}_T} = \frac{1}{\sum\limits_{i=z'}^{8} n_i}. \tag{E.4}$$

Hence, $\dot{Q}_a/\dot{Q}_T$ is a purely geometrical parameter as noted similarly in previous studies (see chapter 5 and Haber *et al.* [89]). Note however that for a space-filling tree, $\dot{Q}_a/\dot{Q}_T$ depends solely on the number of 14-hedra elements rather than actual geometrical dimensions (i.e. diameter, length, etc.). Moreover, $\dot{Q}_a/\dot{Q}_T$ is time-independent, resulting from the fact that alveoli and ducts expand and contract self-similarly in phase. Under heterogeneous ventilation [2] for example, this result may not hold true.

Appendix F

Particle Image Velocimetry

Over the last recent years, particle image velocimetry (PIV) has become a popular technique because it is relatively simple to implement and it provides velocity vector maps, namely two-dimensional measurement fields from a single pair of snapshots of the flow field under investigation. In contrast to other quantitative flow visualization methods such as techniques involving the use of probes to measure local flow properties, PIV is non-intrusive. Detailed reviews on the subject may be found in [79,199,252,286]. An example of a PIV experiment set-up is illustrated in Fig. F.1. Typically, small particles (i.e. "tracer particles") are added to the flow. A power optic source, usually in the form of a laser is required to illuminate the tracer particles within the flow. In PIV, the idea is to track constellations of particles such that a whole field of view is necessary. The laser optic needs to be expanded with a laser expander into a sheet of light as shown in Fig. F.1 so as to enable the CCD camera to capture successive images with short time intervals. CCD cameras differ from conventional cameras in the sense that they are capable of much higher frame rates. CCD cameras are electronic sensors that convert photons into electric charge and subsequently electronic signals. In the setup in Fig. F.1, the CCD camera is connected to a "frame grabber", which is usually an electronic board that is located within a computer. The frame grabber serves as an interface that enables the computer to communicate with the camera or vice versa.

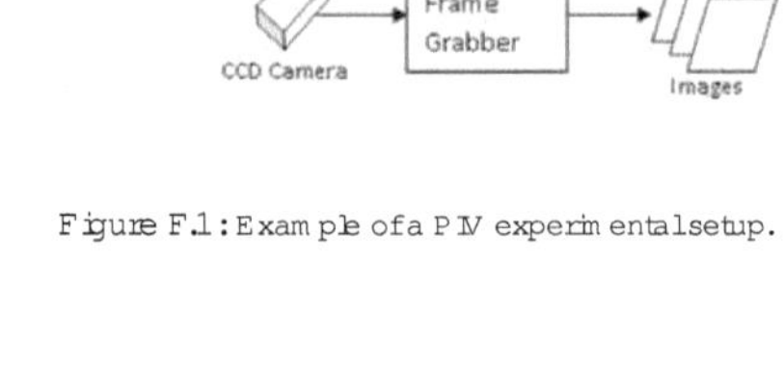

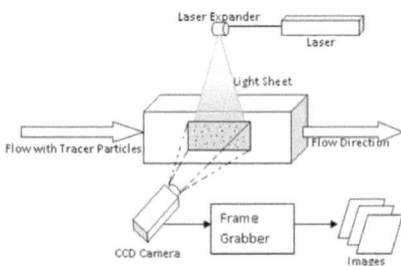

Figure F.1: Example of a PIV experimental setup.

Image Recording Techniques

A number of different methods for image recording exist. In the context of the present thesis, only multi-frame / single exposure and multi-frame double exposure methods are concerned. Multi-frame / single exposure is a method by which a single exposure of the camera produces one complete image or frame whereas multi-frame / double exposure method takes two individual exposures to produce one complete frame. Such recording techniques are schematically illustrated in Fig. F.2. Other image recording techniques exist, such as single frame / double exposure, double frame / double exposure, etc. Multi-frame techniques are, however, the preferred image recording techniques whenever possible as to avoid velocity direction ambiguity and hence reduce the complexity in the valuation process. However, the drawback is the requirement for large data storage capacity. After images have been acquired and stored, the data must be analyzed.

Image Correlation

The successive recorded images are arranged into pairs and compared. Each individual frame is derived into sub-windows known as the interrogation areas (see Fig. F.3). The information or the spatial arrangements of the particles within the individual areas are assumed to be unique and distinct such that an identical interrogation area exists which has been displaced by a given amount. However, the critical criteria to be satisfied is that the local particle displacements are sufficiently smooth between each frame pair, such that the internal spatial particle arrangements remain undistorted.

The image data from the CCD camera is stored as numerical values. Each pixel has a value that represents the intensity (i.e. grey value) of the pixel. For example, an image that has a spatial resolution of 1008 pixels by 1008 pixels is stored in a grid that contains 1016064 numbers. The magnitude of the scale depends on the image quality and is determined by the camera. A 16 bit image has a grey scale distribution from 0 to 4096. The smallest number represents the darkest color which is black, whereas the largest number represents the brightest color, namely white.

As long as the local velocity field is reasonably smooth, the constellations should displace as a whole and without internal distortions. It turns out that the particle constellations are so unique that usually only two exposures are necessary to identify corresponding patterns. The comparison/identification of the

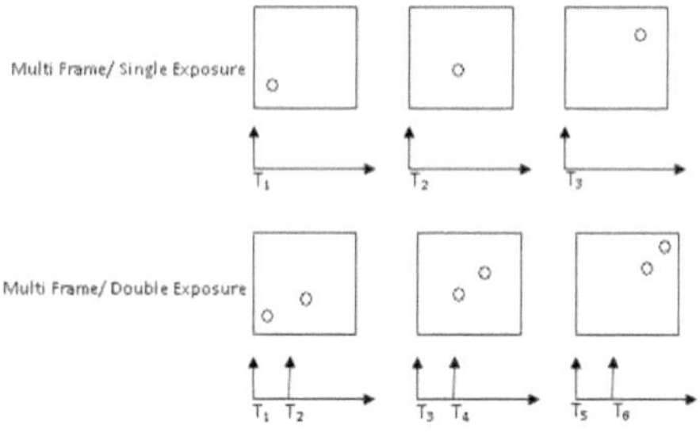

Figure F.2: Comparison of multi-frame techniques.

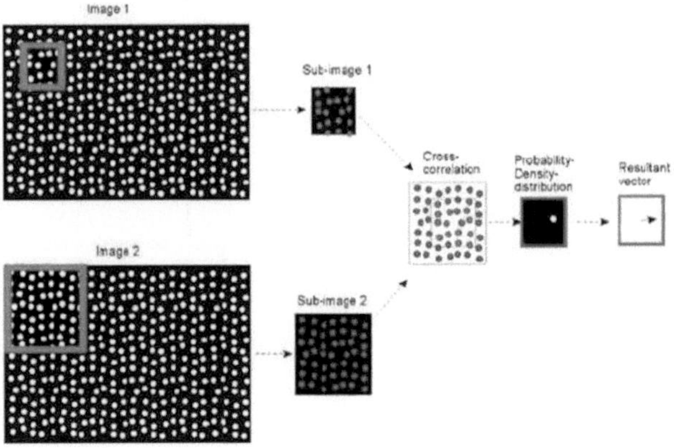

Figure F.3: Diagram of steps in PIV (from Stamhuis [252]). Two sub-images from the same location of two frames are compared in a cross-correlation procedure, resulting in a 2D probability density distribution which located by a peak. A velocity vector, representing the average displacement of the particles in sub-image 1 compared to sub-image 2 is calculated. With kind permission from Springer Science and Business Media.

particle constellations in the two image frames is performed using some form of global similarity criterion inside a local sub-window.

The method of choice is to locally find the best match between the images in a statistical sense. This is accomplished through the use of the discrete cross-correlation function:

$$R_I I(x,y) = \sum_{i=-K}^{K} \sum_{i=-L}^{L} I(i,j) I'(i+x, j+y). \tag{F.1}$$

The variables I and I' are the samples (e.g. intensity values) as extracted from the images where I' is larger than the template I (see Fig. F.3). In essence, the template I is linearly "shifted" around in the sample I' without extending over its edges. For each choice of sample shift (x, y), the sum of the products of all overlapping pixel intensities produces one cross-correlation value $R_I I(x, y)$. Essentially, the cross-correlation function statistically measures the degree of match between the two samples for a given shift. The highest value in the correlation plane can then be used as a direct estimate of the particle image displacement.

For a number of cases it may be useful to quantify the degree of correlation between the two image samples. The standard cross-correlation function in Eq. (F.1) will yield different maximum correlation values for the same degree of matching because the function is not normalized. For example, samples with many (or brighter) particle images will produce much higher correlation values than interrogation windows with fewer (or weaker) particle images. This makes a comparison of the degree of correlation between the individual interrogation windows impossible. Hence, a cross-correlation coefficient function is introduced which normalizes the cross-correlation function of Eq. (F.1) properly:

$$\rho_{kl} = \frac{Cov(p_{i,j}; q_{i+k,j+l})}{\sqrt{Var(p_{i,j}) Var(q_{i+k,j+l})}}, \tag{F.2}$$

where:

$$Cov(x_{i,j}; y_{i,j}) = \frac{1}{(M-1)(N-1)} \sum_{m=0}^{M-1} \sum_{n=0}^{N-1} (x_{i+m,j+n} - \overline{x}_{i,j})(y_{i+m,j+n} - \overline{y}_{i,j}),$$

$$Var(x_{i,j}) = Cov(x_{i,j}; x_{i,j}), \quad (F.3)$$

$$\overline{x}_{i,j} = \frac{1}{MN} \sum_{m=0}^{M-1} \sum_{n=0}^{N-1} p_{i+m,j+n}. \quad (F.4)$$

The value of ρ is in the range $-1 \leq \rho \leq 1$ with $\rho = 1$ being reached in the case of a perfect match. The computational savings come from the fact that the covariance $Cov(x, y)$ may be written as:

$$Cov(x_{i,j}; y_{i+k,j+l}) = \frac{1}{(M-1)(N-1)} \sum_{m=0}^{M-1} \sum_{n=0}^{N-1} x_{i+m,j+n} y_{i+m+k,j+n+l} - \frac{MN}{(M-1)(N-1)} \overline{x}_{i,j} \overline{y}_{i+k,j+l}. \quad (F.5)$$

The first term on the right hand side is a cross-correlation between the two sub-windows and represents the computationally most "costly" part in the evaluation of the correlation coefficient.

Frequency Domain Based Correlation

The alternative to calculating the cross-correlation directly is to take advantage of the correlation theorem which states that the cross-correlation of two functions is equivalent to a complex conjugate multiplication of their Fourier transforms:

$$R_{II} \Leftrightarrow \hat{I} \cdot \hat{I'}^*, \quad (F.6)$$

where $\hat{I}$ and $\hat{I'}^*$ are the Fourier transforms of the function I and I', respectively. In practice the Fourier transform is efficiently implemented for a discrete data using the fast Fourier transform (FFT) which reduced the computation from $O(N^2)$ operations to $O(N \log_2 N)$ operations. The tedious 2D correlation process of Eq. (F.1) can be reduced to computing two 2D FFT's on equal sized samples of the image followed by a complex-conjugate multiplication of the resulting Fourier coefficients. These are then inversely Fourier transformed to produce the actual cross-correlation plane which has the same spatial dimensions as the two input samples. In practice, two real-to-complex, 2D FFT's and one complex-to-real inverse,

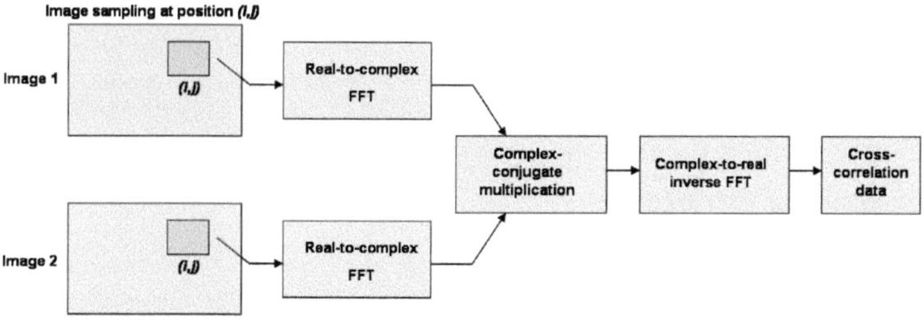

Figure F.4: Implementation of cross correlation using fast Fourier transforms. Adapted from Raffel *et al.* [199].

2D FFT are needed, each of which require approximately half the computation time of standard FFT's (see Fig. F.4).

Peak Detection and Displacement Estimation

One of the most crucial features of digital PIV evaluation is that the position of the correlation peak can be measured to sub-pixel accuracy. Since the input data itself is discretized, the correlation values exist only for integral shifts. The highest correlation value then permits the displacement to be determined with an uncertainty of ±1/2 pixel. However, with the cross-correlation function being a statistical measure of best match, the correlation values themselves also contain useful information.

A variety of methods of estimating the location of the correlation peak have been utilized [199]. Typically, a robust method is to fit the correlation data to some function. Especially for narrow correlation peaks, the approach of using only three adjoining values to estimate a component of the displacement has become widespread. One of the most common of these so-called three-point estimators is the Gaussian peak fit. The reasonable explanation for this is that the particles images themselves, if properly focused, describe functions which are approximated very well by a Gaussian intensity distribution. In particular, the following procedure can be used to detect a correlation peak and obtain a sub-pixel accurate displacement estimate of its location [199]:

- **Step 1:** Locate in the correlation plane, $R = R_{II}$, the maximum correlation value $R_{(i,j)}$ and store its integer coordinates (i, j).
- **Step 2:** Extract the adjoining four correlation values: $R_{(i-1,j)}$, $R_{(i+1,j)}$, $R_{(i,j-1)}$ and $R_{(i1,j+1)}$.
- **Step 3:** Use three points in each direction to apply the three point estimator, e.g. a Gaussian curve:

$$f(x) = Ce^{-\frac{(x_0-x)^2}{k}}, \tag{F.7}$$

with:

$$x_0 = i + \frac{\ln R_{(i-1,j)} - \ln R_{(i+1,j)}}{2\ln R_{(i-1,j)} - 4\ln R_{(i,j)} + 2\ln R_{(i+1,j)}}, \tag{F.8}$$

$$y_0 = j + \frac{\ln R_{(i,j-1)} - \ln R_{(i,j+1)}}{2\ln R_{(i,j-1)} - 4\ln R_{(i,j)} + 2\ln R_{(i,j+1)}}. \tag{F.9}$$

The "peak locking" effect which arises in dealing with sub-pixel interpolation is the tendency of peak position estimates to cluster around integer values. The empirical finding is that a Gaussian peak fit performs better than linear or quadratic interpolation schemes [286].

Estimating Average Velocity Fields

Average velocity fields can be obtained by first measuring instantaneous velocities and then averaging them in either space or time. Estimation of velocity-vector fields using PIV involve, as described above, three steps: (1) Particle image acquisition, (2) Particle image correlation, and (3) correlation peak detection. In order to obtain an average velocity measurement, an averaging operation must be applied. Since the averaging operator is linear, it may be applied after any of the three steps to produce a nonbiased of

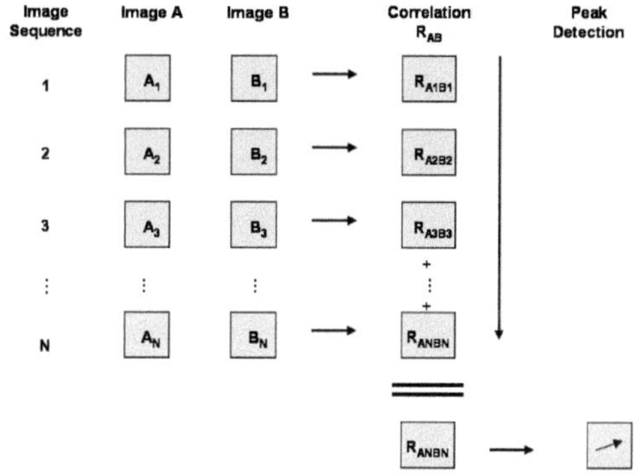

Figure F.5: Diagram depicting the average correlation method to estimate average velocities. Adapted from Meinhart *et al.* [154].

average velocity. However, the particle image correlation and peak detection operations are both nonlinear, and the order in which the averaging operator is applied can dramatically change the quality of the resulting signal.

The method of choice for estimating average displacements is termed the Average Correlation Method [154] and based on calculating instantaneous correlation functions, averaging the correlation function, and then determining the location of the signal peak location. This is illustrated graphically in Fig. F.5. Assuming two single exposure images, *Image A* and *Image B*, separated by a known time delay Δt, the average of instantaneous correlation functions over N realizations can be written formally as [154]:

$$\overline{R}_{AB}(s) = \overline{\int\int A(\underline{x})B(\underline{x}+\underline{s})d^2\underline{x}} = \int\int \overline{A(\underline{x})B(\underline{x}+\underline{s})}d^2\underline{x} \tag{F.10}$$

Since the operations of averaging and integration commute, the average operator can be taken inside of the integral so that:

$$\overline{R}_{AB}(\underline{s}) = \int\int [A_1B_1 + A_2B_2 + A_3B_3 + ... + A_NB_N]\, d^2\underline{x}. \tag{F.11}$$

This type of average produces a much higher signal-to-noise ratio than alternative methods (e.g. Average Velocity Method, Average Image Method). The number of signal terms increases linearly with the number of realizations N. Since the average operator is applied to the correlation function before peak detection, the probability of erroneous measurements is greatly reduced.

Pathline Visualization

Pathline visualizations or streak photographs are a qualitative flow visualization method. Streak photographs are used to visualize pathlines of the flow field. However, the result does not provide quantitative information on the magnitude of the velocity nor the direction of the flow. The formal definition of a pathline is the path that is taken for an individual particle, hence it is possible for two particles to

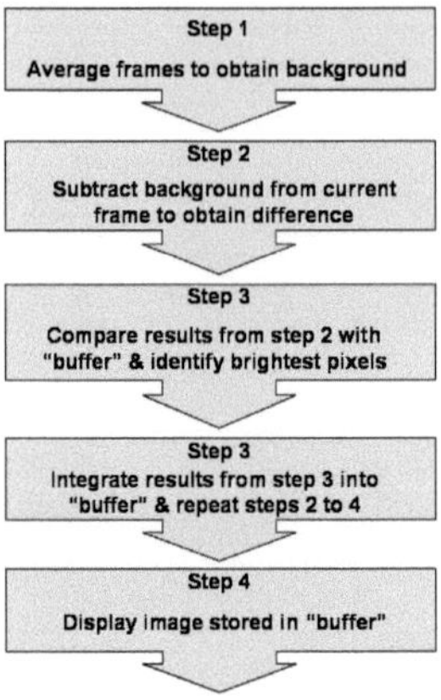

Figure F.6: Flow chart depicting streak algorithm.

pass through the same point but have completely different pathlines. For steady flows, the magnitude and direction of the velocity vectors at all points are fixed, invariant with time. Hence, the pathlines for different particles or fluid elements going through the same point are the same. Moreover, pathlines and streamlines are identical as long as the flows in the context of this thesis are concerned. Streak photography can be achieved either mechanically or numerically. The mechanical way of producing the result is by setting the CCD cameras exposure time longer than necessary thus the tracer particles leave streaks of light instead of being resolved as individual particles on the images. Additionally, it is possible to achieve streak photography results via numerical means without the need to overexpose the images. The most widely implemented streak algorithm is based on the principle of integration multiple frames over time into a single streak image. The concept is outlined in Fig. F.6.

Since the algorithm is based on a repetitive comparison and integration method, it is crucial to first acquire a general background by averaging all the pixel values from the cumulatively available image frames. This procedure serves as the starting point for the procedure followed. The background of each individual image is subtracted from the "current" image to obtain the temporal change in pixel values over time (steps 2 to 4 in Fig. F.6). The background is then subtracted from the "current" image to obtain the temporal change in pixel values over time as described in step 2. The results from step 2 are compared to the information stored in a temporary memory known as the "buffer". The brightest pixels are identified, extracted and integrated into the "buffer". The purpose of the "buffer" is to preserve all the temporal changes in pixel values (which can also be interpreted as the streak displacements). This process is repeated for all the frames and the finalized streak image is produced by displaying the information stored in the "buffer".

Bibliography

[1] M Abramovitz and IA Stegun. *Handbook of Mathematical Functions with Formulas, Graphs, and Mathematical Tables*. Dover, New York, 1972.

[2] RC Anafi and TA Wilson. Airway stability and heterogeneity in the constricted lung. *J. Appl. Physiol.*, 91:1185-1192, 2001.

[3] R Ardila, T Horie, and J Hilderbrandt. Macroscopic isotropy of lung expansion. *J. Appl. Physiol.*, 20:105-115, 1974.

[4] D Aykac and EA Hoffman. Segmentation and analysis of the human airway tree from three-dimensional X-ray CT images. *IEEE Trans. Med. Imaging*, 22:940-950, 2003.

[5] H Bachofen, P Gehr, and ER Weibel. Alterations of mechanical properties and morphology in excised rabbit lungs rinsed with a detergent. *J. Appl. Physiol.*, 47:1002-1010, 1979.

[6] H Bachofen, S Schürch, M Urbinelli, and ER Weibel. Relations among alveolar surface tension, surface area, volume, and recoil pressure. *J. Appl. Physiol.*, 62:1878-1887, 1987.

[7] HJ Bachofen, HJ Hilderbrandt, and M Bachofen. Pressure-volume curves of air and saline-filled excised lungs: Surface tensions *in situ*. *J. Appl. Physiol.*, 29:422-431, 1970.

[8] J Bastacky, CYC Lee, J Goerke, H Koushafar, D Yager, L Kenaga, TP Speed, Y Chen, and JA Clements. Alveolar lining layer is thin and continuous: low-temperature scanning electron microscopy of rat lung. *J. Appl. Physiol.*, 79:1615-1628, 1995.

[9] WD Bennett, JS Brown, KL Zeman, SH Hu, G Scheuch, and K Sommerer. Targeting delivery of aerosols to different lung regions. *J. Aerosol Med.*, 15:179-188, 2002.

[10] E Berggren, M Liljedahl, B Winbladh, B Andreasson, T Curstedt, B Robertson, and J Schollin. Pilot study of nebulized surfactant therapy for neonatal respiratory distress syndrome. *Acta Paediatr.*, 89:460-464, 2000.

[11] S Bernero and HE Fiedler. Application of particle image velocimetry and proper orthogonal decomposition to the study of a jet in a counterflow. *Exp. Fluids*, 29:S274-S281, 2000.

[12] ES Boatman and HB Martin. Electron microscopy of the alveolar pores of kohn. *Am. Rev. Respir. Dis.*, 88:779-784, 1963.

[13] M Bonora, JF Bernaudin, C Guernier, and MC Brahimi Horn. Ventilatory responses to hypercapnia and hypoxia in conscious cystic fibrosis knockout mice cftr/. *Ped. Res.*, 55:738-746, 2004.

[14] C Bowes, G Cumming, K Horsfield, J Loughhead, and S Preston. Gas mixing in a model of the pulmonary acinus with asymmetrical alveolar ducts. *J. Appl. Physiol.*, 52:624-633, 1982.

[15] EA Boyden. The structure of the pulmonary acinus in a child of six years and eight months. *Am. J. Anat.*, 132:275-300, 1971.

[16] JD Brain and JD Blanchard. *Aerosols in Medicine: Principles, Diagnosis and Therapy*,, chapter Mechanisms of Particle Deposition and Clearance, pages 117-156. Elsevier Science Publishers, 1993.

[17] RH Brown, CJ Herold, CA Hirschman, EA Zerhouni, and W Mitzner. In vivo measurements of airway reactivity using high resolution computed tomography. *Am. Rev. Respir. Dis.*, 144:208-212, 1991.

[18] PH Burri, J Dbaly, and ER Weibel. Postnatal growth of the rat lung. I. Morphometry. *Anat. Rec.*, 178:711-730, 1974.

[19] JP Butler and A Tsuda. Effect of convective stretching and folding on aerosol mixing deep in the lung, assessed by approximate entropy. *J. Appl. Physiol.*, 83:800-809, 1997.

[20] P Camner, M Anderson, K Philipson, A Bailey, A Hashish, N Jarvis, M Bailey, and M Svartengren. Human bronchiolar deposition and retention of 6-, 8- and 10-μm particles. *Exp. Lung Res.*, 23:517-535, 1997.

[21] F Carlsson, M Sen, and L Löfdahl. Steady streaming due to vibrating walls. *Phys. Fluids*, 16:1822-1825, 2004.

[22] GA Cavagna, BJ Velasque, R Wetton, and AB DuBois. Alveolar resistance to atelectasis. *J. Appl. Physiol.*, 22:441-452, 1967.

[23] AM Cazabat, F Heslot, SM Troian, and P Carles. Fingering instability of thin spreading films driven by temperature gradients. *Nature*, 346:824-826, 1990.

[24] HK Chang, RT Cheng, and LE Farhi. A model study of gas diffusion in alveolar sacs. *Respir. Physiol.*, 18:386-397, 19873.

[25] HK Chang and LE Farhi. On mathematical analysis of gas transport in the lung. *Respir. Physiol.*, 18:370-385, 1973.

[26] A Chattopadhyay. Molecules in a thin bubble membrane. *Langmuir*, 15:7881-7885, 1999.

[27] A Chattopadhyay. Time-dependent changes in a shampoo bubble. *J. Chem. Educ.*, 77:1339, 2000.

[28] TJ Chung. *Applied Continuum Mechanics*. Cambridge University Press, 1996.

[29] FF Cinkotai. Fluid flow in a model alveolar sac. *J. Appl. Physiol.*, 37:249-251, 1974.

[30] SW Clarke, JG Jones, and DR Oliver. Resistance of two-phase gas-liquid flow in airways. *J. Appl. Physiol.*, 29:464-471, 1970.

[31] JA Clements. Surface phenomena in relation to pulmonary function. *Physiologist*, 5:11-28, 1962.

[32] JK Comer, C Kleinstreuer, and CS Kim. Flow structure and particle deposition patterns in double-bifurcation airway models. Part 2. Aerosol transport and deposition. *J. Fluid Mech.*, 435:55-80, 2001.

[33] JK Comer, C Kleinstreuer, and Z Zhang. Flow structure and particle deposition patterns in double-bifurcation airway models. Part 1. Airflow fields. *J. Fluid Mech.*, 435:25-54, 2001.

[34] Y Couder, JM Chomaz, and M Rabaud. On the hydrodynamics of soap films. *Physica D*, 37:384-405, 1989.

[35] C Crowe, M Sommerfeld, and Y Tsuji. *Multiphase Flows with Droplets and Particles*. CRC Press, Boca Raton, 1998.

[36] G Cummings and SJ Semple. *Disorders of the respiratory system*. Blackwell, Oxford, 1973.

[37] HL Dailey and SN Ghadiali. Fluid-structure analysis of microparticle transport in deformable pulmonary alveoli. *J. Aerosol Sci.*, 38:269-288, 2007.

[38] PJ Dale, FL Mathews, and RF Schroter. Finite element analysis of lung parenchyma. *J. Biomech.*, 13:865-873, 1980.

[39] C Darquenne. A realistic two-dimensional model of aerosol transport and deposition in the alveolar zone of the human lung. *J. Aerosol Sci.*, 32:1161-1174, 2001.

[40] C Darquenne. Heterogeneity of aerosol deposition in a two-dimensional model of human alveolated ducts. *J. Aerosol Sci.*, 33:1261-1278, 2002.

[41] C Darquenne, P Brand, J Heyder, and M Paiva. Aerosol dispersion in human lung: comparison between numerical simulations and experiments. *J. Appl. Physiol.*, 83:966-974, 1997.

[42] C Darquenne and M Paiva. One-dimensional simulation of aerosol transport and deposition in the human lung. *J. Appl. Physiol.*, 77:2889-2898, 1994.

[43] C Darquenne and M Paiva. Two- and three-dimensional simulations of aerosol transport and deposition in alveolar zone of human lung. *J. Appl. Physiol.*, 80:1401-1414, 1996.

[44] C Darquenne, M Paiva, JB West, and GK Prisk. Effect of microgravity and hypergravity on deposition of 0.5 to 3 μm diameter aerosol in the human lung. *J. Appl. Physiol.*, 83:800-809, 1997.

[45] BJ Davidson and N Riley. Cavitation microstreaming. *J. Sound Vib.*, 15:217-233, 1971.

[46] MR Davidson. Lung gas mixing during expiration following an inspiration of air. *Bull. Math. Biol.*, 37:113-126, 1975.

[47] MR Davidson and JM Fitz-Gerald. Flow patterns in models of small airway units of the lung. *J. Fluid Mech.*, 52:161-177, 1972.

[48] MR Davidson and JM Fitz-Gerald. Transport of O_2 along a model pathway through the respiratory region of the lung. *Bull. Math. Biol.*, 36:275-303, 1974.

[49] CN Davies. Breathing of half-micron aerosols II. Interpretation of experimental results. *J. Appl. Physiol.*, 32:601-611, 1972.

[50] FHC De Jongh, MJG Rinkel, and HWM Hoeijmakers. Aerosol deposition in the upper airways of a child. *J. Aerosol Med.*, 19:279-289, 2006.

[51] E Denny and RC Schroter. The mechanical behavior of a mammalian lung alveolar duct model. *ASME J. Biomech. Eng.*, 117:245-261, 1995.

[52] E Denny and RC Schroter. Viscoelastic behavior of a lung alveolar duct model. *ASME J. Biomech. Eng.*, 122:143-151, 2000.

[53] E Denny and RC Schroter. A model of non-uniform lung parenchyma distortion. *ASME J. Biomech. Eng.*, 39:652-663, 2006.

[54] R DiFelice. The voidage function for fluid-particle interaction systems. *Int. J. Multiphase Flow*, 14:61-85, 1994.

[55] A Einstein. Die von der Molekularkinetischen Theorie der Wärme geforderte Bewegung von in ruhenden Flüssigkeiten suspendierten Teilchen. *Ann. Phys.*, 17:549-560, 1905.

[56] AM Elshabka and TJ Chung. Numerical solution of three-dimensional stream function vector compoenents of vorticity transport equation. *Comput. Methods Appl. Mech. Engrg.*, 170:131-153, 1999.

[57] C Elze and A Hennig. Die inspiratorische Vergrösserung von Volumen und Oberfläsche der menschlichen Lunge. *Z. Anat. Entwicklungsgesch.*, 119:457-469, 1956.

[58] LA Engel. Gas mixing within the acinus of the lung. *J. Appl. Physiol.*, 54:609-618, 1983.

[59] ML Everard. Aerosol therapy: regimen and device compliance in daily practice. *Paediatr. Respir. Rev.*, S7:S80-S82, 2006.

[60] EE Faridy. Effect of ventilation on movement of surfactant in airways. *Respir. Physiol.*, 27:323-334, 1976.

[61] WJ Federspiel and JJ Fredberg. Axial dispersion in respiratory bronchioles and alveolar ducts. *J. Appl. Physiol.*, 64:2614-2621, 1988.

[62] M Felici, M Filoche, and B Sapoval. Diffusional screening in the human pulmonary acinus. *J. Applp. Physiol.*, 94:2010-2016, 2002.

[63] M Felici, M Filoche, C Strausc, T Similowski, and B Sapoval. Diffusional screening in real 3D human acini: a theoretical study. *Respir. Physiol. Neurobiol.*, 145:279-293, 2005.

[64] JH Ferziger and M Peric. *Computational Methods for Fluid Dynamics. Third Edition.* Springer Verlag, 2001.

[65] A Fick. Über Diffusion. *Ann. Phys. Leipzig*, 170:59-86, 1955.

[66] W H Finlay. *The Mechanics of Inhaled Pharmaceutical Aerosols. An Introduction*. Academic Press, 2001.

[67] W H Finlay, CF Lange, M King, and D Speert. Lung delivery of aerosolized Dextran. *Am. J. Resp. Crit. Care Med.*, 161:91-97, 2000.

[68] RW Fox and AT McDonald. *An Introduction to Fluid Mechanics*. John Wiley & Sons, Inc., 1998.

[69] DG Frazer, KC Weber, and GN Franz. Evidence of sequential opening and closing of lung units during inflation-deflation of excised rat lungs. *Respir. Physiol.*, 61:277-288, 1985.

[70] YC Fung. Does the surface tension make the lung inherently unstable? *Circ. Res.*, 37:497-502, 1975.

[71] YC Fung. A model of the lung structure and its validation. *J. Appl. Physiol.*, 64:2132-2141, 1988.

[72] YC Fung. *Biomechanics: Motion, Flow, Stress, and Growth*. Springer Verlag, 1990.

[73] YC Fung and SS Sobin. Theory of sheet flow in lung alveoli. *J. Appl. Physiol.*, 26:472-488, 1969.

[74] P Gehr, M Geiser, V Im Hof, and S Schürch. Surfactant-ultrafine particle interactions: what we can learn from PM_{10} studies. *Phil. Trans. R. Soc. Lond. A*, 358:2707-2718, 2000.

[75] P Gehr and S Schürch. Surface forces displace particles deposited in airways toward the epithelium. *News Physiol. Sci.*, 7:1-5, 1992.

[76] P Gehr, S Schürch, Y Berthiaume, V Im Hof, and M Geiser. Particle retention in airways by surfactant. *J. Aerosol Med.*, 3:27-43, 1990.

[77] M Geiser, V Im Hof, W Siegenthaler, R Grunder, and P Gehr. Ultrastructure of the aqueous lining layer in hamster airways: is there a two-phase system? *Microsc. Res. Tech.*, 36:428-437, 1997.

[78] M Geiser, S Schürch, and P Gehr. Influence of surface chemistry and topography of particles on their immersion into the lung's surface-lining layer. *J. Appl. Physiol.*, 94:1793-1801, 2003.

[79] M Gharib and D Dabiri. *Flow Visualization. Techniques and Examples*, chapter Digital Particle Image Velocimetry, pages 123-147. Imperial College Press, 2000.

[80] J Gil, H Bachofen, P Gehr, and ER Weibel. Alveolar volume-surface area relation in air- and saline-filled lungs fixed by vascular perfusion. *J. Appl. Physiol.*, 47:990-1001, 1979.

[81] J Gil, H Bachofen, P Gehr, and ER Weibel. The alveolar volume-to-surface-area relationship in air-and-saline-filled lungs fixed by vascular perfusion. *J. Appl. Physiol.*, 47:990-1001, 1979.

[82] J Gil and ER Weibel. Extracellular lining of bronchioles after perfusion-fixation of rat lungs for electron microscopy. *Anat. Rec.*, 169:185-189, 1971.

[83] J Gil and ER Weibel. Morphological study of pressure-volume hysteresis in rat lungs fixed by vascular perfusion. *Respir. Physiol.*, 15:190-213, 1972.

[84] G Gormley and J Wu. Observation of acoustic streaming near Albunex spheres. *J. Acoust. Soc. Am.*, 104:3115-3118, 1998.

[85] P Gravesen, J Branebjerg, and OS Jensen. Microfluidics - a review. *J. Micromech. Microeng.*, 3:168-182, 1993.

[86] M Green. How big are the bronchioles? *St. Thomas's Hospital Gazette*, 63:136-139, 1965.

[87] S Haber, JP Butler, H Brenner, I Emanuel, and A Tsuda. Shear flow over a self-similar expanding pulmonary alveolus during rhythmical breathing. *J. Fluid Mech.*, 405:243-268, 2000.

[88] S Haber and A Tsuda. The effect of flow generated by a rhythmically expanding pulmonary acinus on aerosol dynamics. *J. Aerosol Sci.*, 29:309-322, 1998.

[89] S Haber, SD Yitzhak, and A Tsuda. Gravitational deposition in a rhythmically expanding and contracting alveolus. *J. Appl. Physiol.*, 95:657-671, 2003.

[90] B Haefeli-Bleuer and ER Weibel. Morphometry of the human pulmonary acinus. *Anat. Rec.*, 220:401-414, 1988.

[91] JR Hammersley and DE Olson. Physical models of the pulmonary airways. *J. Appl. Physiol.*, 72:2404-2414, 1992.

[92] JE Hansen and EP Ampaya. Human air space shapes, sizes, areas, and volumes. *J. Appl. Physiol.*, 38:990-995, 1975.

[93] JE Hansen, EP Ampaya, GH Bryant, and JJ Navin. Branching patterns of airways and air spaces of a single human terminal bronchiole. *J. Appl. Physiol.*, 38:983-989, 1975.

[94] JH Happel and H Brenner. *Low Reynolds Number Hydrodynamics*. Kluwer, 1983.

[95] L Harrington, G Kim Prisk, and C Darquenne. Importance of the bifurcation zone and branch orientation in simulated aerosol deposition in the alveolar zone of the human lung. *J. Aerosol Sci.*, 37:37-62, 2006.

[96] JW Harris and H Stocker. *Handbook of Mathematics and Computational Science*. Springer Verlag, 1998.

[97] FS Henry, JB Butler, and A Tsuda. Kinematically irreversible acinar flow: a departure from classical dispersive aerosol transport theories. *J. Appl. Physiol.*, 92:835-845, 2002.

[98] W R Hess. Das Prinzip des kleinsten Kraftverbrauches im dienste häm odynamischer Forschung. *Archiv Anat. Physiol.*, 1914:1-62, 1914.

[99] J Heyder, JD Blanchard, HA Feldman, and JD Brain. Convective mixing in human respiratory tract: estimates with aerosol boli. *J. Appl. Physiol.*, 64:1273-1278, 1988.

[100] J Heyder, J Gebhart, and G Scheuch. Interaction of diffusional and gravitational particle transport in aerosols. *Aerosol Sci. Tech.*, 4:315-326, 1985.

[101] JL Higdon. Stokes flow in arbitrary two-dimensional domains: shear flow over ridges and cavities. *J. Fluid Mech.*, 159:195-226, 1985.

[102] MJM Hill. On a spherical vortex. *Phil. Trans. Roy. Soc. London*, 185:213-245, 1894.

[103] FC Hiller. Health implications of hygroscopic particle growth in the human respiratory tract. *J. Aerosol Med.*, 4:1-23, 1991.

[104] BA Hills. An alternative view of the role(s) of surfactant and the alveolar model. *J. Appl. Physiol.*, 87:1567-1583, 1999.

[105] FG Hopppin and J Hildebrandt. *Bioengineering Aspects of the Lung*, chapter Mechanical Properties of the Lung, pages 83-162. Marcel Dekker, New York, 1977.

[106] K Horsfield and G Cumming. Morphology of the bronchial tree in man. *J. Appl. Physiol.*, 24:373-388, 1968.

[107] K Horsfield, G Dart, DE Olson, GF Filley, and G Cumming. Models of the human bronchial tree. *J. Appl. Physiol.*, 31:207-217, 1971.

[108] K Horsfield, W Kemp, and S Phillips. An asymmetrical model of the airways of the dog lung. *J. Appl. Physiol.*, 52:21-26, 1982.

[109] ICRP. *Human Respiratory Tract Model for Radiological Protection, Publication 66*. Pergamon Press, New York, NY, 1994.

[110] H Ikura, K Shimizu, J Ikezeo, T Nagareda, and N Yagi. In vitro evaluation of normal and abnormal lungs with ultra-hi-resolution CT. *J. Thorac. Imaging*, 19:8-15, 2004.

[111] V Im Hof, P Gehr, V Gerber, MM Lee, and S Schürch. In vivo determination of surface tension in the horse and in vitro model studies. *Respir. Physiol.*, 109:81-93, 1997.

[112] C Isenberg. *The Science of Soap Films and Soap Bubbles*. Dover, 1992.

[113] J Jacquot, A Hayem, and C Galabert. Functions of proteins and lipids in airway secretions. *Eur. Respir. J.*, 5:286-290, 1992.

[114] SL Jae. *Two-Dimensional Signal and Image Processing*. Englewood Cliffs NJ: PTR Prentice Hall, 1990.

[115] HM Janssens, JC De Jongste, W CJ Hop, and HAWM Tiddens. Extra-fine particles improve lung delivery of inhaled steroids in infants. *Chest*, 123:2083-2088, 2003.

[116] A Karl, FS Henry, and A Tsuda. Low Reynolds number viscous flow in an alveolated duct. *ASME J. Biomech. Eng.*, 126:420-429, 2004.

[117] DE Kataoka and SM Troian. Patterning liquid flow on the microscopic scale. *Nature*, 402:794-797, 1999.

[118] KH Kilburn. A hypothesis for pulmonary clearance and its implications. *Am. Rev. Respir. Dis.*, 98:449-463, 1968.

[119] CS Kim and MA Eldridge. Aerosol deposition in the airway model with excessive mucus secretions. *J. Appl. Physiol.*, 59:1766-1772, 1985.

[120] M King, HB Chang, and ME Weber. Resistance of mucus-lined tubes to steady and oscillatory flow. *J. Appl. Physiol.*, 52:1172-1176, 1982.

[121] M Kojic and A Tsuda. A simple model for gravitational deposition of non-diffusing particles in oscillatory laminar pipe flow and its application to small airways. *J. Aerosol Sci.*, 35:245-261, 2004.

[122] J Kolb and WL Nyborg. Small-scale acoustic streaming in liquids. *J. Acoust. Soc. Am.*, 28:1237-1242, 1956.

[123] CW Kotas, M Yoda, and PH Rogers. Visualization of steady streaming near oscillating spheroids. *Exp. Fluids*, 42:111-121, 2007.

[124] W Kreyling and G Scheuch. *Particle Lung Interactions*, chapter Clearance of Particles Deposited in the Lungs, pages 323-376. Marcel Dekker, New York, 2000.

[125] PK Kundu and IM Cohen. *Fluid Mechanics*. Academic Press; third edition, 2004.

[126] H Lamb. *Hydrodynamics, Sixth Edition*. Dover Publications, 1993.

[127] CA Lane. Acoustical streaming in the vicinity of a sphere. *J. Acoust. Soc. Am.*, 27:1082-1086, 1955.

[128] PS Laplace. *Mécanique céleste*. PhD thesis, Impr. Imperiale, 1836.

[129] BL Laube. In vivo measurements of aerosol dose and distribution: clinical relevance. *J. Aerosol Med.*, S1:S77-S99, 1996.

[130] CP Lee and TG Wang. Outer acoustic streaming. *J. Acoust. Soc. Am.*, 88:2367-2375, 1990.

[131] MM Lee, S Schürch, SH Roth, X Jiang, S Cheng, S Bjarnason, and FH Green. Effects of acid aerosol exposure on the surface properties of airway mucus. *Exp. Lung Res.*, 21:835-851, 1995.

[132] G Lenneweit and D Auerbach. Detachment phenomena in low Reynolds number flows through sinusoidally constricted tubes. *J. Fluid Mech.*, 387:129-150, 1999.

[133] CW Leong and JM Ottino. Experiments on mixing due to chaotic advection in a cavity. *J. Fluid Mech.*, 209:463-469, 1989.

[134] VG Levich. *Physicochemical Hydrodynamics*, chapter Motion Induced by Capillarity, pages 372-394. Prentice-Hall, 1972.

[135] JF Lewis, M Ikegami, AH Jobe, and B Tabor. Aerosolized surfactant treatment of preterm lambs. *J. Appl. Physiol.*, 70:869-876, 1991.

[136] J Lighthill. *Mathematical Biofluiddynamics*. Society for Industrial Mathematics, 1975.

[137] J Lighthill. Acoustic streaming. *J. Sound Vib.*, 61:391-418, 1978.

[138] A Linhartova, W Caldwell, and AE Anderson. A proposed alveolar model for adult human lungs: the regular dodecahedron. *Anat. Rec.*, 214:266-272, 1986.

[139] RH Liu, J Yang, MZ Pindera, M Athavale, and P Grodzinski. Bubble-induced acoustic micromixing. *Lab Chip*, 2:151-167, 2002.

[140] H Loeschke. Die Morphologie des normalen und emphysematosen Acinus der Lunge. *Beit. Path. Anat.*, 68:213, 1921.

[141] AM Lucas and LC Douglas. Principles underlying ciliary activity in the respiratory tract. *Arch. Otolaryngol.*, 20:518-541, 1934.

[142] V Ludviksson and EN Lightfoot. The dynamics of thin liquid films in the presence of surface-tension gradients. *AIChE J.*, 17:1166-1173, 1971.

[143] JL Lumley. *Stochastic Tools in Turbulence.* Academic Press London, 1970.

[144] PT Macklem. Airway obstruction and collateral ventilation. *Physiol. Rev.*, 51:368-436, 1971.

[145] M Malpighi. *De pulmonibus epistolae II as borelum.* PhD thesis, Bonon, 1661.

[146] P Marmottant and S Hilgenfeldt. A bubble-driven microfluidic transport element for bioengineering. *Proc. Natl. Acad. Sci. USA*, 101:9523-9527, 2004.

[147] T Martonen and Y Yang. *Inhalation Aerosols*, chapter Deposition Mechanics of Pharmaceutical Particles in Human Airways, pages 3-27. Marcel Dekker, Inc., 1996.

[148] M Matsuda, YC Fung, and SS Sobin. Collagen and elastin fibers in human pulmonary alveolar mouths and ducts. *J. Appl. Physiol.*, 63:1185-1194, 1987.

[149] B Mauroy, M Filoche, ER Weibel, and B Sapoval. An optimal bronchial tree may be dangerous. *Nature*, 427:633-636, 2004.

[150] MR Maxey and JJ Riley. Equation of motion for a small rigid sphere in a nonuniform flow. *Phys. Fluids*, 26:883-889, 1983.

[151] AE McNamera, NL Muller, M Okazawa, J Arntorp, BR Wiggs, and PD Dare. Airway narrowing in excised canine lungs measured by high-resolution computed tomography. *J. Appl. Physiol.*, 73:307-316, 1992.

[152] J Mead, T Takishima, and D Leith. Stress distribution in lungs: a model of pulmonary elasticity. *J. Appl. Physiol.*, 28:596-608, 1970.

[153] J Mead, JL Whittenberger, and EP Radford. Surface tension as a factor in pulmonary volume-pressure hysteresis. *J. Appl. Physiol.*, 10:191-196, 1957.

[154] CD Meinhart, ST Wereley, and JG Santiago. A PIV algorithm for estimating time-averaged velocity fields. *J. Fluids Eng.*, 122:285-289, 2000.

[155] RR Mercer and JD Crapo. Three-dimensional reconstruction of the rat acinus. *J. Appl. Physiol.*, 63:785-794, 1987.

[156] RR Mercer, ML Russell, and JD Crapo. Alveolar septal structure in different species. *J. Appl. Physiol.*, 77:1060-166, 1994.

[157] H Miki, JP Butler, RA Rogers, and JL Lehr. Geometric hysteresis in pulmonary surface-to-volume ratio during tidal breathing. *J. Appl. Physiol.*, 75:1630-1636, 1993.

[158] WS Miller. *The Lung, Second Edition.* Springfield IL, CC Thomas, 1947.

[159] F Moren, MB Dolovich, MT Newhouse, and SP Newman. *Aerosols in Medicine. Principles, Diagnosis, and Therapy.* Elsevier, Amsterdam, 1993.

[160] RM Moroney, RM White, and RT Howe. Ultrasonically induced microtransport. In *Proceedings of the IEEE Workshop on Micro Electro Mechanical Systems, MEMS 95 Amsterdam*, page 277282, 1991.

[161] PE Morrow. Factors determining hygroscopic aerosol deposition in airways. *Physiol. Rev.*, 66:330-376, 1986.

[162] CD Murray. The physiological principle of minimal work. I. The vascular system and the cost of blood. *Proc. Natl. Acad. Sci. USA*, 12:207-214, 1926.

[163] Division of Medical Sciences National Research Council, Subcommittees on Airborne Particles. *Airborne Particles.* Baltimore, MD: University Park, 1979.

[164] VA Nierstrasz and G Frens. Marginal regeneration and the Marangoni effect. *J. Colloid Interface Sci.*, 215:28-35, 1999.

[165] KR Nightingale, PJ Kornguth, and GE Trahey. The use of acoustic streaming in breast lesion diagnosis: a clinical study - Preliminary results in the breast. *Ultrasound Med. Biol.*, 25:75-87, 1999.

[166] N Nowak, PP Kakade, and AV Annapragada. Computational fluid dynamics simulation of airflow and aerosol deposition in human lungs. *Ann. Biomed. Eng.*, 31:374-390, 2003.

[167] JF Nunn. *Nunns Applied Respiratory Physiology*. Butterworth-Heinemann Ltd., 1993.

[168] WL Nyborg. Acoustic streaming near a boundary. *J. Acoust. Soc. Am.*, 30:329-339, 1958.

[169] WL Nyborg. *Nonlinear Acoustics*, chapter Acoustic Streaming, pages 207-231. Academic Press, 1998.

[170] F Orsos. The frameworks of the lung and their physiological and pathological significance. *Beiträge zur Klinik der Tuberkulose und spezifieschen Tuberkuloseforschung*, 87:568-609, 1836.

[171] CW Oseen. Über die Stokessche Formel und über die verwandte Aufgabe in der Hydrodynamik. *Arkiv Math. Astron. Fys.*, 6:No.29, 1910.

[172] Y Otani, JP Butler, H Emi, and A Tsuda. *Aerosol Inhalation: Recent Research Frontiers*, chapter Flow-induced mixing at low Reynolds number in an expanding and contracting alveolus model, pages 187-193. Kluwer Academic Publishers, 1996.

[173] JM Ottino. *The Kinematics of Mixing: Stretching, Chaos, and Transport*. Cambridge University Press, 1989.

[174] E Özsoy, P Rambaud, A Stitou, and ML Riethmüller. Vortex characteristics in laminary cavity flow at very low Mach number. *Exp. Fluids*, 38:133-145, 2005.

[175] M Paiva. Computation of the boundary conditions for diffusion in the human lung. *Comp. Biomed. Res.*, 5:585-595, 1972.

[176] M Paiva. Gas transport in the human lung. *J. Appl. Physiol.*, 35:401-410, 1973.

[177] M Paiva and LA Engel. Pulmonary interdependence of gas transport. *J. Appl. Physiol.*, 47:296-305, 1979.

[178] M Paiva and LA Engel. The anatomical basis for the sloping N_2 plateau. *Respir. Physiol.*, 44:325-337, 1981.

[179] M Paiva and LA Engel. Model analysis of gas distribution within human lung acinus. *J. Appl. Physiol.*, 56:418-425, 1984.

[180] M Paiva and LA Engel. Theoretical studies of gas mixing and ventilation distribution in the lung. *Physiol. Rev.*, 67:750-796, 1987.

[181] F Pan and A Acrivos. Steady flows in rectangular cavities. *J. Fluid Mech.*, 28:643-655, 1967.

[182] RL Panton. *Incompressible Flow*. John Wiley & Sons, 1996.

[183] W Park, EA Hoffman, and M Sonka. Segmentation of intrathoracic airway trees: a fuzzy logic approach. *IEEE Trans. Med. Imaging*, 489-497:1997, 17.

[184] H Parker, K Horsfield, and G Cumming. Morphology of distal airways in the human lung. *J. Appl. Physiol.*, 31:386-391, 1971.

[185] JM Pedersen and KE Meyer. POD analysis of flow structures in a scale model of a ventilated room. *Exp. Fluids*, 33:940-949, 2002.

[186] TJ Pedley. Viscous boundary layers in reversing flow. *J. Fluid Mech.*, 74:59-79, 1976.

[187] TJ Pedley. Pulmonary fluid dynamics. *Annu. Rev. Fluid Mech.*, 9:229-274, 1977.

[188] TJ Pedley, RC Schroter, and MF Sudlow. Energy losses and pressure drop in models of human airways. *Respir. Physiol.*, 9:371-386, 1970.

[189] TJ Pedley, RC Schroter, and MF Sudlow. The prediction of pressure drop and variation of resistance within the human bronchial airways. *Respir. Physiol.*, 9:387-405, 1970.

[190] TJ Pedley, RC Schroter, and MF Sudlow. Flow and pressure drop in systems of repeatedly branching tubes. *J. Fluid Mech.*, 46:365-383, 1971.

[191] CG Phillips and SR Kaye. On the asymmetry of bifurcations in the bronchial tree. *Respir. Physiol.*, 107:85-98, 1997.

[192] CG Phillips, SR Kaye, and RC Schroter. A diameter-based reconstruction of the branching pattern of the human bronchial tree. *Respir. Physiol.*, 98:193-217, 1994.

[193] A Podgorski and L Gradon. An improved mathematical model of hydrodynamical self-cleansing of pulmonary alveoli. *Ann. Occup. Hyg.*, 37:347-365, 1993.

[194] M Pokorski, M Izumizaki, and I Homma. Transient O_2-dependent effect of CO_2 on ventilation in the anesthetized mouse. *J. Physiol. Pharmacol.*, 56:447-454, 2005.

[195] C Pozrikidis. Shear flow over a plane wall with an axisymmetric cavity or a circular orifice of finite thickness. *Phys. Fluids*, 6:68-79, 1994.

[196] HD Prange. Laplace's law and the alveolus: a misconception of anatomy and a misapplication of physics. *Advan. Physiol. Edu.*, 27:34-40, 2003.

[197] NJ Pritchard, DE Hughes, and AR Peacocke. The ultrasonic degradation of biological macromolecules under conditions of stable cavitation I. Theory, methods and application to deoxyribonucleic acid. *Biopolymers*, 4:259-274, 1966.

[198] OG Raabe, HC Yeh, GM Schum, and FF Phalen. *Tracheobronchial Geometry: Human, Dog, Rat, Hamster*. Albuquerque, NM: Lovelace Foundation for Medical Education and Research, 1976.

[199] M Raffel, C Willert, and J Kompenhans. *Particle Image Velocimetry: A Practical Guide*. Springer Verlag, 1998.

[200] N Rashidnia and R Balasubramaniam. Thermocapillary migration of liquid droplets in a temperature gradient in a density matched system. *Exp. Fluids*, 11:167-174, 1991.

[201] R Reifenrath. The significance of alveolar geometry and surface tension in the respiratory mechanics of the lung. *Respir. Physiol.*, 24:115-137, 1975.

[202] JM Reinhardt, ND D'Souza, and EA Hoffman. Accurate measurement of intrathoracic airways. *IEEE Tans. Med. Imaging*, 16:820-827, 1997.

[203] HS Rhee, JR Koseff, and RL Street. Flow visualization of a recirculating flow by rheoscopic liquid and liquid crystal techniques. *Exp. Fluids*, 2:57-64, 1984.

[204] N Riley. Steady streaming. *Annu. Rev. Fluid Mech.*, 33:43-65, 2001.

[205] NP Robinson, H Kyle, SE Webber, and JG Widdicombe. Electrolyte and other chemical concentrations in tracheal airway surface liquid and mucus. *J. Appl. Physiol.*, 66:2129-2135, 1989.

[206] FL Roman, J Faro, and S Velasco. A simple experiment for measuring the surface tension of soap solutions. *Am. J. Phys.*, 69:920-921, 2001.

[207] L Rosenhead. *Laminar Boundary Layers*. Dover Publications, 1963.

[208] FS Rosenthal, JD Blanchard, and PJ Anderson. Aerosol bolus dispersion and convective mixing in human and dog lungs and in physical models. *J. Appl. Physiol.*, 73:862-873, 1992.

[209] T Rösgen. Optimal subpixel interpolation in particle image velocimetry. *Exp. Fluids*, 35:252-256, 2003.

[210] M Roth Kleiner, TM Berger, MR Tarek, PH Burri, and JC Schittny. Neonatal dexamethasone induces premature microvascular maturation by focal fusion of alveolar capillaries. *Dev. Dyn.*, 233:1261-1271, 233.

[211] SF Ryan, C Dumais, and A Ciannella. The structure of the interalveolar septum of the mammalian lung. *Anat. Rec.*, 165:467-483, 1969.

[212] M Sackmann, M Delius, T Sauerbruch, J Holl, W Weber, E Ippisch, U Hagelauer, O Wess, W Hepp, W Brendel, and et al. Shock-wave lithotripsy of gallbladder stones. The first 175 patients. *N Engl. J. Med.*, 318:393-397, 1988.

[213] RM Sadri and JM Floryan. Accurate evaluation of the loss coefficient and the entrance length of the inlet region of a channel. *J. Fluids Eng.*, 124:685-693, 2002.

[214] B Sapoval, M Filoche, and ER Weibel. Smaller is better-but not too small: A physical scale for the design of the mammalian pulmonary acinus. *Proc. Natl. Acad. Sci. USA*, 99:10411-10416, 2002.

[215] TK Sarma and A Chattopadhyay. Simultaneous measurement of flowing fluid layer and film thickness of a soap bubble using a uv-visible sprectrophotometer. *Langmuir*, 17:6399-6403, 2001.

[216] V Sauret, PM Halson, IW Brown, JS Fleming, and AG Bailey. Study of the three-dimensional geometry of the central conducting airways in man using computed tomographic (CT) images. *J. Anat.*, 200:123-134, 2002.

[217] EM Scarpelli. *Pulmonary Physiology: Fetus, Newborn, Child and Adolescent*, chapter Pulmonary mechanics and ventilation, pages 257-280. Lea & Febiger, 2nd edition, 1990.

[218] G Scheuch, MJ Kohlhaeufl, P Brand, and R Siekmeier. Clinical perspectives on pulmonary systemic and macromolecular delivery. *Advanced Drug Delivery Reviews*, 58:996-1008, 2006.

[219] L Schiller and A Neumann. Über die grundlegenden Berechnungen bei der Schwerkraftaufbereitung. *Verein Deutscher Ingenieure*, 77:318, 1933.

[220] JC Schittny and PH Burri. *Lung Development and Regeneration*, chapter Morphogenesis of the Mammalian Lung: Aspects of Structure and Extracellular Matrix Components, pages 275-317. Marcel Dekker Inc., 2004.

[221] JC Schittny, V Djonov, A Fine, and PH Burri. Programmed cell death contributes to postnatal lung development. *Am. J. Respir. Cell Mol. Biol.*, 18:786-793, 1998.

[222] JC Schittny, M Paulsson, C Vallan, PH Burri, N Kedei, and D Aeschlimann. Protein cross-linked mediated by tissue transglutaminase correlates with the maturation of extracellular matrices during lung development. *Am. J. Respir. Cell. Mol. Biol.*, 17:334-343, 1997.

[223] E Schlenker, Y Shi, C Johnson, and JW Wipf. Acetazolamide affects breathing differently in ICR and C57 mice. *Respir. Physiol. Neurobiol.*, 152:119-127, 2006.

[224] JP Schreider and OG Raabe. Structure of the human respiratory acinus. *Am. J. Anat.*, 162:221-232, 1981.

[225] KG Schüepp, J Jauernig, HM Janssens, HAWM Tiddens, DA Straub, R Stangl, M Keller, and JH Wildhaber. In vitro determination of the optimal particle size for nebulized aerosol delivery to infants. *J. Aerosol Med.*, 18:225-235, 2005.

[226] KG Schüepp, D Straub, A Möller, and JH Wildhaber. Deposition of aerosols in infants and children. *J. Aerosol Med.*, 17:153-156, 2004.

[227] H Schulz, P Heilmann, A Hillebrecht, J Gebhart, M Meyer, J Piiper, and J Heyder. Convective and diffusive gas transport in canine intrapulmonary airways. *J. Appl. Physiol.*, 72:1557-1562, 1992.

[228] S Schürch, P Gehr, V Im Hof, M Geiser, and F Green. Surfactant displaces particles toward the epithelium in airways and alveoli. *Respir. Physiol.*, 80:17-32, 1990.

[229] S Schürch, M Geiser, MM Lee, and P Gehr. Particles at the airway interfaces of the lung. *Colloids and Surfaces*, 15:339-353, 1999.

[230] JA Schuster, RM Rubsamen, PM Lloyd, and LJ Lloyd. The AERx aerosol delivery system. *Pharm. Res.*, 3:354-357, 1997.

[231] LE Scriven and CV Sternling. The Marangoni effects. *Nature*, 187:186-188, 1960.

[232] GAF Seber. *Multivariate Observations*. John Wiley & Sons, 1984.

[233] T Sera, H Fujioka, H Yokota, A Makinouchi, R Himeno, RC Schroter, and K Tanishita. Three-dimensional visualization and morphometry of small airways from microfocal X-ray computed tomography. *J. Biomech.*, 36:1587-1594, 2003.

[234] T Sera, N Yagi, and K Uesugi. Three-dimensional visualization of intact mouse lung by synchrotron radiation CT. In *Proceedings of the 26th Annual International Conference of the IEEE EMBS*, 2004.

[235] RK Shah and AL London. *Laminar Flow Forced Convection in Ducts*. Academic Press, New York, 1978.

[236] PN Shankar. The eddy structure in stokes flow in a cavity. *J. Fluid Mech.*, 250:371-383, 1993.

[237] PN Shankar. Three-dimensional eddy structure in a cylindrical container. *J. Fluid Mech.*, 342:97-118, 1997.

[238] PN Shankar and MD Deshpande. Fluid mechanics in the driven cavity. *Annu. Rev. Fluid Med.*, 32:93-136, 2000.

[239] C Shen and JM Floryan. Low Reynolds number flow over cavities. *Phys. Fluids*, 28:3191-3202, 1985.

[240] FS Sherman. *Viscous Flow*. McGraw-Hill, 1990.

[241] X Shi, RW Martin, S Vaezy, and LA Crum. Quantitative investigation of acoustic streaming in blood. *J. Acoust. Soc. Am.*, 111:1110-1121, 2002.

[242] AF Simone and JS Ultman. Longitudinal mixing by the human larynx. *Respir. Physiol.*, 49:187-203, 1982.

[243] DE Sims, JA Westfall, AL Kiorpes, and MM Horne. Preservation of tracheal mucus by nonaqueous fixative. *Biotech. Histochem.*, 66:173-180, 1991.

[244] L Sirovich. Turbulence and the dynamics of coherent structures. Part 1: Coherent structures. *Q. Appl. Math.*, 45:561-590, 1987.

[245] AS Slutsky, FM Drazen, RH Ingram Jr, RD Kamm, AH Shapiro, JJ Fredberg, SH Loring, and J Lehr. Effective pulmonary ventilation with small-volume oscillations at high frequency. *Science*, 209:609-671, 1980.

[246] GC Smaldone, RJ Perry, WD Bennett, MS Messina, J Zwang, and J Ilosite. Interpretation of "24 hour retention" in studies of mucociliary clearance. *J. Aerosol Sci.*, 1:1-20, 1986.

[247] FF Spinosa and RD Kamm. Thin layer flows due to surface tension gradients over a membrane undergoing nonuniform, periodic strain. *Ann. Biomed. Eng.*, 25:913-925, 1997.

[248] TM Squires and SR Quake. Microfluidics: fluid physics at the nanoliter scale. *Rev. Mod. Phys.*, 77:977-1026, 2005.

[249] W Stahlhofen, J Gebhart, G Rudolf, and G Scheuch. Measurement of lung clearance with pulses of radioactively labelled particles. *J. Aerosol Sci.*, 17:333-338, 1986.

[250] D Stamenovic and JC Smith. Surface forces in lungs. I. Alveolar surface tension-lung volume relationships. *J. Appl. Physiol.*, 60:1341-1350, 1986.

[251] D Stamenovic and JC Smith. Surface forces in lungs. III. Alveolar surface tension and elastic properties of lung parenchyma. *J. Appl. Physiol.*, 60:1358-1362, 1986.

[252] EJ Stamhuis. Basics and principles of particle image velocimetry (PIV) for mapping biogenic and biologically relevant flows. *Aquatic Ecology*, 40:463-479, 2006.

[253] M Stampanoni, G Borchet, P Wyss, R Abela, BD Patterson, S Hunt, D Vermeulen D, and P Rüegsegger. High resolution x-ray detector for synchrotron based microtomography. *Nucl. Instr. and Meth. A*, 491:291-301, 2002.

[254] NC Staub and WF Storey. Relation between morphological and physiological events in lung studied by rapid freezing. *J. Appl. Physiol.*, 17:381-390, 1962.

[255] GP Stelter, JE Hansen, and DG Fairchhild. A three-dimensional reconstruction of lung parenchyma. *Am. Rev. Respir. Dis.*, 94:79-85, 1966.

[256] W Stöber, PE Morrow, and G Morawietz. Alveolar retention and clearance of insoluble particles in rats simulated by a new physiologically oriented compartmental kinetics model. *Fund. Appl. Toxicol.*, 15:329-349, 1990.

[257] GG Stokes. On the effect of the internal friction of fluids on the motion of pendulums. *Cambridge Philos. Trans.*, 9:8-106, 1851.

[258] HA Stone, A Nadim, and SH Strogatz. Chaotic streamlines inside drops immersed in steady stokes flows. *J. Fluid Mech.*, 232:629-646, 1991.

[259] JT Stuart. Double boundary layers in oscillating viscous flow. *J. Fluid Mech.*, 24:562-576, 1966.

[260] S Taneda. Visualization of separating stokes flows. *J. Phys. Soc. Japan*, 46:1935-1942, 1979.

[261] TH Tawhai, AJ Pullan, and PJ Hunter. Generation of an anatomically based three-dimensional model of the conducting airways. *Ann. Biomed. Eng.*, 28:793-802, 2000.

[262] R Theunissen, N Buchmann, P Corieri, ML Riethmuller, and C Darquenne. Experimental investigation of aerosol deposition in alveolar lung airways. In 13th *Int. Symp. on Applications of Laser Techniques to Fluid Mechanics, Lisbon, Portugal, 26-29 June*, 2006.

[263] P Tho, R Manasseh, and A Ooi. Cavitation microstreaming patterns in single and multiple bubble systems. *J. Fluid Mech.*, 576:191-233, 2007.

[264] PJ Thomson. Drug delivery to the small airways. *Am. J. Respir. Crit. Care Med.*, 157:S199-S202, 1998.

[265] A Tippe and A Tsuda. Recirculating flow in an expanding alveolar model: experimental evidence of flow-induced mixing of aerosols in the pulmonary acinus. *J. Aerosol Sci.*, 31:979-986, 1999.

[266] M Tobak and DJ Peake. Topology of three-dimensional separated flows. *Annu. Rev. Fluid Mech.*, 14:61-85, 1982.

[267] A Tsuda, JP Butler, and JJ Fredberg. Effects of alveolated duct structure on aerosol kinetics I. Diffusional deposition in the absence of gravity. *J. Appl. Physiol.*, 76:2497-2509, 1994.

[268] A Tsuda, JP Butler, and JJ Fredberg. Effects of alveolated duct structure on aerosol kinetics II. Gravitational sedimentation and inertial impaction. *J. Appl. Physiol.*, 76:2510-1516, 1994.

[269] A Tsuda, WJ Federspiel, PA Grant, and JJ Fredberg. Axial dispersion of inert species in alveolated channels. *Chem. Eng. Sci.*, 46:1419-1426, 1991.

[270] A Tsuda, FS Henry, and JP Butler. Chaotic mixing of alveolated duct flow in rhythmically expanding pulmonary acinus. *J. Appl. Physiol.*, 79:1055-1063, 1995.

[271] A Tsuda, Y Otani, and JP Butler. Acinar flow irreversibility caused by perturbations in reversible alveolar wall motion. *J. Appl. Physiol.*, 86:977-984, 1999.

[272] A Tsuda, RA Rogers, PE Hydon, and JB Butler. Chaotic mixing deep in the lung. *Proc. Natl. Acad. Sci. USA*, 99:10173-10178, 2002.

[273] JS Ultman. *Gas Mixing and Distribution in the Lung*, chapter Gas transport in the conducting airways, pages 36-136. Dekker, New York, 1985.

[274] PA Valberg and JD Brain. Lung surface tension and air space dimensions from multiple pressure-volume curves. *J. Appl. Physiol.*, 43:730-738, 1977.

[275] A Van As and IWebster. The morphology of mucus in mammalian pulmonary airways. *Environ. Res.*, 7:1-12, 1974.

[276] C Van Ertbruggen, C Hirsch, and M Paiva. Anatomically based three-dimensional model of airways to simulate flow and particle transport using computational fluid dynamics. *J. Appl. Physiol.*, 98:970-980, 2005.

[277] S Verbanck and M Paiva. Model simulations of gas mixing and ventilation distribution in the human lung. *J. Appl. Physiol.*, 69:2269-2279, 1990.

[278] JH Vincent. On the practical significance of electrostatic lung deposition of isometric and fibrous aerosols. *J. Aerosol Sci.*, 16:511-519, 1985.

[279] K von Neergaard. Neue Auffassungen über einen Grundbegriff der Atemmechanik: Die Retraktionsfraft der Lunge, abhängig von der Oberflächenspannung in den Alveolen. *Z. Ges. Exp. Med.*, 66:373-394, 1929.

[280] HH Wei, H Fujioka, RB Hirschl, and JB Grotberg. A model of flow and surfactant transport in an oscillatory alveolus partially filled with liquid. *Phys. Fluids*, 17:031510, 2005.

[281] ER Weibel. *Morphometry of the Human Lung*. Springer-Verlag Berlin, 1963.

[282] ER Weibel. *The Pathway for Oxygen*. Harvard University Press, 1984.

[283] ER Weibel and Bw Knight. A morphometric study on the thickness of the pulmonary air-blood barrier. *J. Cell Biol.*, 21:367-384, 1964.

[284] ER Weibel, B Sapoval, and M Filoche. Design of peripheral airways for efficient gas exchange. *Respir. Physiol. Neuro.*, 148:3-21, 2005.

[285] JB West. *Respiratory Physiology. The Essentials*. Lippincott Williams & Wilkins, 2005.

[286] C Willert and M Gharib. Digital particle image velocimetry. *Exp. Fluids.*, 10:181-193, 1991.

[287] R Wilson and JD Spengler. *Particles in Our Air: Concentration and Health Effects*. Harvard University Press, 1996.

[288] TA Wilson. Mechanics of the pressure-volume curve of the lung. *Ann. Biomed. Eng.*, 9:439-449, 1981.

[289] TA Wilson. Surface tension-surface area curves calculated from pressure-volume loops. *J. Appl. Physiol.*, 53:1512-1520, 1982.

[290] TA Wilson and H Bachofen. A model for the mechanical structure of the alveolar duct. *J. Appl. Physiol.*, 52:1064-1070, 1982.

[291] RK Wolff. *Aerosol Inhalation: Recent Research Frontiers*, chapter Experimental Investigation of Deposition and Fate of Particles: Animal Models and Interspecies Differences, pages 247-263. Kluwer Academic Publishers, Norwell MA, 1996.

[292] JR Womersley. Method for the calculation of velocity rate of flow and viscous drag in arteries when the pressure gradient is known. *J. Physiol.*, 127:553-563, 1955.

[293] SA Wood, EA Zerhouni, JD Hoford, EA Hoffman, and EA Mitzner. Measurement of three-dimensional lung structures by using computed tomography. *J. Appl. Physiol.*, 79:1687-1697, 1995.

[294] J Wu and G Du. Streaming generated by a bubble in an ultrasound field. *J. Acoust. Soc. Am.*, 101:1899-1907, 1997.

[295] J Wu, JP Ross, and JF Chiu. Reparable sonoporation generated by microstreaming. *J. Acoust. Soc. Am.*, 111:1460-1464, 2002.

[296] D Yager, T Cloutier, H Feldman, J Bastacky, JM Drazen, and RD Kamm. Airway surface liquid thickness as a function of lung volume in small airways of the guinea pig. *J. Appl. Physiol.*, 77:2333-2340, 1994.

[297] M Yi, HH Bau, and H Hu. Peristaltically induced motion in a closed cavity with two vibrating walls. *Phys. Fluids*, 14:184-197, 2002.

[298] CP Yu. On equation of gas transport in the lung. *Respir. Physiol.*, 23:257-266, 1975.

[299] CP Yu and S Rajaram. Diffusional deposition in a model alveolus. *J. Aerosol Sci.*, 9:521-525, 1978.

[300] Z Zhang and C Kleinstreuer. Transient airflow structures and particle transport in a sequentially branching lung airway model. *Phys. Fluids*, 14:862-880, 2002.

[301] Z Zhang, C Kleinstreuer, and CS Kim. Flow structure and particle transport in a triple bifurcation airway model. *J. Fluids Eng.*, 123:320-330, 2001.

[302] H Zhao, SS Sadhal, and EH Trinh. Internal circulation in a drop in an acoustic field. *J. Acoust. Soc. Am.*, 106:3289-3295, 1999.

MIX
Papier aus verantwortungsvollen Quellen
Paper from responsible sources
FSC® C105338

Printed by Books on Demand GmbH, Norderstedt / Germany